Lecture Notes of the Institute for Computer Sciences, Social Informatics and Telecommunications Engineering 362

More information about this series at http://www.springer.com/series/8197

Juan Ye · Michael J. O'Grady ·
Gabriele Civitarese · Kristina Yordanova (Eds.)

Wireless Mobile Communication and Healthcare

9th EAI International Conference, MobiHealth 2020
Virtual Event, November 19, 2020
Proceedings

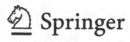
Springer

Editors
Juan Ye 🆔
School of Computer Science
University of St Andrews
St Andrews, UK

Gabriele Civitarese
Department of Computer Science
University of Milan
Milan, Italy

Michael J. O'Grady
School of Computer Science
and Information Technology
University College Dublin
Dublin, Dublin, Ireland

Kristina Yordanova 🆔
Faculty of Computer Science
and Electrical Engineering
University of Rostock
Rostock, Germany

ISSN 1867-8211 ISSN 1867-822X (electronic)
Lecture Notes of the Institute for Computer Sciences, Social Informatics
and Telecommunications Engineering
ISBN 978-3-030-70568-8 ISBN 978-3-030-70569-5 (eBook)
https://doi.org/10.1007/978-3-030-70569-5

This Springer imprint is published by the registered company Springer Nature Switzerland AG
The registered company address is: Gewerbestrasse 11, 6330 Cham, Switzerland

Preface

We are delighted to introduce the proceedings of the ninth edition of the European Alliance for Innovation (EAI) International Conference on Wireless Mobile Communication and Healthcare (MobiHealth). This conference brought together researchers, developers and practitioners around the world who are leveraging and developing mobile and wearable technology for health monitoring and management.

The technical program of MobiHealth 2020 consisted of 13 full papers from the main conference and 10 full papers from two workshops on Medical Artificial Intelligence and on Digital Healthcare Technologies for the Global South. The main conference tracks were: Track 1 – Wearable Technologies; Track 2 – Health Telemetry; Track 3 – Mobile Sensing and Assessment; and Track 4 - Machine Learning in eHealth Applications. Aside from the high-quality technical paper presentations, the technical program also featured two keynote speeches. The two keynote speakers were Prof. Pan Hui from Hong Kong University of Science and Technology and Prof. Ali Hessami from Vega Systems Ltd., UK

Coordination with the steering chairs, Imrich Chlamtac and James C. Lin, was essential for the success of the conference. We sincerely appreciate their constant support and guidance. It was also a great pleasure to work with such an excellent organizing committee team for their hard work in organizing and supporting the conference. In particular, the Technical Program Committee, led by our TPC Chair, Dr. Xiang Su, completed the peer-review process of technical papers and made a high-quality technical program. We are also grateful to the Conference Manager, Kristina Petrovicova, for her support and to all the authors who submitted their papers to the MobiHealth 2020 conference and workshops.

We strongly believe that the MobiHealth conference provides a good forum for all researchers, developers and practitioners to discuss all scientific and technological aspects that are relevant to mobile health systems. We also expect that future MobiHealth conferences will be as successful and stimulating, as indicated by the contributions presented in this volume.

November 2020

Juan Ye
Michael O'Grady
Gabriele Civitarese

Conference Organization

Steering Committee

Chair

Imrich Chlamtac   Bruno Kessler Professor, University of Trento, Italy

Founding Chair

James C. Lin   University of Illinois at Chicago, USA

Members

Dimitrios Koutsouris	National Technical University of Athens, Greece
Janet Lin	University of Illinois at Chicago, USA
Arye Nehorai	Washington University in St. Louis, USA
Konstantina S. Nikita	National Technical University of Athens, Greece
George Papadopoulos	University of Cyprus, Cyprus
Oscar Mayora	FBK e-Health, Italy

Organizing Committee

General Chair

Juan Ye   University of St Andrews, UK

General Co-chairs

Michael O'Grady   University College Dublin, Ireland
Gabriele Civitarese   University of Milan, Italy

TPC Chair and Co-chair

Xiang Su   University of Helsinki, Finland

Local Chair

Kasim Terzić   University of St Andrews, UK

Workshops Chair

Lei Fang   University of St Andrews, UK

Publicity and Social Media Chair

Mauro Dragone   Heriot-Watt University, UK

Publications Chair

Kristina Yordanova   University of Rostock, Germany

Web Chair

Martin Schiemer   University of St Andrews, UK

Technical Program Committee

Dominique Schreurs	KU Leuven, Belgium
Emmanouil Spanakis	Institute of Computer Science – FORTH, Greece
Fedor Lehocki	Slovak University of Technology in Bratislava, Slovakia
Ilias Maglogiannis	University of Piraeus, Greece
Kalle Tammemäe	Tallinn University of Technology, Estonia
Maxim Zhadobov	Institute of Electronics and Telecommunications of Rennes (IETR), France
Nima TaheriNejad	Institute for Computer Technology, TU Wien, Austria
Nizamettin Aydin	Yıldız Technical University, Turkey
Omer Inan	Georgia Institute of Technology, USA
Ouri Wolfson	University of Illinois at Chicago, USA
Panagiotis Kosmas	King's College London, UK
Paolo Perego	Politecnico di Milano, Italy
Tian Hong Loh	National Physical Laboratory, UK
John O'Donoghue	Imperial College London, UK
Frank Krüger	University of Rostock, Germany
Lei Fang	University of St. Andrews, UK
Ai Jiang	University of St. Andrews, UK
Andrea Rosales	University of St. Andrews, UK
Zhicheng Yang	Ping an Technology, US Research Lab, USA
Levent Görgü	University College Dublin, Ireland
Jie Wan	Nantong University, China
Riccardo Presotto	University of Milan, Italy
Aqeel Kazmi	Trinity College Dublin, Ireland
Kasim Terzić	University of St Andrews, UK
Martin Schiemer	University of St Andrews, UK

Contents

Mobile Sensing and Assessment

Machine Learning in eHealth Applications

**EAI International Workshop on Digital Healthcare Technologies
for the Global South**

Mobile Sensing and Assessment

Experiences in Designing a Mobile Speech-Based Assessment Tool for Neurological Diseases

Louis Daudet[1(✉)], Christian Poellabauer[1], and Sandra Schneider[2]

[1] Department of Computer Science and Engineering, University of Notre Dame,
Notre Dame, USA
{ldaudet,cpoellab}@nd.edu
[2] Department of Communicative Sciences and Disorders, Saint Mary's College,
Notre Dame, USA
sschneider@saintmarys.edu
http://m-lab.cse.nd.edu/

Abstract. Mobile devices contain an increasing number of sensors, many of which can be used for disease diagnosis and monitoring. Thus along with the ease of access and use of mobile devices there is a trend towards developing neurological tests onto mobile devices. Speech-based approaches have shown particular promise in detection of neurological conditions. However, designing such tools carries a number of challenges, such as how to manage noise, delivering the instructions for the speech based tasks, handling user error, and how to adapt the design to be accessible to specific populations with Parkinson's Disease and Amyotrophic Lateral Sclerosis. This report discusses our experiences in the design of a mobile-based application that assesses and monitors disease progression using speech changes as a biomarker.

Keywords: Speech analysis · Portable diagnostics · Proof of concept · Experience report · Mobile health

1 Introduction

Neurodegeneration is the process through which the neurons and neuronal structures are compromised, hindering their proper functions, or even leading to their death. This neurodegenerative process is the cause of many diseases such as Alzheimer's Disease, Huntington's Disease, Parkinson's Disease (PD) [1] and Amyotrophic Lateral Sclerosis (ALS) [2]. Although there exist some treatments for these diseases aimed at slowing down their progress or helping with their symptoms [3,4], they remain incurable. As these diseases progress, patients struggle with a variety of symptoms such as speech disorders, tremors, difficulties with movement coordination, cognitive decline, and sensory issues [5–7]. An estimated 10 million people live with PD [8], while ALS is thought to impact 6

© ICST Institute for Computer Sciences, Social Informatics and Telecommunications Engineering 2021
Published by Springer Nature Switzerland AG 2021. All Rights Reserved
J. Ye et al. (Eds.): MobiHealth 2020, LNICST 362, pp. 3–17, 2021.
https://doi.org/10.1007/978-3-030-70569-5_1

people out of 100 000. Furthermore, with the aging of the population worldwide, the impact of these diseases is on the rise. For example, the United Nations predicts that, due to aging, the number of people with ALS worldwide is expected to go up 69% between 2015 and 2040, going from about 223,000 to 377,000 people [9]. Besides the tragic effects these diseases have on a human level, they also have a significant financial impact. The worldwide cost of dementia alone, with both PD and ALS being contributing diseases [10,11], is 614 billion dollars, or 1% of the world GDP [12].

There has been a trend towards mobile-based health assessments, as mobile devices are often constantly with their users, but also featuring an increasing array of sensors that can be used to extract valuable health data. In [13], the authors present the various sensors and mobile developments made that can be used by medical professionals to diagnose and monitor conditions such as asthma, hypertension, or diabetes. Specifically, speech has been used in several mobile based health assessment tools. The field of mobile health is finding new applications for all of these developments in mobile technologies, as shown in [14]. When trying to develop mobile health applications, specific challenges need to be taken into account. In [15], the authors list privacy concerns and usability as some of the main difficulties to be addressed. With a traditional test done in a medical setting, the privacy of the patients data is handled by the strict regulations and policies in place. But with a mobile application, the data is being collected from the patients' devices, and needs to be stored and transmitted securely at all times, adding to the complexity of device based assessments. Usability is also complicated by the small screen sizes, the complex inputs, and the sometimes slow interaction speeds of some lower end mobile devices. Similarly, in [16], the authors considered several categories of challenges when designing mobile-based health applications. For the application itself, the two main challenges were the user interface (i.e., how to make sure that the layout of the graphical elements help and not overwhelm the patients), and the design of the task (i.e., how to handle interruptions such as phone calls, how to handle the test being performed in different types of environments). They also noted that several challenges came from the devices' hardware, such as the screen size (i.e. how to be read by different populations on smaller screens, how to account for variations in screen size), the input (i.e. how to handle various types of input scheme), and the network (i.e. how to deal with sometimes spotty or even nonexistent connectivity).

We created a mobile-based application designed to detect the presence of PD and ALS using speech analysis. The application uses speech based tests, adapted from existing speech language pathology tests, to collect speech samples from participants. Using several metrics extracted from these speech samples, we then developed models to identify features that would help with the classification of participants with PD and ALS. As we designed and developed our application however, we met several challenges that we had to address, such as user prompts, noise handling, data safety, speech sample capture, and user error. This paper describes details of our application and the challenges we met when developing it.

2 Related Work

There has been extensive research in speech features and using speech as a biomarker to detect neurodegenerative diseases. In [17], the authors showed that variation in the fundamental frequency (F0) could be used to differentiate between healthy and PD patients. Moreover, in [18], the authors found that changes in F0's variability could lead to an early diagnosis of PD. In this longitudinal study, which followed a PD patient for eleven years, including seven years pre-diagnosis, they were able to detect abnormal variability in F0 five years before the diagnosis was made. The work in [19] also identified specific speech metrics that are affected by PD. The authors showed that besides the variability of fundamental frequency already discussed above, breathiness and asthenia (weakness) were the two metrics most impacted by PD. These two metrics were measured by subjective means using the GRBAS scale, an auditory-perceptual evaluation method for hoarseness. The Diadochokinetic (DDK) rate and maximum phonation time, both measured objectively by a computer, were also found to be different (shorter) in PD patients.

Similar to our project, in [20], the authors used a 'quick vocal test' to assess which of the participants in their sample, 46 native speaking Czech, had PD. Their vocal test was made up of three different parts: a sustained phonation task, a DDK task, and a running speech task. Although they were able to get a classification performance of 85%, they used eight metrics from the frequency domain such as jitter, shimmer, and variability of fundamental frequency, to reach that result with only 24 PD patients. This means an average of only three participants per significant metrics, which is below the five to ten recommended to avoid overfitting [21, 22].

PD is not the only disease that has been shown to impact the production of speech. In [23], the authors found that ALS affected the speech of the patient by causing abnormal pitch (either too low or too high), limited pitch range, high harmonics-to-noise ratios, and increased nasality, among others symptoms.

From these studies' results, we were encouraged in our hypothesis that different neurodegenerative diseases impact the speech of the patients in specific ways, thereby different speech metrics patterns could assist with the diagnosis of specific neurological diseases. These related efforts on PD detection are different from our system since for one they only rely on a subset of the speech-based tasks contained in our application. They also limited their research to the detection of PD while we have a broader approach that allows for the detection of various neurodegenerative diseases.

3 Application Design

3.1 Overview and Workflow

Developed on iOS, our application is used to collect metadata and speech samples from participants with neurodegenerative diseases PD and ALS, as they have been shown to have a strong impact on speech [17, 18, 23]. This paper focuses on the design and functionality of the application itself, as well as the challenges involved in them, up to the upload of the data to our servers. The analysis of the data made on the servers is outside of the scope of this paper.

Our application consists of a practitioner questionnaire, which includes an optional feedback form, for research purposes to assess the ease of using the application, a participant questionnaire, and a series of speech-based tasks, and an optional participant feedback form. The workflow of the application can be seen in Fig. 1. The workflow is composed of four main steps, detailed below in different subsections.

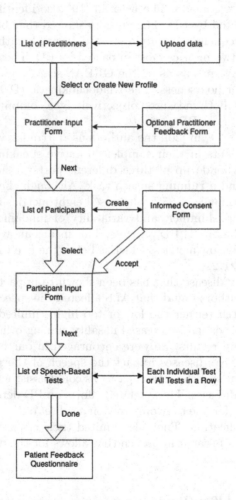

Fig. 1. The workflow of the mobile application

Step 1: The practitioner input/selection. The first screen of the application is the list of first and last names of practitioners registered on the device for selection. It also has two buttons, one to upload the device's data to our cloud servers, and one to create a new practitioner profile. The profile creation page asks for a for basic information (i.e. name, degree, institution), and has an option for the practitioner to submit feedback back to us.

Step 2: The participant input/selection. The participant questionnaire collects the participant's personal and medical information. In order to access the questionnaire, the participant first has to read through and agree to the consent form for our study.

The personal information section consists of asking the participant their name, gender, birth date, and native language. As for the practitioner, we hash the first name, last name and birth date, to create a unique ID for the participant.

The age, gender, and native language are relevant when extracting metrics from the speech samples. The questions about the native language and the strength of the accent serve two purposes. For our initial data collection, it allows us to exclude participants with an accent, as their accents would have been an extra parameter that biased our model. With more data being collected in the future for different accents, we will be able to create specific models for people with different accents. We also ask if the participant has undergone speech therapy of any kind, as it might impact the characteristics of the speech recordings.

The medical information section asks if the participants have an hearing impairment, so that we can assist them if they have difficulties hearing the prompts from the speech based tasks. We also record what cognitive changes if any, have been experienced by the participant, if the participant has been experiencing any unusual movements, or if the participant has felt more emotional or anxious than usual. We also ask if the participant have any problem with their speech. These questions are there for us to see if there is any correlation between the answers obtained from the participants about their self-assess well being, and the metrics extracted from their speech samples.

Finally, we ask what type of disease has the participant has been diagnosed with, and when. For the participants with PD, we also ask when did the participant took the last dose of their treatment. PD having a very regular medication cycle, we want to show a correlated impact on the metrics extracted from the speech samples, by collecting data from the same participants at different point of their medication cycle.

Step 3: The speech-based tasks. The speech-based tasks constitute the core of our application. Fourteen tasks were designed based on de facto standards in the field of speech-language pathology. A summary of the speech based tasks can be seen in the list below.

– Vowel Tests

- Vowel 'Ah' with Timer
- Vowel 'Ah' without Timer
- Vowel 'Eh' with Timer
- Vowel 'Eh' without Timer

Participants with speech impairments will have trouble maintaining a constant pitch or power throughout, or will exhibit vocal fry and breathiness. Two different vowels are being used, 'ah' and 'eh'. We chose these tasks because they have been shown to be a good indicator to detect jitter and shimmer [24,25], and have been used in research to monitor the evolution of PD in patients [26]. Both the time and non timed version of the task are used, in order to see if a difference can be seen in the way control, ALS and PD populations managed running out of air while performing this task.

– DDK Rate

- Repetitions of monosyllabic words. ("Pa"/"Ta"/"Ka") and Repetition of a polysyllabic word. ("PaTaKa") for 5 s intervals

Measure the Alternating Motion Rate (AMR) and Sequential Motion Rate (SMR). The DDK rate is the number of iterations per second a participant is able to produce correctly over a five second window. This permits the assessment of oral motor skills by giving a measure of the participant's ability to make rapid speech movement using different parts of the mouth. This task has been shown to capture differences in control, PD and ALS populations [19,27,28].

– Grandfather Passage

- Reading the grandfather passage

The text of the grandfather's passage was designed to contain almost every phoneme in the English language, thus allowing us to see whether the participants have some difficulties with specific phonemes. As an aside, the history of this text is interesting in its own right [29]. This task has been used in the past to detect acoustic characteristics in speech [30,31], and characteristics specific of PD and Multiple Sclerosis (MS) patients [32].

– Monosyllabic Words & Increasing Syllabic Words

- List of easy words. (mom, Bob, peep, bib, tot, deed, kick, gag, fife, sis, zoos, church, shush, lull, roar)
- Increased syllabic count task. (cat, catnip, catapult, catastrophe/please, pleasing, pleasingly/thick, thicken, thickening)

Here, we test to see at which point, if any, the participants either struggle or become unable to produce the correct word. We look for a "breakdown" in their ability to sequence the words correctly in order to rule out a "motor planning" issue versus a specific motor issue. This task was designed to assess the production of every consonant and vowel in the English language [33–36].

– Picture Description

• Describing a picture presented on the screen

Checking the participant capacity to handle volitional speech, with the extra cognitive load it entails to construct the sentences. A picture is chosen at random from ten possible pictures, and the participants are asked to describe it using any words of their choosing. With this, we are able to both measure the ease of the participants to select and program words on their own, with the extra stress it involves with word finding, semantics, syntax and pragmatic language features. by measuring features such as the rate of word production, the size of the dictionary used (number of different words), and the complexity of the words chosen.

– Multisyllabic Words

• List of complex words. (participate, application, education, difficulty, congratulations, possibility, mathematical, opportunity, statistical analysis, Methodist episcopal church)

Can the participant handle the complex motor patterns required to go from the front to the back of the mouth when saying these words.

– Sentences

• Sentences. (We saw several wild animals, My physician wrote out a prescription, The municipal judge sentenced the criminal, The supermarket chain shut down because of poor management, Much more money must be donated to make this department succeed)

Can the participant program the whole sentence while handling the formation of complex words that compose it. Part of the sentences used in this task were designed by Dr. Julie Liss from Arizona State University. Her goal with these sentences was to determine the type of dysarthria of participants based on rhythmicity of speech while uttering these sentences [37]. These sentences are: In this famous coffee shop they serve the best doughnuts in town, The chairman decided to pave over the shopping center garden, The standards committee met this afternoon in an open meeting.

– Automatic Speech Production

• Iterate the days of the week
• Iterate the months of the year
• Count from 1 to 30

Test the participants' automatic speech production, and their endurance in producing speech. It is considered automatic speech, as opposed to volitional or imitative speech, as the participants do not repeat the words like with the other tasks so far, but do not have to truly think about the words they are saying either, like in the picture description task, since they are part of sequences that are deeply ingrained into the participants' minds for having used them since childhood. The endurance part of the task comes from the length these tasks have, especially the first one. With some diseases, such as ALS, producing speech over such a long list of words in a row can be difficult.

3.2 Challenges in Design

We began data collection with a first version of the application for 28 days in November 2015 before implementing an improved V2 of our application. With this first version, a total of 1260 recordings have been made, corresponding to 103 min recorded, but with unfortunately 34% of these recordings which could not be used. We identified challenges that were addressed in subsequent versions; these challenges being discussed in the remainder of this paper.

User Handicap. The first issue we ran into was the difficulty for some participants, particularly ALS ones, to perform all of the tasks. They often did not have the endurance to go through all of the tests without having to take long pauses to recuperate, In order to deal with this, we added the option to skip tasks, and modified the tasks' order. This order is designed to allow the ALS patients to perform as many tasks as possible before they had to stop the testing. The screen listing the speech based tasks can be seen in Fig. 2.

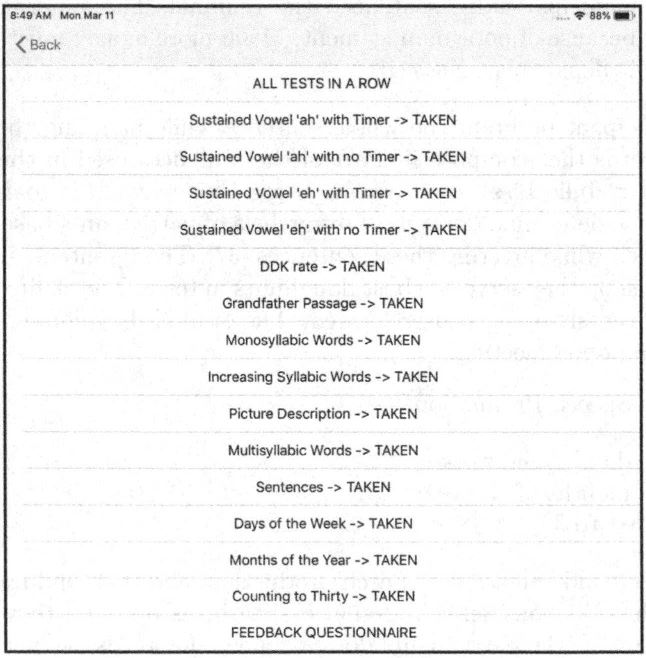

Fig. 2. The list of tasks after completion of a series

User Prompts. Each task needs audible instructions to explain to the participants what they are to do. Using a text-to-speech software avoid introducing any bias for participants that would try to mimic the speech patterns of a human voice. However, text-to-speech voice was reported as confusing for a lot of participants and had a clear negative impact on the application's usage, as participants did not understand the prompts. Instructions provided by a human voice are now used, that we made as even toned and accented as possible.

For the sustained vowel task, the challenge is to have the participant understand that the sound has to be sustained for a relatively long time. We displayed a long 'aaaaaaaaah' across the device's screen, and had a small arrow going under its length in 5 s. However, not everyone understood exactly what sound they were expected to make, which was solved by using audible prompts. Also, many participants did not understand that they were to start when the arrow under the text started moving nor were they able to know exactly how long the task was going to run for, and had trouble managing their breath to maintain voicing throughout. So a timer is now used, indicating how long the task is going to run for, and how much of it is left at all times, as can be seen in Fig. 3.

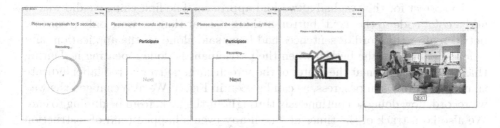

Fig. 3. From left to right: timer for timed tasks (here, the sustained vowel), screen while the participants listen to a word, screen when the participants repeat a word, picture description task while device in portrait mode, picture description task when device has been switched to landscape mode

For the DDK test, special care had to be taken, as here we needed the application to explain what specific sounds to produce, and the fact that these sounds needed to be produced as fast as possible, but not too fast that it hindered the proper production of the expected sounds. The initial design would show the words go across the screen, but for one, people would read 'Pa' several different ways, and, more importantly, the participants would, try to match the speed of the text on the screen rather than reaching their own maximum speed. Like in the sustained vowel task, an audible prompt is now used to indicate the proper pronunciation and a timer is now used to indicate how long remains on the test.

With this grandfather passage, the difficulty is to choose how to display the text. The ability to choose the font, and potentially make the page scrollable would introduce too much variables from participant to participant. So we chose to instead use a fixed font that would be as big as possible as to fit the whole text on the screen. After testing this design, feedback from the practitioners taught us that it would be easier for most participants if the font was a bit smaller and instead the line spacing a bit bigger, so these modifications were integrated into the application.

Clipping of the Recordings. Another challenge with the design of the speech-based tasks was to deal with participants not being timed properly with the application's prompts, talking before the end of the instructions, or going to the next task, or part of a task, as they are still completing the previous one. We thought it would be best to make one recording per word or sentence, making it easier to know what words contained each recordings. After the end of each instruction, a new recording would start, and end when the participant pressed the 'next' button that was on the screen. After some data collection, it became clear that a lot of clipping was happening, from people that would start to talk a little bit before the instruction's recording was done, or tap the next button while they were still talking. This lead to a lot of recordings either too clipped for use, or empty all together. Out of all the recordings that are not usable, 42% of them where due to this issue.

To correct for this, we had a two-fold approach. The first thing we did was to add a color code to the 'next' button making it clear that we were only recording between after the word or sentences had been said aloud by the application, and before the press of the button when the participant is done repeating it. During that time, the button at the center of the screen turns red and a red label indicate that a recording is in progress, as can be seen in Fig. 3. We also changed the way we record, now doing so continuously throughout the task, from beginning to end. We also keep track of the times at which any events happen (end of instruction sound file being played, button being tapped by user, etc.). With this, we are able to know when in the sound file we can find the participant talking. To deal with what clipping still happens in spite of the clearer color coding during the task, we can also crop the sound file for each word or sentences a few 10s of a second before and after the timing information recorded the participant to be talking, insuring that we capture all of the speech sample.

User Error. Another big challenge was handling incorrect inputs from the participants. As seen in Fig. 3, there are two buttons present at the upper right corner of the screen during each task: 'Skip' and 'Stop'. When pressing skip, the practitioner signals that the task was either avoided altogether or that the participant could not complete it. This allows for a task series to be completed even by participant who do not have the capacities to go through all the tasks. When pressing the stop button, the task currently being performed is canceled and the application goes back to the list of tasks. The recordings for that task is not saved, nor are the meta-data about the task, which thus remains as non-taken on the screen with the list of tasks. When doing all the tasks in a row, we added a transition screen in between tasks to redo a specific task without having to stop the series. This screen gives the option, at the end of every task, to either proceed to the next one if all went well, or redo it if the first attempt was not performed properly, without leaving the current series.

After a test series is completed, and all the tasks as marked as taken, the practitioner can still, if needed, redo any of the task that might not have been properly performed by the participant. The data previously collected for that task would then be overwritten by the new recording. This way, the data from tasks that needed redoing are not kept, keeping the data collected as clean as possible. By default, the task series are automatically reset at the end of each day, so that if a task series exists for the selected participant, and it has been started on a day prior to the current one, this task series is closed and a new one is created at the current time and date.

Data Handling. As our application is dealing with medical data, privacy and security are of the utmost importance. It is imperative that the data be kept secured on the device, as well as on the backend servers, and in transit from the former to the later. On the device, the data is kept encrypted by iOS which prevent the data to be accessed by anyone without the device's password.

Initially, our application's data was stored in flat text files. This was easy to implement but made analysing the data complex as dedicated scripts had to be written to query the data. Starting with V2 of the application, we now use a SQLite database through iOS Core Data, allowing the data to be queried using SQL.

To increase the security of the participant's private information, we upload the anonymous information from the participant on a different server than the rest of the data collected. This allows for an extra layer of security: even if one of the server were to be breached, the data of each server would not be useful for an attacker without to data from the other as they would either get access to a list of name with no associated information, or to completely anonymized data. When uploading, the application first separate the anonymous information from the participants (first and last name of the participants), together with the unique ID generated for each participants. The anonymous data is then sent through an encrypted connection to an AWS server. The rest of the data is sent, still through an encrypted connection, to a different server hosted by the Center for Research Computing (CRC) at Notre Dame. Both servers are located behind firewalls to prevent unallowed access.

4 Conclusion and Future Work

Data has been recorded between November 2015 and March 2019. The V2 has been implemented from December 2015 while V3 was used from August 2018. A total of 70 individuals were tested, including control group, ALS suffering individuals and Parkinsons suffering individuals, and team members testing the application. Out of those 70 individuals we excluded all the tests and all bad recordings, which let us with a total of 64 individuals having contributed usable recordings. Each individual has been recorded under a single version of the application, none has tested different versions of the application. The average number of recordings per participant is 26, while the average total recording of an individual is almost 7 min. Of all 64 participants, 56% were men and 44% were female, while the distribution per pathology can be seen in Fig. 4.

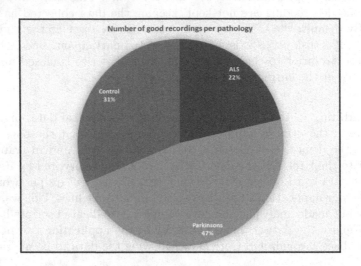

Fig. 4. Distribution of the participants per pathology

A total of 509 min of recordings have been made, out of them 446 min are considered 'good', i.e. can be properly analysed. For most individuals all recording was conducted within a single day, while it was organized in 2 or even 3 d for around 20% of them.

To determine the quality of the recordings, we created a small iOS application that allowed us to efficiently check each of the recordings manually. For each recording, we could set a boolean to indicate if the recording could be used in our analysis, and a comment to indicate why not (no sound, loud ambient noise, participant did not understand the test...). With each version of the application, the percentage of good recordings kept on going higher. Through this data collection process, learning from our errors, we have been able to overcome each of the challenges detailed in this paper. From more than a third of the recordings not fit for analysis, we achieved to go under the 10% threshold with less than 8% of poor quality recordings in the current version of the application, which we consider acceptable, as can be seen in Fig. 5. With each version, the incremental improvements made allowed for the application to perform better. In its current state, it is able to record more accurately, prompting the users clearly and without introducing biases, collecting more metadata for a richer and easier analysis of the recordings.

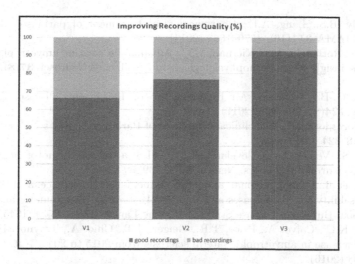

Fig. 5. Proportion of bad recordings per version of the application

With the data that we have now collected, we are working on building statistical and machine learning models to classify the recordings with high accuracy. We will first work on extracting metrics from each of the recordings, both from the time and frequency domain. In the time domain, these could be the number of utterance per second for the DDK test, or the number of words per second, total time per sentences, amount of time in between each words for the sentences tests, and grandfather passage. These can be measured by using Sphinx [38] to measure the start and end of each words in the tests. For the frequency domain, a large array of metrics will be extracted using python and praat [39], such as the shimmer, jitter, average pitch, variance in intensity, breathiness... All these metrics will then serve as the basis for our modelling work to classify each recording as control, PD or ALS. The work is currently in progress and will be presented as part of a future paper.

Acknowledgment. This research was supported in part by GE Health and the National Football League through the GE/NFL Head Health Challenge. The research was further supported in part by the National Science Foundation under Grant Number IIS-1450349.

The authors wish to thanks Dr. Julie Stierwalt from the Mayo clinic, Rochester, MI, Dr. Kim Winter from the Hospital for Special Care, New Britain, CT, and the Rock Steady Boxing program participants and leaders, especially Don Sheliga and Morgan Books.

References

1. Poewe, W., et al.: Parkinson disease. Nat. Rev. Dis. Primers **3**(1), 1–21 (2017)
2. Kiernan, M.C., et al.: Amyotrophic lateral sclerosis. Lancet **377**(9769), 942–955 (2011)

3. Connolly, B.S., Lang, A.E.: Pharmacological treatment of parkinson disease: a review. JAMA **311**(16), 1670–1683 (2014)
4. Vucic, S., Rothstein, J.D., Kiernan, M.C.: Advances in treating amyotrophic lateral sclerosis: insights from pathophysiological studies. Trends Neurosci. **37**(8), 433–442 (2014)
5. Tysnes, O.-B., Storstein, A.: Epidemiology of Parkinson's disease. J. Neural Transm. **124**(8), 901–905 (2017)
6. Sveinbjornsdottir, S.: The clinical symptoms of Parkinson's disease. J. Neurochem. **139**, 318–324 (2016)
7. Boillée, S., Velde, C.V., Cleveland, D.W.: ALS: a disease of motor neurons and their nonneuronal neighbors. Neuron **52**(1), 39–59 (2006)
8. Vos, T., et al.: Global, regional, and national incidence, prevalence, and years lived with disability for 310 diseases and injuries, 1990–2015: a systematic analysis for the Global Burden of Disease Study 2015. The Lancet **388**(10053), 1545 (2016)
9. Arthur, K.C., Calvo, A., Price, T.R., Geiger, J.T., Chio, A., Traynor, B.J.: Projected increase in amyotrophic lateral sclerosis from 2015 to 2040. Nat. Commun. **7**, 12408 (2016)
10. Ringholz, G., Appel, S.H., Bradshaw, M., Cooke, N., Mosnik, D., Schulz, P.: Prevalence and patterns of cognitive impairment in sporadic ALS. Neurology **65**(4), 586–590 (2005)
11. Strong, M.J., et al.: Consensus criteria for the diagnosis of frontotemporal cognitive and behavioural syndromes in amyotrophic lateral sclerosis. Amyotrophic Lateral Sclerosis **10**(3), 131–146 (2009)
12. World Health Organization, et al.: Dementia: A Public Health Priority. World Health Organization (2012)
13. Sim, I.: Mobile devices and health. New Engl. J. Med. **381**(10), 956–968 (2019)
14. Silva, B.M., Rodrigues, J.J., de la Torre Díez, I., ópez-Coronado, M.L., Saleem, K.: Mobile-health: a review of current state in 2015. J. Biomed. Inf. **56**, 265–272 (2015)
15. Zhang, C., Zhang, X., Halstead-Nussloch, R.: Assessment metrics, challenges and strategies for mobile health apps. Issues Inf. Syst. **15**(2) (2014)
16. Al-Saadi, T.A., Aljarrah, T.M., Alhashemi, A.M., Hussain, A.: A systematic review of usability challenges and testing in mobile health. Int. J. Acc. Financ. Rep. **5**(2), 1–14 (2015)
17. Rusz, J., Cmejla, R., Ruzickova, H., Ruzicka, E.: Quantitative acoustic measurements for characterization of speech and voice disorders in early untreated Parkinson's disease. J. Acoust. Soc. Am. **129**(1), 350–367 (2011)
18. Harel, B., Cannizzaro, M., Snyder, P.J.: Variability in fundamental frequency during speech in prodromal and incipient Parkinson's disease: a longitudinal case study. Brain Cogn. **56**(1), 24–29 (2004)
19. Midi, I., Dogan, M., Koseoglu, M., Can, G., Sehitoglu, M., Gunal, D.: Voice abnormalities and their relation with motor dysfunction in Parkinson's disease. Acta Neurol. Scand. **117**(1), 26–34 (2008)
20. Rusz, J., et al.: Acoustic assessment of voice and speech disorders in Parkinson's disease through quick vocal test. Mov. Disord. **26**(10), 1951–1952 (2011)
21. Peduzzi, P., Concato, J., Kemper, E., Holford, T.R., Feinstein, A.R.: A simulation study of the number of events per variable in logistic regression analysis. J. Clin. Epidemiol. **49**(12), 1373–1379 (1996)
22. Vittinghoff, E., McCulloch, C.E.: Relaxing the rule of ten events per variable in logistic and cox regression. Am. J. Epidemiol. **165**(6), 710–718 (2007)

23. Green, J.R., et al.: Bulbar and speech motor assessment in ALS: challenges and future directions. Amyotrophic Lateral Sclerosis Frontotemporal Degeneration 14(7–8), 494–500 (2013)
24. Brockmann, M., Drinnan, M.J., Storck, C., Carding, P.N.: Reliable jitter and shimmer measurements in voice clinics: the relevance of vowel, gender, vocal intensity, and fundamental frequency effects in a typical clinical task. J. Voice 25(1), 44–53 (2011)
25. Horii, Y.: Jitter and shimmer differences among sustained vowel phonations. J. Speech, Lang. Hear. Res. 25(1), 12–14 (1982)
26. Tsanas, A., Little, M.A., McSharry, P.E., Ramig, L.O.: Accurate telemonitoring of Parkinson's disease progression by noninvasive speech tests. IEEE Trans. Biomed. Eng. 57(4), 884–893 (2010)
27. Canter, G.J.: Speech characteristics of patients with Parkinson's disease: III. articulation, diadochokinesis, and over-all speech adequacy. J. Speech Hear. Disord. 30(3), 217–224 (1965)
28. Tjaden, K., Watling, E.: Characteristics of diadochokinesis in multiple sclerosis and Parkinson's disease. Folia Phoniatrica et Logopaedica 55(5), 241–259 (2003)
29. Reilly, J., Fisher, J.L.: Sherlock holmes and the strange case of the missing attribution: a historical note on "the grandfather passage". J. Lang. Hear. Res. (2012)
30. Vogel, A.P., Maruff, P., Snyder, P.J., Mundt, J.C.: Standardization of pitch-range settings in voice acoustic analysis. Behav. Res. Methods 41(2), 318–324 (2009)
31. Zraick, R.I., Wendel, K., Smith-Olinde, L.: The effect of speaking task on perceptual judgment of the severity of dysphonic voice. J. Voice 19(4), 574–581 (2005)
32. Tjaden, K., Sussman, J.E., Wilding, G.E.: Impact of clear, loud, and slow speech on scaled intelligibility and speech severity in Parkinson's disease and multiple sclerosis. J. Speech, Lang. Hear. Res. 57(3), 779–792 (2014)
33. Duffy, J.R., et al.: Temporal acoustic measures distinguish primary progressive apraxia of speech from primary progressive aphasia. Brain Lang. 168, 84–94 (2017)
34. Strand, E.A., McNeil, M.R.: Effects of length and linguistic complexity on temporal acoustic measures in apraxia of speech. J. Speech, Lang. Hear. Res. 39(5), 1018–1033 (1996)
35. Odell, K., McNeil, M.R., Rosenbek, J.C., Hunter, L.: Perceptual characteristics of vowel and prosody production in apraxic, aphasic, and dysarthric speakers. J. Speech, Lang. Hear. Res. 34(1), 67–80 (1991)
36. Haley, K.L., Overton, H.B.: Word length and vowel duration in apraxia of speech: the use of relative measures. Brain Lang. 79(3), 397–406 (2001)
37. Liss, J.M., LeGendre, S., Lotto, A.J.: Discriminating dysarthria type from envelope modulation spectra. J. Speech, Lang. Hear. Res. 53(5), 1246–1255 (2010)
38. Huggins-Daines, D., Kumar, M., Chan, A., Black, A.W., Ravishankar, M., Rudnicky, A.I.: PocketSphinx: a free, real-time continuous speech recognition system for hand-held devices. In: 2006 IEEE International Conference on Acoustics, Speech and Signal Processing, 2006. ICASSP 2006 Proceedings, vol. 1, p. I. IEEE (2006)
39. Styler, W.: Using praat for linguistic research. University Colorado at Boulder Phonetics Lab (2017)

Patient-Independent Schizophrenia Relapse Prediction Using Mobile Sensor Based Daily Behavioral Rhythm Changes

Bishal Lamichhane[1]($\boxtimes$), Dror Ben-Zeev[2], Andrew Campbell[3],
Tanzeem Choudhury[4], Marta Hauser[5], John Kane[5], Mikio Obuchi[3],
Emily Scherer[3], Megan Walsh[5], Rui Wang[3], Weichen Wang[3], and Akane Sano[1]

[1] Rice University, Houston, USA
bishal.lamichhane@rice.edu
[2] University of Washington, Seattle, USA
[3] Dartmouth College, Hanover, USA
[4] Cornell University, Ithaca, USA
[5] Northwell Health, New Hyde Park, USA

Abstract. A schizophrenia relapse has severe consequences for a patient's health, work, and sometimes even life safety. If an oncoming relapse can be predicted on time, for example by detecting early behavioral changes in patients, then interventions could be provided to prevent the relapse. In this work, we investigated a machine learning based schizophrenia relapse prediction model using mobile sensing data to characterize behavioral features. A patient-independent model providing sequential predictions, closely representing the clinical deployment scenario for relapse prediction, was evaluated. The model uses the mobile sensing data from the recent four weeks to predict an oncoming relapse in the next week. We used the behavioral rhythm features extracted from daily templates of mobile sensing data, self-reported symptoms collected via EMA (Ecological Momentary Assessment), and demographics to compare different classifiers for the relapse prediction. Naive Bayes based model gave the best results with an F2 score of 0.083 when evaluated in a dataset consisting of 63 schizophrenia patients, each monitored for up to a year. The obtained F2 score, though low, is better than the baseline performance of random classification (F2 score of 0.02 ± 0.024). Thus, mobile sensing has predictive value for detecting an oncoming relapse and needs further investigation to improve the current performance. Towards that end, further feature engineering and model personalization based on the behavioral idiosyncrasies of a patient could be helpful.

Keywords: Mobile sensing · Ubiquitous computing · Schizophrenia · Relapse prediction

© ICST Institute for Computer Sciences, Social Informatics and Telecommunications Engineering 2021
Published by Springer Nature Switzerland AG 2021. All Rights Reserved
J. Ye et al. (Eds.): MobiHealth 2020, LNICST 362, pp. 18–33, 2021.
https://doi.org/10.1007/978-3-030-70569-5_2

1   Introduction

Schizophrenia is a chronic mental disorder affecting about 20 million people worldwide [11]. Patients with schizophrenia perceive reality abnormally and show disturbances in their thoughts and behaviors. Some of the associated symptoms are delusions, hallucinations, disordered thinking, incoherent speech (putting together words that do not make sense), disorganized motor functions, social withdrawal, appearances of lack of emotions, etc. [1,10]. A patient with schizophrenia is generally treated with antipsychotic drugs and psycho-social counseling. These patients are treated as out-patients, in the general non-serious cases, and they visit the clinic for routine mental health assessment. During the visit, the patient's symptoms are tracked and medications/therapies are adapted. Questionnaires such as BPRS (Brief Psychiatric Rating Scale) [15] are used to keep track of the symptoms. A patient with schizophrenia under a treatment regimen might sometimes experience a relapse, an acute increase of schizophrenia symptoms and degrading mental health. The routine clinical visits and BPRS based assessments are meant to keep track of symptoms and prevent any likely relapses. However, the clinical visits happen only every few months and a patient might have a relapse in between the visits.

A relapse has severe consequences for both the patients and their caregivers (e.g. their family), even endangering their lives in some cases. So it is important to detect an oncoming relapse and provide timely interventions for prevention. It might be possible to use mobile sensing to predict an oncoming relapse by detecting behavioral and emotional changes associated with schizophrenia symptoms. Mobile sensors like accelerometer, GPS, ambient light sensors, microphones, etc. can capture various aspects of a person's behavior. These can then be complemented by questionnaires (e.g. Ecological Momentary Assessments - EMA), delivered through a mobile application, to assess the person's self-reported symptoms, behavior and feeling and build a relapse prediction model. Mobile sensing would be a low-cost and scalable solution for relapse prediction compared to other alternatives such as the pharmacological approach [12].

In this work, we investigated mobile sensing based schizophrenia relapse prediction using mobile sensing. Relapse prediction is framed as a binary classification problem, associating an upcoming period as relapse or non-relapse based on the features observed in the current period. We extracted daily behavioral rhythm based features from mobile sensing data, which was also effective in predicting self-reported schizophrenia symptoms in our previous work [17], complemented by self-reported symptoms collected through EMA and demographics features, and evaluated different classifiers for relapse prediction. Daily template based rhythm features were found to outperform feature sets proposed in previous works for relapse prediction. Further, our proposed model is a sequential prediction model trained and evaluated in a patient-independent setting. Such a relapse prediction model, closer to a clinical deployment solution, has not been investigated in previous works. Our work establishes the basic feasibility of using mobile sensing for schizophrenia relapse prediction and identifies related challenges, to be addressed in future work. The paper is organized as follows.

In Sect. 2, we present some of the related works on relapse prediction in the context of schizophrenia and other mental disorders. In Sect. 3, the dataset and methodology used for developing the relapse prediction model are discussed. This is followed by Sect. 4 where we present the evaluation results of the developed model. These results are discussed in Sect. 5 and we present our conclusions in Sect. 6.

2   Related Work

Several previous works have investigated the prediction of relapses in the context of mental disorders and substance addiction. The authors in [4] studied the prediction of psychotic symptoms relapses based on the linguistic and behavioral features inferred from the Facebook post. The prediction model was evaluated to have a specificity of 0.71 in a study of 51 participants. The work thus showcased the potential of behavior profiling for relapse prediction in the context of mental disorders. In [9], the authors are aiming to use mobile sensing based features such as sleep quality, sociability, mobility, and mood changes to predict the relapse of depressive episodes. Mobile sensing and social behavior (online or offline social behavior) have also been found to be helpful in predicting relapses of substance addictions. The authors in [22] analyzed social media posts and social network influences to predict the relapse of opioid usages. Similarly, the authors in [5] discussed the relevance of several contextual information such as sleep deprivation, affect, environment, and location, derivable from mobile sensing, for predicting relapse of alcoholism.

Some earlier works have already investigated schizophrenia relapse prediction based on mobile sensing. For example, the authors in [2] investigated the relation of schizophrenia relapse with mobility and behavioral features derived from mobile sensing. In their study population of 17 patients, 5 patients had a relapse. The authors analyzed the anomaly of mobility and sociability features in this population and found increased incidences of an anomaly in weeks leading up to relapse. The anomaly was defined as the deviation of features from an expected pattern. Though this work is one of the pioneering works on mobile sensing based schizophrenia relapse prediction, generating novel qualitative insights, the authors did not develop any prediction model probably due to the limited size of the study population. The authors in [6] also explored the usage of mobile sensing based features for schizophrenia relapse prediction. Sociability features based on outgoing calls and messages were found to be significantly different before a relapse, compared to a non-relapse period. This insight is helpful to predict an oncoming relapse. However, the others only provided qualitative analysis and no predictive models were evaluated. In contrast to these two earlier works which offered qualitative analysis only, we proposed and evaluated relapse prediction models in our work.

Relapse prediction models have been investigated in a previous work of [18,19]. The authors evaluated the potential of mobile sensing based features to predict an oncoming relapse. The authors also framed relapse prediction as a binary classification task, classifying an oncoming period as either relapse or non-relapse. Mobility, sociability, and EMA features were computed for each epoch of the day (morning, afternoon, evening, and night) and features from N days (comparing for different values of N) were used to predict if there was going to be a relapse in the next day. Several machine learning models were evaluated for relapse prediction. Using 3-fold cross-validation, SVM (rbf kernel) was found to give the best performance with an F1-score of 0.27. The study population consisted of 61 patients with schizophrenia where 27 instances of relapse were reported in 20 patients. We used the same dataset for our evaluations and build upon the work of the authors to generate further insights on a mobile sensing based relapse prediction model. The authors in [18] established that the mobile sensing based behavioral features indeed have an association with an upcoming relapse. However, there was likely a look-ahead bias in their evaluations due to k-fold random cross-validation that was used. Within k-fold cross-validation, mobile sensing data from the future is also used for building a prediction model for a given test patient, while the model is being evaluated using the currently observed data. In contrast to this approach, we developed a sequential relapse prediction model evaluated in a patient-independent setting. The relation between current/past mobile sensing data and future relapses is first modeled from the patients in the training set only. The trained model is then used to predict, sequentially over time, if the mobile sensing data from the patient in the test set indicate an oncoming relapse. This approach of modeling brings the evaluation closer to clinical deployment. Further, unlike the work in [18], we do not impose any knowledge of relapse location to create the feature extraction/evaluation windows. Its implication is that a sliding window approach to relapse prediction has to be used, leading to a higher number of feature extraction windows to be evaluated. Naturally, this leads to a higher chance of incurring false positives during prediction and reduced classification performance. Nonetheless, such an evaluation would better reflect a real clinical deployment scenario. Finally, we used the daily behavioral rhythm features extracted from the daily template, composed of the hourly averages of the mobile sensing data, to characterize the behavioral patterns of a patient. Thus, finer temporal resolution is retained for feature extraction compared to the work of [18] where features were extracted for each of the 6-hour periods of the day (6 am–12 pm, 12 pm–6 pm, 6 pm–12 am, and 12 am–6 am).

3   Methods

In this section, we describe the dataset and methodology that has been used to develop our proposed relapse prediction model.

3.1   Dataset

We used the dataset from the CrossCheck project [6, 19–21] (available at https://www.kaggle.com/dartweichen/crosscheck) for the development and evaluation of a relapse prediction model. The dataset consists of data from a clinical trial where 75 schizophrenia patients were monitored for up to a year with the Crosscheck system [3] continuously collecting passive sensing data from patients' smartphones. The number of patients and the monitoring period are significantly larger than those in previous works on schizophrenia patient monitoring [2]. The data collected were: accelerometer, light levels, sound levels, GPS, and call/sms log. Further, the Crosscheck system also routinely obtained self-assessments from patients with EMA (Ecological Momentary Assessment) [16]. These EMA, which were obtained up to three times in a week, consisted of 10 questions to assess patients' current emotional and behavioral state. The questions asked were, for instance, *Have you been feeling calm?*, *Have you been social?* etc. Patients could answer the EMA questions with four options: *Not at all, A little, Moderately, Extremely*. EMA obtained at a low frequency, e.g. every few days only, makes it less burdensome for the patients. In the dataset, data from 63 patients were made available for analysis. The mean age and education years of these patients were: 37.2 years (min: 18 years, max: 65 years) and 9.4 years (min: 5 years, max: 14 years) respectively. Among the 63 patients, 20 patients had a relapse and there were 27 instances of relapse in total (some patients had multiple relapses) as annotated by clinical assessors [18, 19].

3.2   Relapse Prediction Model

We developed machine learning models that can predict if there is an oncoming relapse in the next week (prediction window) based on the mobile sensing data from recent 4 weeks (feature extraction window). A sliding window with a stride of 1 week is used for feature extraction, thus obtaining a sequential prediction for each week of monitoring. This approach of relapse prediction is shown in Fig. 1. We trained and evaluated the model in a patient-independent setting, using leave-one-patient-out cross-validation. The features that were used for our relapse prediction model are described next.

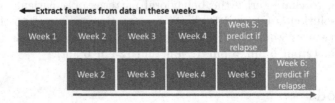

Fig. 1. Relapse prediction approach in our model. Features are extracted from 4 weeks of data to predict an oncoming relapse in the next week. A prediction for each week is produced with a sliding window of stride length 1 week.

3.3 Features

A summary of all the features extracted from the daily template (composed of hourly averages) of mobile sensing data, EMA, and demographics data are shown in Table 1. In this section, we describe how these different features are extracted.

Table 1. Different features extracted from the mobile sensing, EMA, and demographics for relapse prediction. Features are extracted from six mobile sensing signal using their daily template representation and 10 items of the EMA.

Daily Rhythm features
Mean daily template (mDT) features: *mean, standard deviation, maximum, range, skewness, kurtosis*
Standard deviation template (sDT) features: *mean*
Absolute difference between mDT and mxDT: *maximum*
Distance between normalized mDT(current) and mDT(previous)
Weighted distance between normalized mDT(current) and mDT(previous)
Distance between normlized mxDT(current) and mDT(previous)
Daily averages: *mean, standard deviation*
EMA features
EMA item values: *mean, standard deviation*
Demographics
Age, Education years

Daily Rhythm Features. Six mobile sensing signals, obtained continuously throughout the day, were derived from the dataset for daily template based rhythm feature extraction. The signals derived were: accelerometer magnitude (magnitude from 3-axis accelerometer signal recordings), (ambient) light levels, distance traveled (from GPS), call duration (from call log), sound levels, and conversation duration. These signals were derived from the raw mobile sensor recordings as in [18]. We obtained a daily template for each of the mobile sensing signals by computing the hourly averages of the signal in a given day of monitoring (thus the template consists of 24 points corresponding to each hour of the day). The templates capture daily rhythmic behaviors which are relevant for monitoring behavioral changes in schizophrenia patients [17]. An example of a daily template obtained for the light level signal is shown in Fig. 2. Five categories of features were extracted from the daily templates of mobile sensing signals.

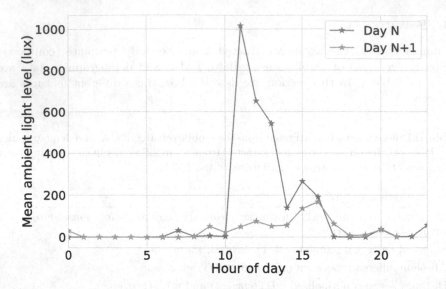

Fig. 2. An example showing the daily template for the ambient light levels in two consecutive days, obtained from the hourly averages of the light levels recorded from the smartphone of a patient for the given days. Daily templates were obtained for six different signal modalities available: accelerometer magnitude, light levels, distance, conversation, sound levels, and call duration. These templates were then characterized to obtain daily template features used for relapse prediction.

   (i) Mean daily template features: Since we used a feature extraction window of 4 weeks, there are 28 daily templates of each of the mobile sensing signals in a given feature extraction window. The daily templates of a mobile sensing signal across the 4 weeks were averaged to obtain the mean daily template (mDT). An example is shown in Fig. 3. The obtained mDT was then characterized by six statistical features: mean, maximum, standard deviation, range, skewness, and kurtosis.

  (ii) Deviation daily template features: Just like the mean daily template which was obtained by averaging the 28 daily templates in a feature extraction window, deviation daily template (dDT) was obtained by taking the standard deviation of the daily templates (deviation of each of the points in the template) across the 28 days, for each patient. The mean of the obtained dDT was then extracted as a feature to characterize the signal variability in a given feature extraction window.

 (iii) Maximum daily template features: Maximum daily template (mxDT) was obtained similarly as mDT and dDT by taking the maximum of the hourly average points across 28 days in the daily templates, within a feature extraction window. For computing features from mxDT, the difference between mDT and mxDT was obtained and the maximum absolute difference ($\text{maxDiff} = max(|mDT - mxDT|)$) was extracted as a feature

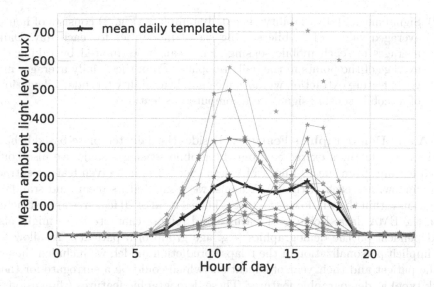

Fig. 3. Mean daily template obtained by averaging the daily templates of the days within a feature extraction window.

characterizing the maximum deviation from the mean in a given feature extraction window.

(iv) Template distance features: To characterize the changes between successive feature extraction windows, we computed features based on the distance between the templates for the current and the previous feature extraction window. In particular, distance based on mDT and mxDT were used. First, we normalized mDT and mxDT of a feature extraction window with their respective maximum value. Then the distance between the normalized mDTs (mDT for the current and the previous feature extraction window) was computed as a feature with:

$$dist_{mDT} = \sum_{i=1}^{24}((mDT_{norm}(curr)[i] - mDT_{norm}(prev)[i])^2)$$

A weighted version of $dist_{mDT}$, considering the points in the template between 9 AM–9 PM only, was also extracted as a feature to characterize the differences seen in the main part of the day. The weighted distance was computed as:

$$wdist_{mDT} = \sum_{i=9}^{21}((mDT_{norm}(curr)[i] - mDT_{norm}(prev)[i])^2)$$

The mxDT based distance feature was computed between the normalized mxDT and mDT as:

$$dist_{mxDT} = \sum_{i=1}^{24}((mxDT_{norm}(curr)[i] - mDT_{norm}(prev)[i])^2)$$

(v) Signal mean and variability: The daily template (Fig. 2) consists of hourly averaged values of mobile sensing signal modalities for each day. Daily averages for each mobile sensing signal can be estimated by taking the average of the points in the daily template. From these daily averages in a given feature extraction window, mean and variability (standard deviation) of a mobile sensing signal were computed as features.

EMA and Demographics Features. Besides the daily template-based behavioral rhythm features extracted from the mobile sensing signals, we also computed features from the 10-item EMA data (Sect. 3.1) in a given feature extraction window. For each of the EMA items, we computed its mean and standard deviation within the window as features. Thus a total of 20 features are extracted from the EMA data. Behavioral features and relapse characteristics might also be dependent on the demographics (e.g. age group of a patient). To allow for the implicit personalization of the relapse prediction model, we included the age of the patient and their year of education (which could be a surrogate for their work type) as demographic features. These demographic features (dimension 2) were appended alongside the EMA features (dimension 20) and daily template features (dimension 78) for each of the feature extraction window to characterize the behavioral patterns in a given window.

3.4 Classification

Dataset Size. With our feature extraction and prediction window sizes (Sect. 3.2), we obtained a total of 2386 feature extraction windows from the entire dataset. Of these, 23 windows were labeled as preceding (by a week) an incidence of relapse. Some of the relapse incidents got excluded from the analysis as they were too early in the monitoring period or there was no monitoring data around the relapse dates. When a feature extraction window was identified as preceding a relapse, then the next feature extraction window was obtained after a cool-off period of 28 days (similar to the cool-off period concept used in [18]). This was done to prevent any feature extraction window from being corrupted by monitoring data during the actual relapse which might include hospitalization or other interventions.

Model Validation. We used leave-one-patient-out cross-validation for the validation of the relapse prediction model. Data from all the patients, except from one (hold-out set), was used to train a classifier for relapse prediction. The trained model was then evaluated using the data from the hold-out patient. This process was repeated with a different patient in the hold out set every time. Leave-one-patient-out for model validation reflects a clinical deployment scenario where a trained model is expected to provide predictions for a new unseen patient. The trained model could be adapted for the new patient with different model personalization strategies.

Classifiers. As our dataset size is fairly small, a simple classifier could be more suited for the classification task. Therefore we chose to evaluate Naive Bayes based classification for relapse prediction. We also evaluated other classifiers for comparison. In particular, we evaluated Balanced Random Forest (BRF) [8] and EasyEnsemble (EE) classifier [14]. These classifiers were selected since they are suited for learning in an imbalanced dataset (The ratio of relapse to non-relapse is ~1:100 in our classification task and is thus imbalanced). Isolation Forest (IF) [13], a one-class classifier commonly used for outlier detection, was also evaluated. In the IF based classification, the relapse class was treated as the outlier class. The number of trees for BRF, EE, and IF was empirically set to 51, 101, and 101 respectively. We also evaluated a classification baseline by randomly predicting relapse or non-relapse for each week of prediction in the test set (within the leave-one-patient-out cross-validation setting). The ratio of relapse to non-relapse in these random predictions was matched to the ratio in the training set. The random predictions for 1000 independent runs were averaged to obtain the baseline results.

Feature Transformation: There are different flavors of Naive Bayes classifier, each imposing an assumption on the distribution of the underlying features. We used the Categorical Naive Bayes model since features can be easily transformed to be categorical with simple transformations. We transformed each of the features extracted (Sect. 3.3) into 15 categories (empirically chosen) based on the bin membership of each feature values in its histogram. The histogram is constructed from the training data only. These transformed features were then used in a categorical Naive Bayes classification model. The categorization of features quantizes the behavioral patterns and relapses could be linked as a shift in the categorized levels. Feature transformation with categorization was found to be beneficial (better classification performance) for use with the other classifiers considered (BRF, EE, and IF). Thus we employed feature transformation in the classification pipeline irrespective of the classifier used.

Feature Selection: Since we extracted a large number of features and our dataset size is relatively small, we evaluated the classification pipeline with a patient-specific feature selection strategy. A training sub-sample, consisting of all the data points labeled as relapse in the training set and N non-relapse data points from the training set patients closest in age to the patient in the test set, is selected. From this training sub-sample, M top features are identified. We used mutual information based criterion between features and the target label to select the top M features. The machine learning model for relapse prediction was then trained using these selected M features only. In our leave-one-patient-out cross-validation, different feature sets would be automatically selected depending upon the patient currently in the test set. The value of N was set to 100 (so that non-relapse data from at least two patients are included in the training subset) and M was set to 5 (which gave the best performance from the considered values: 3, 5, 10, 15, and 20). The underlying hypothesis for the age-based training sub-sample creation is that the patients from a similar age group would have similarities in their behavior and thus the feature-target relations would translate within the age groups.

3.5 Evaluation Metric

We evaluated the relapse prediction model using F2 score metric which is defined as:

$$F2 = \frac{5 * precision * recall}{4 * precision + recall}$$

where $precision = \frac{TP}{TP+FP}$ and $recall = \frac{TP}{TP+FN}$ (TP: Number of True positives, FP: Number of False positives, FN: Number of False Negatives). F2 score gives higher priority to recall compared to precision. In the context of the relapse prediction task, this translates to higher importance assigned for correctly predicting an oncoming relapse which is more important than the associated trade-off of avoiding a false alarm.

4   Results

Classifier Comparison. We evaluated the classification performance with different machine learning models using leave-one-patient-out cross-validation. The obtained results are given in Table 2. Naive Bayes based classification gives the best classification performance with an F2 score of 0.083.

Table 2. Comparison of different classifiers for relapse prediction models. Features from the daily template of mobile signal data, EMA, and demographics are used for the classifier.

Method	F2-score	Precision	Recall
Naive Bayes	**0.083**	0.22	0.086
Balanced Random Forest	0.042	0.01	0.47
EasyEnsemble	0.034	0.007	0.43
Isolation Forests	0.045	0.01	0.39
Random classification baseline	0.020 ± 0.024	0.010 ± 0.012	0.026 ± 0.032

Feature Comparison. In our work, we computed daily template based rhythm features to characterize behavioral patterns and changes. We compared the classification performance obtained with this feature set to that obtained using the feature set from [18] where features are computed with lower temporal resolution. To optimize the classification pipeline using the feature set from [18], we selected the best parameter (training subset size for feature selection N, and the number of selected features M) using grid search. Similarly, the demographic features were also added as it improved the classification performance. The obtained results using Naive Bayes model, which provided the best performance in both of the feature sets, are given in Table 3.

Table 3. Comparison of feature sets for the relapse prediction task. The features based on the daily templates, where the hourly averages of the mobile sensing signal are retained, are compared with the features from [18] where features are computed with a lower temporal resolution (6 h).

Feature set	F2-score
Daily template based, EMA, demographics (this work)	**0.083**
Feature set from [18]	0.065

Modality Comparison. The template features were obtained from 6 mobile sensor signals to characterize the behavioral patterns, and the EMA based features were extracted to further characterize the emotional state of the patient. We analyzed the classification performance obtained with the individual modalities (feature set from 6 mobile sensor signals and EMA). The demographic information is also included in the feature set for this analysis and we used the Naive Bayes based classification pipeline. The obtained result is given in Fig. 4, showing the top three modalities with the highest classification performance. Distance traveled was found to provide the best classification performance, followed by the EMA and the call duration modalities. An example of the call duration time-series for a patient who had three instances of relapse is shown in Fig. 5. Increased call duration activity are seen closer to the relapse dates.

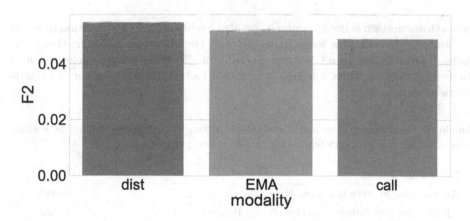

Fig. 4. F2 score obtained with different signal modalities (top 3 modalities) for the relapse prediction task. Distance traveled (dist) is found to be most relevant for relapse prediction followed by EMA and call duration (call).

Impact of Feature Selection and Demographics Features. We implemented our relapse prediction model using mutual information based feature selection. We evaluated the performance of the Naive Bayes based classifier when

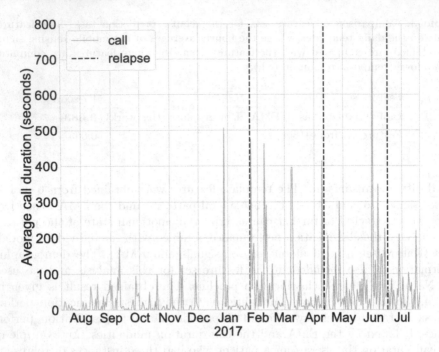

Fig. 5. An example showing the call duration time-series for a patient who has had three relapses. Increased activity in call duration signal is seen near the relapse dates, though there are other similar activities in few non-relapse periods too.

no feature selection is used. Similarly, we also evaluated the classification pipeline without the demographic features, to quantify the impact of including those features. The obtained result is given in Table 4. Both the feature selection and inclusion of demographic features were found to be advantageous for the classification performance.

Table 4. Comparison of different evaluation setting to assess the impact of feature selection and demographics feature on classification performance.

Evaluation setting	F2-score
All features, Feature selection, Naive Bayes model	**0.083**
All features, No feature selection, Naive Bayes model	0.036
All except demographic features, Feature selection, Naive Bayes model	0.058

5 Discussion

We investigated mobile sensing based schizophrenia relapse prediction using patient-independent evaluation in this work. Our implementation of the relapse prediction model is closer to clinical deployment and builds upon the insights from the previous work in [18] where mobile sensing based features were found to be associated with an upcoming relapse. We used features extracted from the daily template of the mobile sensing data, EMA, and demographics. The mobile sensing data and EMA characterized behavioral and emotional rhythmic patterns while the demographics information helped to personalize the prediction models. We obtained an F2 score of 0.083 with Naive Bayes based classifier for relapse prediction. Though this classification performance is low, it is still much higher than the random classification baseline (F2 score of 0.02). Thus, mobile sensing data has predictive value for schizophrenia relapse prediction even when employed in a patient-independent sequential prediction model, close to a clinical deployment scenario. Nonetheless, the lower F2 score obtained indicates that the relapse prediction task based on mobile sensing is difficult, and more improvements need to be done. Towards this effort, we will investigate more discriminatory features derived from the mobile sensing data (e.g. novel mobility features as presented in [7]) in future work.

We evaluated different classifiers for the relapse prediction task. The simpler Naive Bayes based classifier outperformed relatively complex Balanced Random Forest and EasyEnsemble classifiers (Table 2). This could be because our dataset size is small and complex models had difficulties generalizing. We also evaluated a one-class classification (outlier detection) technique to detect relapses using Isolation Forests. Though the obtained performance was better than the random classification baseline, one-class classifier resulted in a slightly lower F2 score than those obtained with the two-class Naive Bayes classifier. This shows that supervised classification is helpful for relapse prediction, probably because the dataset size is not large enough for unsupervised approaches to automatically learn a good generalized model of the non-relapse cases.

In our work, we used daily templates composed of hourly averages of mobile sensing data to extract features characterizing behavioral patterns. This feature set was found to provide better performance when compared to the features from [18] where features were computed per 6-hour epochs of the day (Table 3). A higher temporal resolution might be better to characterize finer nuances in the behavioral patterns, leading to the higher classification performance obtained. Similarly, individual signal modalities were found to provide lower classification performance (Fig. 4) compared to the classification performance obtained with multiple modalities combined together. This shows that a multi-modal assessment of behavior is important for the relapse prediction task. With a single modality, the observed behavioral pattern of an individual might be noisy and incomplete. However, with the inclusion of multiple modalities, the resulting feature dimension is also large. When the dataset is small, as in our case, feature selection is important to reduce the feature dimension (Table 4). In our relapse prediction model, the feature selection aids for model personalization since the selected features are made dependent on the age group. Further, demographic features are also directly provided as input in the model for implicit personalization. Both of these approaches were found to be helpful for classification

(Table 4). Other feature personalization approaches need to be investigated in future work. Behavioral patterns before a relapse might manifest differently in different patients. A relapse prediction model that can adaptively personalize to the best signal modalities for a given patient, in a given period, might lead to improved classification performance.

6 Conclusion

Mobile sensing could be used for detecting behavioral and emotional changes associated with an oncoming schizophrenia relapse. In this work, we developed a relapse prediction model based on the features extracted from the daily template of the mobile sensing data, EMA, and demographics. Our relapse prediction model, trained in a patient-independent setting and providing a sequential relapse prediction, is closer to a clinical deployment scenario. The developed model was found to give much better performance than a random classification baseline. Thus, we conclude that the behavioral and emotional changes detected using mobile sensing have predictive value for detecting an oncoming schizophrenia relapse. The classification performance currently obtained for relapse prediction is still low and much room for improvement exists. Relapse prediction task is particularly challenging due to the limited instances of relapse incidences which makes it difficult to develop a generalized model that works across different patients. Even within the same patient, different relapse incidences might manifest differently in terms of observed behavioral and emotional changes. We will continue the investigation of optimal features and classification framework that uniquely addresses the challenges of the relapse prediction task in future work.

References

1. Andreasen, N.C., Flaum, M.: Schizophrenia: the characteristic symptoms. Schizophr. Bull. **17**(1), 27–49 (1991)
2. Barnett, I., Torous, J., Staples, P., Sandoval, L., Keshavan, M., Onnela, J.P.: Relapse prediction in schizophrenia through digital phenotyping: a pilot study. Neuropsychopharmacology **43**(8), 1660–1666 (2018)
3. Ben-Zeev, D., et al.: Crosscheck: integrating self-report, behavioral sensing, and smartphone use to identify digital indicators of psychotic relapse. Psychiatr. Rehabil. J. **40**(28368138), 266–275 (2017)
4. Birnbaum, M.L., et al.: Detecting relapse in youth with psychotic disorders utilizing patient-generated and patient-contributed digital data from facebook. NPJ Schizophr. **5**(1), 17 (2019)
5. Bishop, F.M.: Relapse prediction: a meteorology-inspired mobile model. Health Psychol. Open **3**(2), 2055102916665934 (2016)
6. Buck, B., et al.: Relationships between smartphone social behavior and relapse in schizophrenia: a preliminary report. Schizophr. Res. **208**, 167–172 (2019)

7. Canzian, L., Musolesi, M.: Trajectories of depression: unobtrusive monitoring of depressive states by means of smartphone mobility traces analysis. In: Proceedings of the 2015 ACM International Joint Conference on Pervasive and Ubiquitous Computing, pp. 1293–1304. UbiComp2015, Association for Computing Machinery, New York (2015). https://doi.org/10.1145/2750858.2805845. https://doi.org/10.1145/2750858.2805845
8. Chao, C., Liaw, A., Breiman, L.: Using random forest to learn imbalanced data. University of California, Berkeley, Technical report (2004)
9. Faith, M., et al.: Remote assessment of disease and relapse in major depressive disorder (RADAR-MDD): a multi-centre prospective cohort study protocol. BMC Psychiatry **19**(1), 72 (2019)
10. Jablensky, A.: The diagnostic concept of schizophrenia: its history, evolution, and future prospects. Dialogues Clin. Neurosci. **12**(20954425), 271–287 (2010)
11. James, S.L., et al.: Global, regional, and national incidence, prevalence, and years lived with disability for 354 diseases and injuries for 195 countries and territories, 1990–2017: a systematic analysis for the global burden of disease study 2017. Lancet **392**(10159), 1789–1858 (2018)
12. Lieberman, J.A., et al.: Prediction of relapse in schizophrenia. Archiv. General Psychiatry **44**(7), 597–603 (1987)
13. Liu, F.T., Ting, K.M., Zhou, Z.: Isolation forest. In: 2008 Eighth IEEE International Conference on Data Mining, pp. 413–422, December 2008
14. Liu, X., Wu, J., Zhou, Z.: Exploratory undersampling for class-imbalance learning. IEEE Trans. Syst. Man, Cybern. Part B (Cybern.) **39**(2), 539–550 (2009)
15. Overall, J.E., Gorham, D.R.: The brief psychiatric rating scale. Psychol. Rep. **10**(3), 799–812 (1962)
16. Shiffman, S., Stone, A.A., Hufford, M.R.: Ecological momentary assessment. Ann. Rev. Clin. Psychol. **4**, 1–32 (2008)
17. Tseng, V.W.S., et al.: Using behavioral rhythms and multi-task learning to predict fine-grained symptoms of schizophrenia. Sci. Rep. **10**(1), 15100, September 2020. https://doi.org/10.1038/s41598-020-71689-1. https://doi.org/10.1038/s41598-020-71689-1
18. Wang, R., et al.: Methods for predicting relapse episodes in schizophrenia using mobile phone sensing. In: 2020 IEEE International Conference on Pervasive Computing and Communications (PerCom) (2020)
19. Wang, R.: Mental Health Sensing Using Mobile Phones. Ph.D. thesis, Dartmouth College (2018)
20. Wang, R., et al.: Crosscheck: toward passive sensing and detection of mental health changes in people with schizophrenia. In: Proceedings of the 2016 ACM International Joint Conference on Pervasive and Ubiquitous Computing, pp. 886–897. UbiComp2016, Association for Computing Machinery, New York (2016)
21. Wang, R., et al.: Predicting symptom trajectories of schizophrenia using mobile sensing. Proc. ACM Interact. Mob. Wearable Ubiquitous Technol. **1**(3), 1–24 (2017)
22. Yang, Z., Nguyen, L., Jin, F.: Predicting opioid relapse using social media data (2018). https://arxiv.org/pdf/1811.12169.pdf

Understanding E-Mental Health for People with Depression: An Evaluation Study

Kim Janine Blankenhagel[1]($\boxtimes$), Johannes Werner[1], Gwendolyn Mayer[2],
Jobst-Hendrik Schultz[2], and Rüdiger Zarnekow[1]

[1] Technical University Berlin, Straße des 17. Juni 135, 10623 Berlin, Germany
k.blankenhagel@tu-berlin.de
[2] Heidelberg University Hospital, Im Neuenheimer Feld, 69120 Heidelberg, Germany

Abstract. Depression is widespread and, despite a wide range of treatment options, causes considerable suffering and disease burden. Digital health interventions, including self-monitoring and self-management, are becoming increasingly important to offer e-mental health treatment and to support the recovery of people affected. SELFPASS is such an application designed for the individual therapy of patients suffering from depression. To gain more insights, this study aims to examine e-mental health treatment using the example of SELFPASS with two groups: healthy people and patients suffering from depression. The analysis includes the measurement of the constructs Usability, Trust, Task-Technology Fit, Attitude and Intention-to-use, the causal relationships between them and the differences between healthy and depressive participants as well as differences between participants' evaluations at the beginning and at the end of the usage period. The results show that the Usability has the biggest influence on the Attitude and the Intention-to-use. Moreover, the study reveals clear differences between healthy and depressive participants and indicates the need for more efforts to improve compliance.

Keywords: eHealth · Digital mental health · Depression · Individual therapy · Self-management · Structural equation modelling · ANOVA

1 Introduction

Depression is a severe and widespread disease with considerable effects on people's well-being and quality of life [1]. Although evidence-based treatments such as psychotherapy are available for depressive disorders, a significant portion of people afflicted with such disorders do not receive treatment [1] or wait a long time for treatment to begin [2]. At the same time, a large portion of the world's population uses the Internet, with much of this usage being focused on health [3]. Consequently, self-monitoring and self-management are becoming increasingly important [1], and digital health interventions have proven to be a promising way of supporting people with depression [4]. These can be an effective complement to personal psychotherapy or pharmacological treatment and are particularly suitable for people who have insufficient access to psychological

J. Ye et al. (Eds.): MobiHealth 2020, LNICST 362, pp. 34–51, 2021.
https://doi.org/10.1007/978-3-030-70569-5_3

treatment or do not wish to get in personal contact with a psychotherapist [5]. To seize this potential, a web-based therapeutic platform for patient-individualized therapy and self-management called SELFPASS has been developed for people suffering from depression. So far, web intervention research has mainly focused on the effectiveness of therapy and changes in symptom severity [6], but little research (quantitative or qualitative) has been conducted on gathering more insights about those systems in terms of their acceptance or attitudes towards them. To close this gap, we analyze the underlying factors that affect people's decision to use e-mental health applications to manage depression. The aim is to examine the Usability, Trust, Task-Technology Fit, Attitude and Intention-to-use of those applications using the example of SELFPASS. Of particular interest are the causal relationships between the above-mentioned constructs and the differences between healthy and depressive participants as well as differences between the beginning and the end of the usage period.

2 Background

The background section consists of a practical and a theoretical part. Section *SELFPASS* outlines the SELFPASS application, and section *Theoretical Background* presents the theoretical foundation of the study.

2.1 SELFPASS

SELFPASS is a therapeutic platform designed for the individual therapy and self-management of patients suffering from depression. It is based on a combination of algorithms for a daily self-assessment and analysis of the patient's biosignal data and environmental information. SELFPASS enables therapy by offering self-assessment of the severity of the patient's mental distress and by suggesting practical steps for self-management. This takes into account the integrated biosignal data (for example, heart rate) and current environmental information (for example, weather). Depending on his/her individual situation, the patient receives individualized guidance for self-management and therapeutic interventions. The structure of the therapy sessions varies according to the degree of severity indicated. SELFPASS is designed for depressive people, who have received a diagnosis by a medical institution and are now waiting for personal therapy. We conducted this study with a SELFPASS prototype, which did not contain a link to biosignal data or environmental information. Instead, the participants in the study were able to use the self-assessment and various interventions (diary, activity plan, relaxation exercises and so on).

2.2 Theoretical Background

We have focused on the measurement of five constructs (Usability, Trust, Task-Technology Fit, Attitude, and Intention-to-use), which are of crucial importance for the evaluation of eHealth technologies. The term "Usability" describes the degree to which a product can be used by a particular user in a certain context with effectiveness, efficiency and satisfaction [7]. The usability of technology plays a significant role in increasing its acceptance and creating user loyalty, which is especially important in the healthcare sector [8]. Usability factors remain one of the major obstacles to the adoption of health technologies, emphasizing the necessity of usability evaluations [9]. Trust "indicates a positive belief about the perceived reliability of, dependability of, and confidence in a person, object or process" [10]. In addition, trust in technology is a key factor in establishing a satisfactory relationship between the user and product in any interactive situation [11]. Trust is a component of Trust and Mistrust, where Mistrust is the complement of Trust [12]. We decided to integrate the positive part of Trust into our study and excluded Mistrust. Goodhue and Thompson proposed the Task-Technology Fit theory to highlight the importance of an adequate correspondence between the characteristics of technologies and user tasks for achieving the desired effects in terms of individual performance [13]. Therefore, the technology must be a good fit with the tasks it supports in order to have a positive impact. We have used the two very established constructs Attitude and Intention-to-use, known from the Technology Acceptance Model (TAM) [14], to assess technology usage.

The five constructs presented above are not only an evaluation standard in themselves but are also linked to each other in certain relationships. TAM, as a widespread innovation adoption model, explains the use of new technology and outlines the Attitude construct having a positive effect on the Intention-to-use construct [14]. Furthermore, the literature shows that the Usability, Trust and Task-Technology Fit constructs have a positive effect on the Attitude and Intention-to-use constructs [15–17].

Due to the high importance of the above-mentioned constructs for the success of eHealth interventions, it is crucial for research and practice to thoroughly analyze them with respect to new platforms such as SELFPASS.

3   Method

Between February and May 2019, study participants were recruited in Berlin and Heidelberg (Germany), and the survey took place in the same period. Participants were acquired offline at the University Hospital in Heidelberg and at the Technical University in Berlin through personal information sessions pertaining to SELFPASS and to participation in the study. Furthermore, the study was made public through online forums and in order to attract more participants we used snowball sampling. Those deemed to be eligible included adult people with German language skills and, with respect to the participants in Berlin, those who had access to the Internet and owned an Internet-enabled device. In Heidelberg, patients were provided with an Internet connection and tablets to access SELFPASS. For each participant, the survey took place over a period of five consecutive days, during which the participants used SELFPASS daily for a period of around 30 min. Each day, participants were asked to log in, complete the self-assessment and try at least one intervention. They were also encouraged to test SELFPASS critically by skipping some of the interventions or stopping them altogether and noticing anything conspicuous as a result. At the end of the first day (point in time - T1) and the fifth day (point in time - T2), the participants completed a questionnaire to assess SELFPASS. All participants participated on a voluntary basis, and the procedures of the study were approved by the Ethics Committee of the Heidelberg University. Furthermore, the study is listed in the registry of clinical trials.

3.1   Research Model and Hypotheses

We have conducted an empirical study on SELFPASS in order to first examine the causal relationships between the following five constructs Usability (USA), Trust (TR), Task-Technology Fit (TTF), Attitude (ATT) and Intention-to-use (INT).

The hypotheses regarding the causal relationships are derived from the literature and shown in Table 1:

Table 1. Research hypotheses

Research hypotheses	Path
H1: Usability relates positively to Attitude	USA → ATT
H2: Usability relates positively to Intention-to-use	USA → INT
H3: Trust relates positively to Attitude	TR → ATT
H4: Trust relates positively to Intention-to-use	TR → INT
H5: Task-Technology Fit relates positively to Attitude	TTF → ATT
H6: Task-Technology Fit relates positively to Intention-to-use	TTF → INT
H7: Attitude relates positively to Intention-to-use	ATT → INT

Second, we determined differences between the scores of the constructs on the first and on the last day of the trial period (T1 and T2) as well as differences between the scores obtained by healthy participants and by those suffering from depression.

3.2   Questionnaire Design and Data Collection

The survey scheduled for T1 comprised relevant socio-demographic and demographic questions as well as questions related to the participants' experiences with digital technologies. Depression symptoms were measured using the Patient Health Questionnaire 9 (PHQ-9) [18] to verify whether the participant was suffering from depression. All participants with low PHQ-9-scores (smaller than ten) were classified as not depressive while the rest (PHQ-9 greater than or equal to 10) were classified into the comparison group whose members suffered from depression. Additionally, the five constructs Usability, Trust, Task-Technology Fit, Attitude and Intention-to-use were first assessed at T1 and a second time at T2. All constructs have a reflective measurement, because the measured variables do not construct their respective latent variables, instead they measure or manifest them. All used instruments had been previously validated. Usability was evaluated by the SUS (System Usability Scale) [19], which consists of ten items answered on a 5-point Likert rating scale, ranging from "strongly disagree" to "strongly agree". Among them, five are positive statements, and the rest are negative. SUS can provide a single score that ranges from 0 to 100, with higher scores denoting higher usability (scores were manipulated to a 0 to 4 rating and multiplied by 2.5). For the measurement of the Trust construct [12] the 7 Items of Jian et al. were used. They were arranged into a 7-point Likert rating scale and consisted of positive statements. The Task-Technology

Fit [20] comprised of 8 items answered on a 7-point scale, just like Attitude [21] (5 items) and Intention-to-use [22] (3 Items). The answer alternatives to the questions were all formed with unweighted scores. The questionnaires were delivered in German after being translated from the English original. In order to ensure that the content did not lose its original meaning, one of the other authors translated it back from German into English and compared it with the original.

Figure 1 summarizes the methodological procedure.

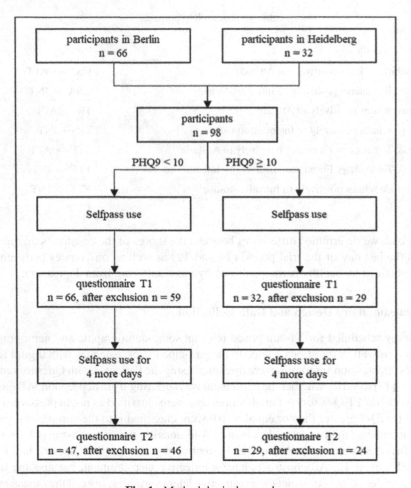

Fig. 1. Methodological procedure

The online questionnaire service SoSciSurvey was used to create and distribute the questionnaires of the study in Berlin. The participants received an email with a web link to the survey. At the clinic in Heidelberg, participants received a paper-pencil-version of the questionnaire, which was handed out to them by the investigator-in-charge. They received 50 Euro for completing the questionnaires. Each questionnaire was anonymous and identified by a unique identification number. A cover letter presenting the study's objectives and a brief overview of the key characteristics of SELFPASS was attached to the questionnaire. The collected data were organized in Microsoft Excel. We excluded questionnaires with incomplete information (more than 20% missing data) and those with an obviously distorted response behavior. In case of missing values in the underlying sample after the exclusion, we applied the method of medium value replacement.

3.3 Statistical Analyses

The data were analyzed in three different ways: descriptive statistics, structural equation modelling (SEM) and analysis of variance (ANOVA) with repeated measures. Descriptive analyses were used for obtaining the summary statistics of all measures and for the study of general characteristics.

We applied partial least squares structural equation modeling (PLS-SEM) to examine the causal relationships between the individual constructs. This approach was deemed suitable due to the complexity of the model and the high number of constructs and indicators involved. SmartPLS 3 was used to validate the measures and to test the research hypotheses. The quality measures factor loadings, composite reliability, displayed average variance and heterotrait-monotrait (HTMT) ratio were used as a basis for the evaluation of the reflective measurement model. To assess the structural model, we used $R2$, path coefficients significance and the effect size.

During the second phase ANOVA was used to compare changes in the constructs at T1 and T2 as well as between the healthy and depressive participants. Mean scores were calculated for all subscales, and the significance level for the tests was alpha = 0.05. Before performing data analysis, we used the Shapiro-Wilk test to assess normality and calculated the Cronbach alpha coefficients to assess the internal consistency of the theoretical constructs. Therefore, SPSS Version 25 was used.

4 Results

A total of 98 participants completed the questionnaire at T1, and 76 completed it at T2. 66 were classified as having no symptoms of depression and 32 as suffering from depression. The demographic data of the participants in this study largely corresponded to the demographics of the population that uses health apps (more females, young and with high education levels) [23]. Therefore, we conclude that we have a representative and relevant sample for this study in terms of early adopters of eHealth applications, but not with respect to the general population. The resulting samples formed the basis for subsequent statistical analysis. Table 2 shows the demographic statistics of the sample, subdivided into healthy participants and those with depression. These include the characteristics of all participants whose questionnaire responses at T1 and/or T2 were included in the analysis.

Table 2. Demographics

		Healthy participants n (%)	Participants suffering from depression n (%)
Gender	Male	31 (51)	11 (37)
	Female	26 (43)	19 (63)
	Not specified	4 (7)	0 (0)
Age	<25	18 (30)	18 (60)
	25–35	29 (48)	6 (20)
	35–45	0 (0)	2 (7)
	>45	8 (13)	4 (13)
	Not specified	6 (10)	0 (0)
Marital status	Single	45 (74)	21 (70)
	Married	10 (16)	4 (13)
	Separated/divorced/widowed	2 (3)	5 (17)
	Not specified	4 (7)	0 (0)
Highest degree	No/lower education	6 (10)	11 (37)
	Moderate/high education	51 (84)	18 (60)
	Not specified	4 (6)	1 (3)
Computer skills	Sufficient	2 (3)	2 (7)
	Moderate	3 (5)	4 (13)
	Good	25 (41)	17 (57)
	Excellent	30 (49)	7 (23)
	Not specified	1 (2)	0 (0)
Job situation	Self-employed	2 (3)	0 (0)
	Apprentice	0 (0)	1 (3)
	University/school	38 (62)	15 (50)
	Employee	16 (26)	11 (37)
	Unemployed	1 (2)	2 (7)
	Pensioners	0 (0)	0 (0)
	Other/not specified	4 (7)	1 (3)

4.1   Structural Equation Modelling – Measurement Model

In order to perform structural equation modelling, we started with a validation of our measurement model. First, we examined the factor loadings and eliminated items if their factor loadings were smaller than 0.7 and if eliminating the item resulted in an increase in the internal consistency reliability [24]. This method led to an elimination of a total of 6 items (all eliminated items pertained to Usability). Thereafter, the considered items had values greater than the minimum value of 0.4 (smallest value being 0.63) and were regarded suitable [24]. Subsequently, we assessed the construct reliability by determining the composite reliability. A construct reliability greater than 0.7 was deemed an acceptable reliability coefficient [25], and Table 3 shows that all the constructs met this criterion and demonstrated their internal consistency. All constructs showed an average variance extracted above 0.5, meaning that on average, the construct explains more than 50% of the variance of its indicators [25]. In discriminant analysis, the results of the HTMT ratio met the discriminatory criterion (being below 0.9) [26]. Thus, the measurement model had acceptable reliability and convergent validity, leading to a viable structural analysis of the model.

Table 3. Validation of the measurement model

Construct	Number of items	Composite reliability	Average variance extracted
USA	4	0.8	0.5
TR	7	0.9	0.6
TTF	8	0.9	0.8
ATT	5	0.9	0.7
INT	3	0.9	0.9

4.2 Structural Equation Modelling – Structural Model Assessment

We estimated the structural model paths and tested the research hypotheses with the entire sample (at T1 and T2, all participants) to identify the main determinants in the usage of SELFPASS. The multi-group analysis did not show significant differences between the causal relationships of T1 and T2 and revealed a significant difference between healthy and depressive participants in only one causal relationship (TTF → INT). All other relationships showed no significant differences. Therefore, it is reasonable to calculate a structural equation model based on all subgroups.

The evaluation of the structural model included the execution of SmartPLS under default settings with 5.000 samples, with a bootstrap of 5.000 resampling iterations and with mean replacement of missing data. All constructs had variance inflation factor (VIF) values less than 5, indicating that there was no multicollinearity problem.

The PLS-SEM model and its loadings are depicted in Fig. 2. The value in parentheses is the p value, the result of calculating the significance of quality to success relationships using the bootstrapping approach.

The model explains 44% of variance for the Attitude construct and 29% of variance for the Intention-to-use construct. The results show that all hypothetical relationships except for H4 and H6 are supported. The path coefficients of these hypotheses are very close to zero. As predicted by H1 and H2, the study finds significant positive impacts of Usability on Attitude and on Intention-to-use. The effect size of both relationships proves to be moderate. Our findings confirm the favorable effect of Trust on Attitude (H3); H5, which predicted a positive relationship between Task-Technology Fit and Attitude, is also confirmed. Regarding H7, Attitude is found to be positively related to Intention-to-use. The last three causal relationships mentioned have small effect sizes. Table 4 shows the results of the modeling.

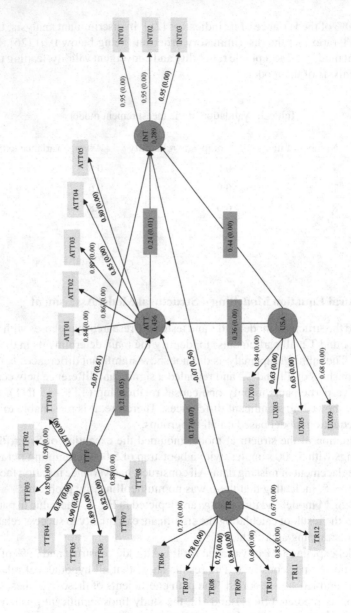

Fig. 2. PLS-SEM model

Table 4. PLS-SEM modelling results

Research hypotheses	Coefficient	P value	Outcome	f^2
H1: USA → ATT	0.357	<0.000[a]	Supported	0.12[c]
H2: USA → INT	0.444	<0.000[a]	Supported	0.13[c]
H3: TR → ATT	0.173	0.069[b]	Supported	0.02[d]
H4: TR → INT	−0.069	0.562	Not supported	0.00
H5: TTF → ATT	0.212	0.052[b]	Supported	0.03[d]
H6: TTF → INT	−0.066	0.612	Not supported	0.00
H7: ATT → INT	0.244	0.006[a]	Supported	0.05[d]

a: $p \leq 0.05$ b: $0.05 < p \leq 0.10$ c: moderate d: small

4.3 ANOVA

The descriptive analysis of the chosen constructs shows an overall good evaluation of the Usability of SELFPASS (SUS approx. 79). Among the four other constructs, the Task-Technology Fit construct receives the best rating on the 7-point Likert scale with a value of approximately 5, closely followed by Attitude and then Trust with an overall rating of approximately 4.7. The Intention-to-use construct was rated worst with an overall rating of approximately 4.0.

Table 5 illustrates the mean value and standard deviation of all constructs and distinguishes between T1 and T2 and the healthy and depressive groups.

Table 5. Descriptive analysis results

	Healthy T1 Mean (SD)	Depressive T1 Mean (SD)	Healthy T2 Mean (SD)	Depressive T2 Mean (SD)
Usability – SUS*	80.83 (12.30)	73.94 (14.23)	79.49 (14.87)	80.30 (9.07)
Trust**	4.81 (1.19)	4.20 (0.86)	5.03 (1.27)	4.69 (0.86)
Task-Technology-Fit**	5.32 (1.18)	4.55 (1.19)	5.18 (1.36)	5.25 (0.92)
Attitude**	5.19 (1.12)	4.38 (1.29)	4.99 (1.31)	4.81 (1.24)
Intention-to-use**	3.84 (2.15)	5.32 (1.37)	2.96 (2.04)	4.74 (1.57)

*Score from 0 to 100. **Score on a 7-point Likert scale

We calculated Cronbach's Alpha at both points in time (see Table 6) in order to determine sufficient reliability for the following analyses. Table 6 indicates, that the reliability of Usability (T1 and T2), Trust (T1 and T2) and Attitude (T1 and T2) can be rated as excellent [27]. The Task-Technology Fit and Intention-to-use construct have high reliability measures, indicating them as redundant items. Since the elimination of individual items did not lead to any significant improvement in reliability, we refrained from doing so.

Table 6. Cronbach alpha coefficients

	Usability (10 items)	Trust (7 items)	Task-technology Fit (8 items)	Attitude (5 items)	Intention-to-use (3 items)
T1	0.82	0.89	0.97	0.91	0.94
T2	0.76	0.87	0.94	0.90	0.97

As this sample is relatively small, we used the Shapiro-Wilk test to verify normal distribution. Turns out, not all constructs are normally distributed. However, we performed an ANOVA because there is no non-parametric equivalent and studies have shown that ANOVA is robust against violations of normality [28]. Table 7 presents the results of the ANOVA.

Table 7. ANOVA results

Construct	Group	P-value	Partial eta-squared
Usability - SUS	Time of measurement (T1 vs. T2)	0.070	0.05
	Condition (healthy vs. depressive)	0.006^a	0.111^c
Trust	Time of measurement (T1 vs. T2)	$<0.000^a$	0.175^d
	Condition (healthy vs. depressive)	0.158	0.030
Task-Technology Fit	Time of measurement (T1 vs. T2)	0.012^a	0.095^c
	Condition (healthy vs. depressive)	$<0.000^a$	0.190^d
Attitude	Time of measurement (T1 vs. T2)	0.383	0.012
	Condition (healthy vs. depressive)	0.018^a	0.085^c
Intention-to-use	Time of measurement (T1 vs. T2)	0.002^a	0.148^d
	Condition (healthy vs. depressive)	0.513	0.007

a: $p \leq 0.05$ c: moderate effect d: strong effect

The analysis of the differences between T1 and T2 and among healthy and depressive participants revealed a total of 6 significant differences from the 10 analyzed ones.

The Usability does not change significantly during the five days of use, but the two groups differ significantly with a moderate effect. Figure 3 depicts clearly that at the beginning the participants suffering from depression rate the Usability of SELFPASS significantly worse than the healthy participants. However, the depressive participants give a considerably better rating after the five days of usage, and their evaluation even exceed that of the healthy participants.

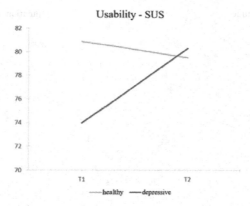

Fig. 3. Usability results

Trust in SELFPASS does not differ significantly between healthy and depressive participants, but there is a noticeable change in the assessment of trust during use, in the sense that trust in SELFPASS increases remarkably (strong effect, see Fig. 4). The Task-Technology Fit shows significant differences between T1 and T2 as well as between healthy and depressive participants. This construct also improves during application with moderate effect, with the increase being observed within the group of depressive participants. At the end of the usage period, the Task-Technology Fit is rated higher by depressive participants than by healthy ones (Fig. 5).

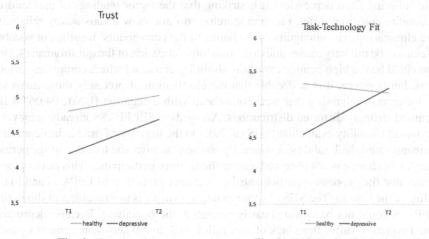

Fig. 4. Trust results   **Fig. 5.** Task-Technology Fit results

The Attitude construct shows a moderate, significant difference with respect to the existing health condition, whereby healthy participants demonstrate higher Attitude values than the depressive ones. The Attitude of the healthy participants decreases over the 5-day usage, while the Attitude of the depressive participants increases. Intention-to-use decreases significantly throughout the five days of usage with a strong effect (Figs. 6 and 7).

Attitude

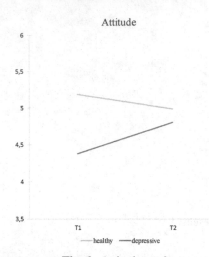

Intention-to-use

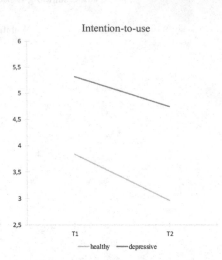

Fig. 6. Attitude results   **Fig. 7.** Intention-to-use results

5 Discussion

The causal relationships described in the PLS-SEM model clearly show that Usability has the greatest influence on Attitude (path coefficient $0.36/f2 = 0.12$) and on Intention-to-use (path co-efficient $0.44/f2 = 0.13$). Therefore, it is fundamentally important to place a high significance on Usability when developing such therapeutic systems for people suffering from depression. It is striking that the factor loadings of the items of the Usability construct differ a lot and therefore do not show a satisfactory reliability before elimination. The ambiguity of the points or the participants' insufficient vocabulary seems to be unlikely causes due to the previous validation of the questionnaires. One reason could be the high complexity of the Usability construct which comprises various aspects. Furthermore, it is noticeable that the elimination of precisely those items led to an increase in reliability that were formulated with a negation (UX02,04,06,08,10) and caused strongly distorted distributions. Altogether, SELFPASS already achieves a good overall Usability evaluation (SUS ca. 79). On the first day of usage, the depressive participants rated the Usability significantly worse than after the five-day usage period, although this change is not observed among the healthy participants. This development indicates that the depressive participants became accustomed to SELFPASS and to the handling of the system. The SUS of approximately 73 at T1 is improvable and shows that SELFPASS could not be operated easily enough at the beginning. Because depressive people frequently suffer from lack of motivation and digital self-management systems show high dropout rates [29, 30], an improvement of compliance could be achieved through a specific Usability adapted to the target group. We should aim to enable effortless and intuitive usage in digital self-management systems for people suffering from depression. Thus, the period of familiarization with the system could be reduced, thereby preventing premature dropout. This finding is in accordance with the literature, which shows that for example guidance regarding key functionalities [31], clearly structured content and overviews [32], warning notices [33] and confirmation or congratulation messages after completed activities [34] are particularly important for people suffering from depression to improve orientation and ease of use.

Trust (path coefficient $0.17/f2 = 0.02$) and Task-Technology Fit (path coefficient $0,21/f2 = 0.03$) have a positive influence on Attitude. The Trust score improves greatly in the course of the five-day usage. This shows that trust in health-related digital platforms is only built up over time and does not come about immediately. Other studies have proven that trust in medical technology empirically differs from the general trust in technology [35]. Therefore, trust seems to be more indispensable if health-related aspects are conveyed technologically [36]. Although the literature attaches a very critical importance to trust in the field of eHealth, SELFPASS achieves an overall moderate to good evaluation with a mean of approximately 4.7. The evaluation of the Task-Technology Fit improves among depressive participants during usage. This suggests that users recognize an added value of SELFPASS while using the platform and shows that SELFPASS fulfils its purpose as a self-management tool for depression. This goes hand in hand with the observation, that this trend is not discernible among the healthy participants. They are healthy and have no psychological strain; therefore, they naturally recognize less benefit and improvement with SELFPASS, which is why the Task-Technology Fit barely changes for them in the course of five days. On the fifth day of us-age, they rate the fit slightly worse than the depressive group; hence, they assess SELFPASS as being less helpful and suitable.

The Attitude construct shows a similar curve progression. Over the period of use, the participants suffering from depression improve their attitude towards SELFPASS while that of healthy participants diminishes slightly. From this, we conclude that people suffering from depression generally have a positive estimation regarding e-mental health applications such as SELFPASS. The coefficient of determination (R2) of Attitude is approximately 0.44 and therefore, explains 44% of the variance. Compared to other studies in the field of eHealth this is a good result [3, 37, 38]. This study is one in which we measure human behavior and naturally in this area, numerous and of-ten not directly measurable, influences come into play. Therefore, smaller R2 values are to be expected here than in other disciplines, such as physics, with exactly measurable variables and low disturbances.

The Attitude construct shows a positive influence on Intention-to-use (path coefficient $0.24/f2 = 0.05$). We had expected this effect, and it is congruent with the literature [14]. The small R2 of Intention-to-use (approximately 0.29) could be explained by the fact that Intention-to-use strongly depends on the subgroup, and depressive and healthy participants have generally different motivations for usage. Strikingly, in this study, healthy participants quit the study rather earlier than the depressive ones. One reason could be the non-existing psychological strain. Intention-to-use decreases over the five-day period, highlighting the necessity to integrate strong elements into e-mental health applications that increase motivation and compliance. Poor compliance is also discussed in the literature as a common obstacle to the use of eHealth applications [5] and gamification is addressed among other things. There is promising evidence that suggests gamification works. Innovative ways need to be found to make digital health interventions entertaining and appealing; these may include, for example, providing meaningful rewards or making the system more social [39]. Undoubtedly combining gamification and the special needs of depressive people in a meaningful way would be a challenging task.

6 Limitations

This study has some limitations. As conducting studies anonymously is a sensitive process, especially in the health-related area, we used an identification code to maintain confidentiality in the collection of the survey data. This in turn did not allow us to confirm whether the participants did in fact use SELFPASS daily in the manner required. Furthermore, we assume that due to the iterative nature of Internet interventions and the varying intensity and duration of time for which the users tested SELFPASS, the intervention exposure was likely to be different for each user. The research used participants' self-reports, and we can't guarantee that the participants correctly articulated their assessments. Since patients of the Heidelberg University Hospital received a fee for participating in the study, but the participants in Berlin did not, distortions cannot be ruled out. The SELFPASS version used was only a prototype and did not have the full range of the functions. A repeated measurement with the completed SELFPASS version could lead to different results, especially in terms of the Task-Technology Fit. Due to feasibility constraints, the resulting sample size was relatively small for such a complex investigation, leading to limited generalizability of the findings to the population as a whole. The small sample size of the group consisting of participants with depression could be a reason why the multi-group analysis of the structural equation modelling did not reveal significant group differences.

7 Conclusion and Future Work

The study contributes to the literature by pinpointing significant effects to help understand the usage of e-mental health applications to manage depression. PLS-SEM structural equation modelling proves that the Usability, Trust and Task-Technology Fit constructs have a positive effect on Attitude towards SELFPASS and that Attitude has a positive influence on Intention-to-use. The Usability has the biggest influence and should therefore be given special consideration in the development of self-management systems for people suffering from depression.

Overall, the ANOVA results reveal clear differences between healthy and depressive participants. The trend observed is that depressive participants generally rate SELFPASS better on the fifth day than on the first, therefore showing that they require a longer period for familiarization with the system compared to the healthy participants. The Intention-to-use decreases in both subgroups during the five-day usage, showing the necessity of further research projects to improve compliance to digital self-management systems for people suffering from depression. Furthermore, an effectiveness study of SELFPASS compared to a waiting list group could be a topic of interest for future research and practice. Whether self-management systems such as SELFPASS will also be suitable for patients suffering from severe depression, and under which conditions, remains largely unknown and also requires further research.

References

1. Hartmann, R., Sander, C., Lorenz, N., Böttger, D., Hegerl, U.: Utilization of patient-generated data collected through mobile devices: insights from a survey on attitudes toward mobile self-monitoring and self-management apps for depression. JMIR Mental Health **6**(4), e11671 (2019). https://doi.org/10.2196/11671
2. Bundespsychotherapeutenkammer BPtK: Ein Jahr nach der Reform der Psychotherapie-Richtlinie, Berlin (2018)
3. Ahadzadeh, A.S., Pahlevan Sharif, S., Ong, F.S., Khong, K.W.: Integrating health belief model and technology acceptance model: an investigation of health-related internet use. J. Med. Internet Res. **17**(2), e45 (2015). https://doi.org/10.2196/jmir.3564
4. Radovic, A., Gmelin, T., Hua, J., Long, C., Stein, B.D., Miller, E.: Supporting our valued adolescents (SOVA), a social media website for adolescents with depression and/or anxiety: technological feasibility, usability, and acceptability study. JMIR Mental Health **5**(1), e17 (2018). https://doi.org/10.2196/mental.9441
5. Lutz, W., et al.: Defining and predicting patterns of early response in a web-based intervention for depression. J. Med. Internet Res. **19**(6), e206 (2017). https://doi.org/10.2196/jmir.7367
6. Andersson, G., Cuijpers, P., Carlbring, P., Riper, H., Hedman, E.: Guided Internet-based vs. face-to-face cognitive behavior therapy for psychiatric and somatic disorders: a systematic review and meta-analysis. World Psychiatry Official J. World Psychiatr. Assoc. (WPA) **13**(3), 288–295 (2014). https://doi.org/10.1002/wps.20151
7. Harrison, R., Flood, D., Duce, D.: Usability of mobile applications: literature review and rationale for a new usability model. J. Interact. Sci. **1**(1), 1 (2013). https://doi.org/10.1186/2194-0827-1-1
8. Kortum, P., Peres, S.C.: Evaluation of home health care devices: remote usability assessment. JMIR Hum. Factors **2**(1), e10 (2015). https://doi.org/10.2196/humanfactors.4570
9. Cho, H., et al.: A mobile health intervention for HIV prevention among racially and ethnically diverse young men: usability evaluation. JMIR mHealth uHealth **6**(9), e11450 (2018). https://doi.org/10.2196/11450
10. Tseng, S., Fogg, B.J.: Credibility and computing technology. Commun. ACM **42**(5), 39–44 (1999). https://doi.org/10.1145/301353.301402
11. Mcknight, D.H., Carter, M., Thatcher, J.B., Clay, P.F.: Trust in a specific technology. ACM Trans. Manage. Inf. Syst. **2**(2), 1–25 (2011). https://doi.org/10.1145/1985347.1985353
12. Jian, J.-Y., Bisantz, A.M., Drury, C.G.: Foundations for an empirically determined scale of trust in automated systems. Int. J. Cogn. Ergon. **4**(1), 53–71 (2000). https://doi.org/10.1207/S15327566IJCE0401_04
13. Goodhue, D.L., Thompson, R.L.: Task-technology fit and individual performance. MIS Q. **19**(2), 213 (1995). https://doi.org/10.2307/249689
14. Davis, F.D.: A Technology Acceptance Model for Empirically Testing New End-User Information Systems: Theory and Results (1986)
15. Burney, S.M.A., Ali, S.A., Ejaz, A., Siddiqui, F.A.: Discovering the correlation between technology acceptance model and usability. IJCSNS Int. J. Comput. Sci. Netw. Secur. **17**(11), 53–61 (2017)
16. Dishaw, M.T., Strong, D.M.: Extending the technology acceptance model with task–technology fit constructs. Inf. Manage. **36**(1), 9–21 (1999). https://doi.org/10.1016/S0378-7206(98)00101-3
17. Zhao, J., Fang, S., Jin, P.: Modeling and quantifying user acceptance of personalized business modes based on TAM, trust and attitude. Sustainability **10**(2), 356 (2018). https://doi.org/10.3390/su10020356

18. Löwe, B., Kroenke, K., Herzog, W., Gräfe, K.: Measuring depression outcome with a brief self-report instrument: sensitivity to change of the Patient Health Questionnaire (PHQ-9). J. Affect. Disord. **81**(1), 61–66 (2004)
19. Brooke, J.: SUS-A quick and dirty usability scale. In: Usability Evaluation in Industry, vol. 189, pp. 4–7 (1996)
20. Lin, T.-C., Huang, C.-C.: Understanding knowledge management system usage antecedents: an integration of social cognitive theory and task technology fit. Inf. Manage. **45**(6), 410–417 (2008). https://doi.org/10.1016/j.im.2008.06.004
21. Ajzen, I.: The theory of planned behavior. Organ. Behav. Hum. Decis. Process. **50**(2), 179–211 (1991). https://doi.org/10.1016/0749-5978(91)90020-T
22. Ajzen, I.: Perceived behavioral control, self-efficacy, locus of control, and the theory of planned behavior 1. J. Appl. Soc. Psychol. **32**(4), 665–683 (2002). https://doi.org/10.1111/j.1559-1816.2002.tb00236.x
23. Zhang, X., Yu, P., Yan, J., Spil, I.T.A.M.: Using diffusion of innovation theory to understand the factors impacting patient acceptance and use of consumer e-health innovations: a case study in a primary care clinic. BMC Health Serv. Res. **15**, 71 (2015). https://doi.org/10.1186/s12913-015-0726-2
24. Hair, J.F., Hult, G.T.M., Ringle, C.M., Sarstedt, M., Richter, N.F., Hauff, S.: Partial Least Squares Strukturgleichungsmodellierung. Eine anwendungsorientierte Einführung. Franz Vahlen, München (2017)
25. Hair, J.F., Sarstedt, M., Ringle, C.M., Mena, J.A.: An assessment of the use of partial least squares structural equation modeling in marketing research. J. Acad. Mark. Sci. **40**(3), 414–433 (2012). https://doi.org/10.1007/s11747-011-0261-6
26. Henseler, J., Ringle, C.M., Sarstedt, M.: A new criterion for assessing discriminant validity in variance-based structural equation modeling. J. Acad. Mark. Sci. **43**(1), 115–135 (2014). https://doi.org/10.1007/s11747-014-0403-8
27. Tavakol, M., Dennick, R.: Making sense of Cronbach's alpha. Int. J. Med. Educ. **2**, 53–55 (2011). https://doi.org/10.5116/ijme.4dfb.8dfd
28. Blanca, M.J., Alarcón, R., Arnau, J., Bono, R., Bendayan, R.: Non-normal data: Is ANOVA still a valid option? Psicothema **29**(4), 552–557 (2017). https://doi.org/10.7334/psicothema2016.383
29. Ryan, C., Bergin, M., Wells, J.S.G.: Theoretical perspectives of adherence to web-based interventions: a scoping review. Int. J. Behav. Med. **25**(1), 17–29 (2017). https://doi.org/10.1007/s12529-017-9678-8
30. Sherdell, L., Waugh, C.E., Gotlib, I.H.: Anticipatory pleasure predicts motivation for reward in major depression. J. Abnorm. Psychol. **121**(1), 51–60 (2012). https://doi.org/10.1037/a0024945
31. Fuller-Tyszkiewicz, M., et al.: A mobile app-based intervention for depression: end-user and expert usability testing study. JMIR Mental Health **5**(3), e54 (2018). https://doi.org/10.2196/mental.9445
32. Good, A., Sambhanthan, A.: Accessing web based health care and resources for mental health: interface design considerations for people experiencing mental illness. In: Marcus, A. (ed.) DUXU 2014. LNCS, vol. 8519, pp. 25–33. Springer, Cham (2014). https://doi.org/10.1007/978-3-319-07635-5_3
33. Stiles-Shields, C., Montague, E., Lattie, E.G., Schueller, S.M., Kwasny, M.J., Mohr, D.C.: Exploring user learnability and learning performance in an app for depression: usability study. JMIR Hum. Factors **4**(3), e18 (2017). https://doi.org/10.2196/humanfactors.7951
34. Tiburcio, M., Lara, M.A., Aguilar Abrego, A., Fernández, M., Martínez Vélez, N., Sánchez, A.: Web-based intervention to reduce substance abuse and depressive symptoms in mexico: development and usability test. JMIR Mental Health **3**(3), e47 (2016). https://doi.org/10.2196/mental.6001

35. Montague, E.N.H., Kleiner, B.M., Winchester, W.W.: Empirically understanding trust in medical technology. Int. J. Ind. Ergon. **39**(4), 628–634 (2009). https://doi.org/10.1016/j.ergon.2009.01.004
36. Wilkowska, W., Ziefle, M.: Understanding trust in medical technologies. In: Proceedings of the 4th International Conference on Information and Communication Technologies for Ageing Well and e-Health : Funchal, Madeira, Portugal, 22–23 March 2018. SCITEPRESS - Science and Technology Publications Lda, Setúbal (2018)
37. Eivazzadeh, S., Berglund, J.S., Larsson, T.C., Fiedler, M., Anderberg, P.: Most influential qualities in creating satisfaction among the users of health information systems: study in seven European union countries. JMIR Med. Inform. **6**(4), e11252 (2018). https://doi.org/10.2196/11252
38. Laugesen, J., Hassanein, K., Yuan, Y.: The impact of internet health information on patient compliance: a research model and an empirical study. J. Med. Internet Res. **17**(6), e143 (2015). https://doi.org/10.2196/jmir.4333
39. Cugelman, B.: Gamification: what it is and why it matters to digital health behavior change developers. JMIR Serious Games **1**(1), e3 (2013). https://doi.org/10.2196/games.3139

Evaluating Memory and Cognition via a Wearable EEG System: A Preliminary Study

Stavros-Theofanis Miloulis[1,2]([⊠]) [iD], Ioannis Kakkos[1] [iD],
Georgios N. Dimitrakopoulos[3] [iD], Yu Sun[4] [iD], Irene Karanasiou[1,5] [iD],
Panteleimon Asvestas[2] [iD], Errikos-Chaim Ventouras[2] [iD], and George Matsopoulos[1] [iD]

[1] Laboratory of Biomedical Optics and Applied Biophysics, School of Electrical and Computer Engineering, National Technical University of Athens, 15780 Athens, Greece
smiloulis@biomig.ntua.gr
[2] Department of Biomedical Engineering, University of West Attica, 17, Ag. Spyridonos Street, 12243 Athens, Egaleo, Greece
[3] Department of Medicine, University of Patras, 26500 Patras, Greece
[4] Key Laboratory for Biomedical Engineering of Ministry of Education of China, Department of Biomedical Engineering, Zhejiang University, Hangzhou 310027, China
[5] Department of Mathematics and Engineering Sciences, Hellenic Military Academy, 80, Varis Koropiou Avenue, 19400 Athens, Kitsi, Greece

Abstract. Human memory comprises one of the most complex brain functions, attracting researchers to unveil the neural mechanisms governing its effective operation. In this respect, the current study examines the application of a wearable single-channel EEG to the interpretation of cognitive operations reflecting memory processes. For this purpose, we implemented a set of tasks for evaluating the participants' processing skills and memory efficiency, in order to examine potential outcomes derived from a specialized cognitive training routine. The employed training method targeted the distinction of automatic and controlled processing and its effects on memory, while we also investigated transfer effects to untrained tasks. Based on the electrophysiological data recorded during the cognitive tasks, we computed measures of induced EEG activity for each frequency band to examine the influence of cognitive training on both task performance and brain activity, as well as whether the EEG metrics could provide insight into the underlying brain processes and augment the interpretation of behavioral outcomes. Ultimately, statistical analysis showed an apparent contribution of EEG in understanding the observed behavioral differences, while our training program had a clear impact on the participants' performance and brain activity. Moreover, we observed the reported distinction between automatic and controlled memory processes which play an integral part in both ageing and cognitive impairments.

Keywords: Memory · Cognitive training · Electroencephalography · Portable EEG · EEG synchronization · Dual process theory

J. Ye et al. (Eds.): MobiHealth 2020, LNICST 362, pp. 52–66, 2021.
https://doi.org/10.1007/978-3-030-70569-5_4

1 Introduction

The human brain is one of the most complicated organs of the human body, working round the clock engaging with stimulus processing and activity coordination [1]. It comprises multiple interconnected units that both specialize in specific functions (e.g. vision) and work collectively in order to serve more convoluted operations such as speech, motion and problem solving. This category also includes memory processes, which have drawn intensive research interest due to the variety of cognitive processes involved (stimulus processing, encoding, storage, consolidation, retrieval) as well as their immense influence on one's personality [2].

In this context, numerous studies have investigated the causes and underlying mechanisms of cognitive decline, focusing on the effects of age and cognitive disorders. To that end, both healthy and cognitively impaired individuals have been recruited in multiple experiments involving the completion of cognitive tasks that gauge cognitive capacity and overall skills [3, 4]. Moreover, a multitude of research works have attempted to implement non-pharmacological interventions in pursuance of maintaining or even restoring cognitive functionality [5, 6]. Indeed, the human brain has been found to behave much like a muscle, in a sense that it can be trained in order to "stay in shape" or even improve its performance [7, 8].

From this standpoint, cognitive training has been implemented for maintaining or improving cognitive capacity and processing skills, as well as for slowing down or even mitigating the effects of age-related or impairment-related decline [7, 9]. For this purpose, researchers have aimed at capitalizing on processes that normally do not diminish with age and remain intact until the last stages of most cognitive disorders. In that spirit, we opted to focus on the distinction between controlled and automatic processing, as described by the dual process theory [10–12]. Specifically, automatic processing is a fast, unconscious and stimulus-driven operation, while controlled processes are conscious and demand more resources, deteriorating with age or under the presence of a cognitive impairment. In addition, on investigating cognitive training outcomes, researchers often analyze potential transfer effects [13], namely performance differences observed in other tasks, closely (near transfer) or remotely (far transfer) related to the trained task.

On studying the above phenomena, electroencephalography (EEG) has emerged as an invaluable tool, since it provides access to physiological activity reflecting cognitive processes, enabling scientists to extract measurable – and therefore objective – information with respect to brain functions [14]. However, high-density recordings employ large-scale devices under laboratory settings, requiring time-demanding setups that lack portability and convenience for the people involved. On that premise, the availability of wearable non-invasive EEG recording devices [15] has allowed their easy application on cognition analyses, greatly augmenting the interpretation of behavioral outcomes [16]. Within this context, we developed a dedicated experimental protocol for assessing cognitive training effects on memory and processing functions based on a combination of EEG-related features and conventional behavioral metrics. In particular, we sought to examine aspects of face-name memory related to familiarity and recollection processes that bear a major role in the study of ageing and dementia effects [17] using a single-channel dry EEG with high portability and user-friendly setup. Considering the fact that very few studies have targeted the EEG aspect of training effects based on dual process theory, our primary goal was to establish the applicability of minimal wearable EEG in studying cognitive training outcomes, as well as to assess the effects of the implemented training routine on brain functions.

2 Materials and Methods

2.1 Participants

Data were acquired from six healthy adults (4 male, 2 female) aged 25–40 years old with homogeneous educational level. All participants were right-handed and reported no history of cognitive disorders or medication intake, as well as normal amount of sleep for two days prior to the experiment. During the pre-experimental screening process, they all scored over 28 at the Montreal Cognitive Assessment (MoCA) [18]. The study was conducted in accordance with the Declaration of Helsinki, while written informed consent was obtained from all individuals.

2.2 Experimental Design

The participants were divided into two groups (training group and control group, each group consisting of two men and one woman) and were requested to complete a series of memory related cognitive tasks, during which they were placed in front of a TV monitor at a distance of 2 m. The experimental protocol (Fig. 1) consisted of three stages, conducted over a 6-day period. During the first stage (pre-training evaluation), the participants were asked to complete a baseline evaluation consisting of a Face-Name Memory (FNM) Test, the Verbal Paired Associates (VBA) Test [19] and an N-back task [20]. During the second stage, beginning from the following day, the training group underwent a 4-day training program involving an application of the Repetition-Lag Procedure [21– 23] for two sessions per day. On the 6th day, a post-training evaluation (3rd stage) took place, where both groups had to repeat the pre-training evaluation tasks. The control group completed only the pre-training and post-training stages, while participants from both groups were asked to not perform any further cognitive exercises (e.g. crosswords) during the 4-day interval between the two evaluation stages.

Single-channel EEG data were recorded during the pre- and post-training stages for all participants, while no recording was conducted during training in an attempt to establish a comfortable training environment. For every task, each trial (stimulus presentation & response intervals) followed a 5-s time interval, representing the reference interval corresponding to baseline EEG activity. In order to avoid overextending the duration of the evaluation stages, we limited the number of trials close to the minimum required based on literature [24, 25], leading to a total duration of approximately 65 min, including three 3-min breaks between two consecutive tasks.

The FNM test comprised the main cognitive task of the experiment, gauging the participants' skills on face recognition and name recall, while the VBA test and the N-back task were employed for examining transfer effects of training, assessing verbal and working memory respectively. Our hypothesis was that the VBA test would reflect near transfer, while the N-back task would reveal potential far transfer effects. Training was conducted using the repetition-lag procedure, focusing on separating automatic and controlled memory processes and strengthening the latter, which are known to decline due to age and cognitive impairment. Finally, it must be emphasized that participants were strongly advised to use the same mnemonic strategy during each task for all sessions (pre-training & post-training), in order to avoid performance differences due to strategy effectiveness.

The 380 images used for the face recognition tasks (FNM & repetition-lag training) were acquired from the FERET, PICS and IMM databases, selecting pictures with neutral facial expressions and no accessories (e.g. glasses or hats), while maintaining a uniform age distribution and a unit ratio of males and females. All images were normalized regarding their dimensions and were converted to grayscale and jpg format. The names that were matched with the faces were derived based on the results of the survey given in [26], consisting of the most frequent male and female names.

Face-Name Memory Test. Our FNM test involved two sessions of a study phase and an immediate recognition phase, as well as a delayed recognition phase. During the study phase, each participant was presented with a series of 15 face-name combinations, which comprised the study list. This step was directly followed by the immediate recognition phase (after 20 s), involving a series of 30 recognition tasks featuring the 15 studied faces and 15 new faces (distractors). On each task, the participant was presented with a face and was asked to respond on whether or not it was part of the study list. Upon a positive response (correct or not) the participant had to also provide a name to match with the face. After each recognition task, visual feedback was provided on the response correctness. Subsequently, after time delay of 20 min, participants again completed a series of recognition tasks with the same stimuli, which corresponded to a delayed recognition phase, during which no response feedback was provided. Based on the respective time windows after the study phase, the immediate and delayed recognition phases were expected to evaluate short-term and long-term memory. The stimuli presentation order was defined pseudorandomly and each stimulus was presented for 5 s followed by a 5-s interstimulus interval, while the response was to be provided within 4 s.

Verbal Paired Associates Test. Similar to the FMN test, the VBA test included two sessions of a study phase and an immediate recall phase, followed by a delayed recognition phase. Instead of faces, the stimuli for this test consisted of word pairs presented on the screen. During a study phase, the participants were presented with a sequence of 15 word pairs (study list), the two words being semantically unrelated and displayed aside one another. Afterwards, during the immediate recall phase, the first (left) word of each pair was shown (representing the cue) and the participant was asked to voice the second word (cued recall), followed by an acoustic feedback. It is noted that only the left word of each pair was given as a cue, corresponding to the priming condition for the VBA test [27]. Twenty minutes after the two sessions of study and immediate recall, a delayed recognition phase was conducted where 45 word pairs were presented and the individuals were asked to recognize whether they were part of the study list. No response feedback was provided. The additional (non-study) word pairs were formed by mixing the original word pairs, teaming the first word of each pair with the second word of another. The stimuli presentation order was pseudorandom and each stimulus was presented for 4 s followed by a 5-s interstimulus interval, while the response was to be provided within 4 s.

N-back Task. During the N-back task, the participants were presented with a sequence of digits, while for each stimulus they had to respond within 2 s on whether this specific digit appeared exactly N positions earlier in the sequence. Thereby, before each new stimulus they had to remember the latest N digits, where the N value echoed the difficulty level of the task. In the current study, we examined 3 distinct difficulty levels ($N_1 = 2$, $N_2 = 3$, $N_3 = 4$) that included 12, 13 and 14 trials for each level respectively. The interstimulus interval was set at 3 s, with 5-s and 20-s intervals between levels and sessions respectively. The digits for each sequence were determined pseudorandomly, ensuring that each N-back level contained at least 4 digit repetitions. Each set of the three difficulty levels was conducted three times and no response feedback was provided.

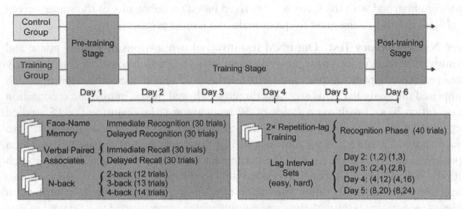

Fig. 1. Experimental Protocol. On the upper part of the figure the three protocol stages are displayed, relative to their duration and group participation. The bottom part depicts the specific tasks of the pre- and post-training stages (left) as well as the training stage (right).

Repetition-Lag Training. For the training method selection, the criteria used by the authors required a relatively uncomplicated method without a steep learning curve that presented relevance with our targeted cognitive processes, namely face recognition and name recall. In addition, we sought a method promoting implicit learning, presenting a record of successful applications as per existing studies. Based on these criteria, we decided to adopt the repetition-lag procedure (adjusted for face recognition), which builds on the dual process theory described in the "Introduction" section.

Each session of the repetition-lag procedure consisted of a study phase and a recognition phase. During the study phase, the participant was presented with a series of 16 study faces and a corresponding name, comprising the study list, which was displayed twice. Each stimulus was presented for 5 s, while the interstimulus interval was set at 5 s. After 1 min the recognition phase was carried out, where each individual was subjected to a series of yes/no recognition tasks. More specifically, we presented a list of faces (without a name) and the participants were to decide (within a response time of 3 s) whether a face belonged to the original study list or not. Whenever a face was recognized, the individual was also asked to provide a name to match with the face (within 5 s), thus completing the face-name recognition. After each recognition task, the individual was provided with visual feedback on whether the responses on face recognition and name recall were correct or incorrect.

However, some of the non-study faces were presented more than once, in an attempt to lure the individual into falsely recognizing them as parts of the study list, failing to recollect that they have indeed seen them before, although not among the study faces they were expected to "learn". These 16 faces were part of the repetition list, while the interval between two consecutive presentations of a repetition item represented the lag interval. The lag interval corresponded to the difficulty level of the recognition phase, since the more items that intervene between two presentations of the same face, the harder it was for the participants to recognize whether they saw this specific face earlier during the recognition phase or as part of the study list. Indicatively, it has been reported that a healthy young adult can achieve lags of about 18–19 [28]. Finally, the recognition phase included 8 additional faces that belonged neither to the study list nor to the repetition list, hence presented only once during the recognition phase, composed the filler list. Therefore, the recognition phase involved a total of 40 trials. If no more than two recognition errors were committed, the lag interval was increased for the next session, which was therefore carried out at a higher difficulty level. Otherwise, the lag interval remains the same for the next session, until the target criterion is met. The basic version of the repetition-lag procedure employs a single lag interval for each session, however some researchers have opted for a set of two lag interval values, both fixed for each session [28]. For the purposes of this study we have adopted the second approach, defining sets of two lag interval values ("easy" and "hard"). In that way, a participant could simultaneously practice with the two values during each session, where the easy value reflects the performance level achieved through the previous session and the hard value represents the elevated new practice level. It should be noted that name recall errors did not impact level progression, as only face recognition errors were taken into account for increasing the lag intervals of the next session. The lag interval sets that were used in this study were based on the research by [28], thus for our 4-day, 2 session-per-day training program we used the following eight sets: (1, 2), (1, 3), (2, 4), (2, 8), (4, 12), (4, 16), (8, 20), (8, 24). Furthermore, every session employed a different study list in order to avoid "learning" faces and instead trigger overall strengthening of face-name encoding and recognition cognitive processes.

The distinctiveness of this procedure in introducing non-target items presented more than once during recognition enables the dissociation of familiarity and recollection memory processes, rendering the method particularly intriguing for the authors. Specifically, each face that is part either of the study list or the repetition lists triggers an automatic familiarity effect to the individual, who has already been presented with this specific face. However, the participant has then to recall the learning context for this face, meaning to remember whether it was presented as a study face or not. This function represents recollection, which has been identified as part of controlled processing, known to decline due to age or cognitive impairment. In conclusion, by receiving feedback on correct/incorrect responses and progressively increasing difficulty, it has been hypothesized that the individuals implicitly (i.e. implicit learning) work on improving their controlled processing skills and therefore their ability to recall contextual information when recognizing familiar faces.

2.3 Data Acquisition and Pre-processing

Physiological recordings were conducted using the MindWave Mobile [29–31], a single-channel wearable EEG device with an Fp1 dry sensor and a reference A1 sensor, able to record 12-bit signals of up to 100 Hz with a sampling rate of 512 Hz. For the purposes of our study we used custom codes developed in MATLAB R2017b using the *EEGLAB* toolbox. For establishing connectivity between MindWave Mobile and MATLAB we used the necessary files provided in [32] as well as the recommended compiler from [33]. The experiment was conducted using two concurrent MATLAB sessions synced with each other, one handling EEG recordings and the other administering the computerized protocol, managing behavioral data and creating the appropriate event markers for the EEG data processing.

Initially, the raw EEG data recorded during the pre-training and post-training stages of the study were band-pass filtered by applying a windowed sinc FIR filter using a Blackman window with a bandwidth of 0.7–40.0 Hz. Subsequently, data were detrended before undergoing a denoising process. Specifically, due to the single-channel recording device, we employed EMD-ICA [34] in order to isolate noisy signal components and reconstruct the original EEG signal using only the desired components. According to this method, we firstly applied Empirical Mode Decomposition (EMD) using the *EMD-LAB* extension of the EEGLAB toolbox [35] in order to separate the one-dimensional EEG signal into four components, constituting the Intrinsic Mode Functions (IMFs). The generated IMFs represent oscillations within the source signal and are by default sorted based on their periodicity and decreasing frequency content. Afterwards, Independent Component Analysis (ICA) was applied on these four modes in order to produce four new signal components. The detection of components attributed to artifacts was based on signal variance, amplitude and frequency content. Finally, the four IMFs were reconstructed for each signal using the remaining components and were subsequently summed to produce the denoised EEG signal. Signals were then segmented into epochs based on event markers and baseline-adjusted relative to a 1-s pre-stimulus baseline.

2.4 Estimation of Synchronization Waveforms

In order to evaluate the participants' cognitive status and processing load during the tasks, we studied the occurrence of event-related synchronization/desynchronization (ERS/ERD) within the electrophysiological activity [36], representing collective increases/decreases in neuronal activity at a given frequency. The main characteristic of these manifestations is that they represent induced activity, meaning they are time-locked but not phase-locked to the stimulus [37]. This method was implemented due to its applicability on our single-channel data as opposed to techniques such as event-related potentials (ERPs), though it should be noted that it requires larger time windows for stimuli presentation and interstimulus intervals – combined with a lower number of EEG epochs – compared to ERP analysis [24, 38].

Our analysis of the induced EEG activity was independently conducted for the five EEG bands (δ: 0.5–4 Hz, θ: 4–8 Hz, α: 8–13 Hz, β: 14–26 Hz, γ: 30–40 Hz), aiming to interpret results based on the known traits of each frequency band. As such, we defined the frequency bands and then calculated the induced band power (IBP) for each reconstructed signal x_f using the inter-trial covariance method on each individual sample j over all trials ($i = 1, \ldots, n$) as follows:

$$IBP(j) = \frac{1}{n-1}\sum_{i=1}^{N}\left[x_f(i,j) - \bar{x}_f(j)\right]^2 \qquad (1)$$

The $\bar{x}_f(j)$ signal corresponds to the mean filtered signal of a specific band across all trials, representing evoked activity. Consequently, removing this signal gives prominence to the non-phase-locked (i.e. induced) activity that does not include evoked potentials.

The occurrence of synchronization or desynchronization within the EEG signal is identified by calculating for each sample j the percentage change P(j) of the IBP(j) relative to the mean IBP of the reference interval $[r_0, r_0 + k]$ recorded for each task.

$$IBP_r = \frac{1}{k}\sum_{j=r_0}^{r_0+k} IBP(j) \qquad (2)$$

$$P(j) = (IBP(j) - IBP_r)/IBP_r \qquad (3)$$

Evidently, positive values correspond to synchronization phenomena (ERS), with negative values reflecting occurrence of desynchronization (ERD). Finally, to address the lack of IBP waveforms smoothness for the extraction of statistical metrics, we applied a moving average filter with a window of 103 samples, corresponding to a recording duration of 0.2 s.

Figure 2 summarizes the processing flow applied on the EEG data, including pre-processing, induced activity waveform extraction and statistical analysis:

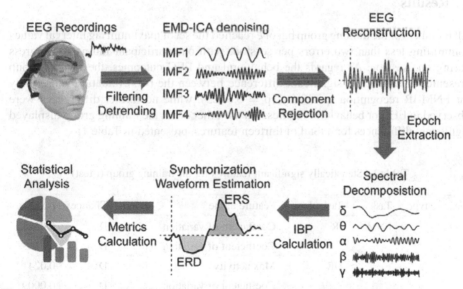

Fig. 2. Data Processing Workflow. Filtering and detrending were followed by the denoising process, where we firstly decomposed the single-channel data and then applied ICA to the resulting IMFs in order to identify and reject noisy components. The initial data channel was then reconstructed, followed by spectral decomposition and estimation of waveforms reflecting induced activity. Based on these waveforms, we extracted statistical measures for every task and each EEG band.

2.5 Statistical Analysis

Following the eventual waveform extraction, for each EEG band and each phase of every cognitive task, we extracted statistical measures of location and variability, consisting of maximum/minimum activity, mean activity, standard deviation, range and coefficient of variation (CV). With the term "activity" we denote the percentage change in the induced band power, reflecting ERS/ERD phenomena. Metrics were extracted for pre-training and post-training data. In addition, we computed behavioral measures describing the participants' performance during the cognitive tasks by calculating quantities describing sensitivity, specificity, accuracy, precision, recall rate and response time for all tasks, namely face recognition, name recall, word recall rate and recognition, as well as N-back recognition.

On comparing pre-training and post-training performances of the training and control groups and taking into account our small groups (3 participants per group), we used a t-test on each group in order to investigate the existence of features that presented a statistically significant difference between the two evaluation stages. T-tests were implemented on each feature data individually, while inference was conducted at a significance level of 5%.

3 Results

All members of the training group but one reached the set of maximum lag interval values committing less than two errors per session, with one participant failing to progress during one session. As regards the behavioral and EEG outcomes, the control group presented a statistically significant difference between the two evaluation stages only for FNM-IR recognition specificity ($p = 0.0423$), while no further differences were observed in EEG or behavioral metrics. On the other hand, the training group displayed significant differences for a total of thirteen features, presented in Table 1:

Table 1. Statistically significant features for the training group (t-test)

Feature type	Task	Task phase	Feature name	Band	Change	p-value
EEG	FNM	IR	Coefficient of variation	α	D	0.0328
			Coefficient of variation	θ	D	0.0363
		DR	Max activity	β	D	0.0241
			Coefficient of variation	δ	D	0.0009
			Max activity	θ	I	0.0399
			Standard deviation	θ	I	0.0458

(continued)

Table 1. (*continued*)

Feature type	Task	Task phase	Feature name	Band	Change	p-value
Behavioral	FNM	IR	Recognition sensitivity		D	0.0153
			Recognition specificity		D	0.0335
			Recognition accuracy		D	0.0206
			Name recall specificity		D	0.0075
	N-back	2-back	Sensitivity		I	0.0257
		3-back	Precision		I	0.0463
		4-back	Accuracy		I	0.0390

*IR: immediate recognition, DR: delayed recognition, I: Increase, D: Decrease

4 Discussion and Future Research

In this study, we developed an experimental protocol aiming to evaluate specific aspects of cognitive skills and investigate the influence of cognitive training in performance by introducing single-channel EEG data acquired via a mobile user-friendly device. Our minimal setup limits pre-processing alternatives, thus we resorted to a specialized single-channel denoising method combined with conventional filtering. Likewise, since extraction of reliable ERPs from cerebral areas of interest (i.e. face recognition) was not possible, we analyzed band synchronization activity that has also been implemented on previous works [39, 40]. This framework aimed to investigate inference capacity within a simplified EEG setup.

At first glance, the EEG contribution to the study of the participants' cognitive performance is evident, since we identified multiple features presenting a statistically significant change, thus confirming our initial assumption that the incorporation of single-channel measures can assist in the interpretation and validation of behavioral results. Moreover, statistical outcomes revealed almost no changes for the control group concerning performance between pre-training and post-training stages, while the training group showed differences on both EEG and behavioral metrics for a variety of features, implying that our cognitive training program had a tangible effect on the participants. Inspecting the related outcomes, we initially comment on the behavioral outcomes and on a second level we attempt to interpret these results by introducing the EEG findings.

As such, Table 1 shows an unexpected overall performance decrease of the training group for the face-name memory test. In an attempt to explain this result, we considered the participants' shared reports on occurrence of mental fatigue after the 3rd training day, as well as their reported bias during the recognition tasks. In particular, having undertaken the 4-day training program trying to avoid false recognition of familiar faces, all participants admitted a lack of confidence during the post-training evaluation, where their performance anxiety often led them into altering their intended responses, resulting to more errors compared to the pre-training evaluation. Taking into the EEG changes into account, we observed that the performance decrease was accompanied by a decrease in the coefficient of variation in the α and θ bands. Mathematically, this corresponds to a decrease in the ratio of standard deviation to the mean value for the induced band power percentage waveform. Interestingly, this may reflect improved processing [41], despite the fact that response bias and fatigue led to a reduced performance. Increases in the θ band (ERS) during the delayed recognition task also reflect a high memory load [42], with the comparison to the pre-training results supporting the participants' self-reports on fatigue occurrence.

Regarding the reduction in the β band maximum activity (ERD), this could simply refer to verbal responses of the participants during recognition [43]. However, since this was not observed during pre-training, it seems more likely that β ERD is related to enhanced cognitive control during long-term memory retrieval [44] (since it was observed during the delayed recognition task) or increased working memory information maintenance [45]. Furthermore, the coefficient of variation decrement in the δ band is also consistent with previous studies, reflecting concentration during task performance [46, 47]. Finally, no indication was provided on whether the improvements in N-back performance should be attributed to transfer effects or mere task experience.

On another note, we must highlight the observed distinction between controlled and automatic processing which was evident on the participants during the training program. Namely, when presented with a repetition face with a lag of over 10, it was clear that the participants recognized the image before promptly recalling the learning context and thus providing a negative response. The former event represented the familiarity effect, followed by the recollection effect where the participants recalled that the specific face was not part of the study list. From the authors' point of view, this observation supports the dual process theory and encourages further investigation of its underlying mechanisms as well of the repetition-lag procedure effects in a future study using electroencephalography to distinguish and compare brain activity during familiarity and recollection processes. On that premise, despite the fact that clear changes were ascertained, fatigue reported by the participants and reflected on the results prevented us from validating the beneficial effect of training, thus we intent to use a modified routine in a future study, distributing training sessions along a wider time period and adding days of rest for the participants. Furthermore, we intend to conduct a deeper analysis regarding the contribution of electroencephalography on reliable cognitive evaluation by recruiting a large number of participants in order to increase statistical power, as well as by utilizing a modified and more targeted experimental design that will allow for the recording of a higher number of EEG epochs in order to extract smoother and more representative activity waveforms, without overextending the experiment duration. In this regard, we also intend to explore the usage of a multi-channel portable EEG headset in order to employ brain connectivity metrics and extract ERPs related to face recognition. The comparison of single-channel vs. multi-channel results is expected to provide evidence with respect to the true applicability extent of single-channel measurements. The potential outcomes could bear considerable value in further comprehending the dual process theory, applying this knowledge on the study of cognitive disorders and the development of non-pharmacological interventions based on objective measures of physiological activity.

5   Conclusion

Summarizing the conducted work, we employed a wireless portable EEG device to assess the outcomes of cognitive training on memory processes. Our framework was able to ascertain the benefits of EEG regarding the evaluation of these complicated functions even in light portable setups, as well as to achieve the manifestation of statistically significant outcomes that could be attributed to training. In particular, we managed to identify changes for a variety of EEG features without the need for a multi-channel recording station that can only be applied on laboratory settings. In addition, we were able to jointly explain EEG and behavioral results, confirming the efficiency of our experimental protocol. Ultimately, the participants that followed the proposed training routine presented multiple differentiations regarding both behavioral and EEG metrics, while the control group showed almost no changes but in one behavioral feature. No EEG differences where observed for the members of the control group, as opposed to the training group that displayed activity alterations. Building on these outcomes, we intend to extend our study utilizing a refined experimental protocol employing advanced EEG analytics for gaining comprehensive insight into the cognitive mechanisms of human memory and the dual process theory.

Acknowledgments. The research work was supported by the Hellenic Foundation for Research and Innovation (H.F.R.I.) under the "First Call for H.F.R.I. Research Projects 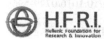 to support Faculty members and Researchers and the procurement of high-cost research equipment grant" (Project Number: 1540).

References

1. Carter, R.: The Brain Book. Dorling Kindersley Limited, London (2009)
2. Straube, B.: An overview of the neuro-cognitive processes involved in the encoding, consolidation, and retrieval of true and false memories. Behav. Brain Funct. **8**(1), 35 (2012). https://doi.org/10.1186/1744-9081-8-35
3. Mostert, J.C., et al.: Cognitive heterogeneity in adult attention deficit/hyperactivity disorder: a systematic analysis of neuropsychological measurements. Eur. Neuropsychopharmacol. **25**(11), 2062–2074 (2015). https://doi.org/10.1016/j.euroneuro.2015.08.010
4. McTeague, L.M., Huemer, J., Carreon, D.M., Jiang, Y., Eickhoff, S.B., Etkin, A.: Identification of common neural circuit disruptions in cognitive control across psychiatric disorders. AJP **174**(7), 676–685 (2017). https://doi.org/10.1176/appi.ajp.2017.16040400
5. Fritz, N., Cheek, F., Nichols-Larsen, D.: Motor-cognitive dual-task training in neurologic disorders: a systematic review. J. Neurol. Phys. Ther. **39**(3), 142–153 (2015). https://doi.org/10.1097/NPT.0000000000000090
6. Bamidis, P.D., et al.: Gains in cognition through combined cognitive and physical training: the role of training dosage and severity of neurocognitive disorder. Front. Aging Neurosci. **7** (2015). https://doi.org/10.3389/fnagi.2015.00152
7. Bherer, L.: Cognitive plasticity in older adults: effects of cognitive training and physical exercise. Ann. N. Y. Acad. Sci. **1337**(1), 1–6 (2015). https://doi.org/10.1111/nyas.12682
8. Harvey, P.D., McGurk, S.R., Mahncke, H., Wykes, T.: Controversies in computerized cognitive training. Biol. Psychiat. Cogn. Neurosci. Neuroimaging **3**(11), 907–915 (2018). https://doi.org/10.1016/j.bpsc.2018.06.008

9. Hill, N.T.M., Mowszowski, L., Naismith, S.L., Chadwick, V.L., Valenzuela, M., Lampit, A.: Computerized cognitive training in older adults with mild cognitive impairment or dementia: a systematic review and meta-analysis. AJP **174**(4), 329–340 (2016). https://doi.org/10.1176/appi.ajp.2016.16030360
10. Hasher, L., Zacks, R.T.: Automatic and effortful processes in memory. J. Exp. Psychol. Gen. **108**(3), 356–388 (1979). https://doi.org/10.1037/0096-3445.108.3.356
11. Frankish, K.: Dual-process and dual-system theories of reasoning. Philos. Compass **5**(10), 914–926 (2010). https://doi.org/10.1111/j.1747-9991.2010.00330.x
12. Bago, B., De Neys, W.: Fast logic?: Examining the time course assumption of dual process theory. Cognition **158**, 90–109 (2017). https://doi.org/10.1016/j.cognition.2016.10.014
13. Barnett, S.M., Ceci, S.J.: When and where do we apply what we learn? A taxonomy for far transfer. Psychol. Bull. **128**(4), 612–637 (2002). https://doi.org/10.1037/0033-2909.128.4.612
14. Enriquez-Geppert, S., Huster, R.J., Herrmann, C.S.: EEG-Neurofeedback as a tool to modulate cognition and behavior: a review tutorial. Front. Hum. Neurosci. **11** (2017). https://doi.org/10.3389/fnhum.2017.00051
15. Casson, A.J.: Wearable EEG and beyond. Biomed. Eng. Lett. **9**(1), 53–71 (2019). https://doi.org/10.1007/s13534-018-00093-6
16. Submarine Navigation Team Resilience: Linking EEG and Behavioral Models - Ronald Stevens, Trysha Galloway, Cynthia Lamb (2014). https://journals.sagepub.com/doi/abs/10.1177/1541931214581051
17. Jacoby, L.L.: A process dissociation framework: separating automatic from intentional uses of memory. J. Mem. Lang. **30**(5), 513–541 (1991). https://doi.org/10.1016/0749-596X(91)90025-F
18. Nasreddine, Z.S., et al.: The Montreal Cognitive Assessment, MoCA: a brief screening tool for mild cognitive impairment. J. Am. Geriatr. Soc. **53**(4), 695–699 (2005). https://doi.org/10.1111/j.1532-5415.2005.53221.x
19. Uttl, B., Graf, P., Richter, L.K.: Verbal paired associates tests limits on validity and reliability. Arch. Clin. Neuropsychol. **17**(6), 567–581 (2002). https://doi.org/10.1016/S0887-6177(01)00135-4
20. Kane, M., Conway, A., Miura, T., Colflesh, G.: Working memory, attention control, and the N-back task: a question of construct validity . J. Exp. Psychol. Learn. Mem. Cogn. **33**, 615–622 (2007). https://doi.org/10.1037/0278-7393.33.3.615
21. Anderson, N.D., Ebert, P.L., Grady, C.L., Jennings, J.M.: Repetition lag training eliminates age-related recollection deficits (and gains are maintained after three months) but does not transfer: Implications for the fractionation of recollection. Psychol. Aging **33**(1), 93–108 (2018). https://doi.org/10.1037/pag0000214
22. Finn, M., McDonald, S.: Repetition-lag training to improve recollection memory in older people with amnestic mild cognitive impairment. A randomized controlled trial. Neuropsychol. Dev. Cogn. B Aging Neuropsychol. Cogn. **22**(2), 244–258 (2015). https://doi.org/10.1080/13825585.2014.915918
23. Boller, B., Jennings, J.M., Dieudonné, B., Verny, M., Ergis, A.-M.: Recollection training and transfer effects in Alzheimer's disease: effectiveness of the repetition-lag procedure. Brain Cogn. **78**(2), 169–177 (2012). https://doi.org/10.1016/j.bandc.2011.10.011
24. Graimann, B., Huggins, J.E., Levine, S.P., Pfurtscheller, G.: Visualization of significant ERD/ERS patterns in multichannel EEG and ECoG data. Clin. Neurophysiol. **113**(1), 43–47 (2002). https://doi.org/10.1016/s1388-2457(01)00697-6
25. Klimesch, W., Russegger, H., Doppelmayr, M., Pachinger, T.: A method for the calculation of induced band power: implications for the significance of brain oscillations. Electroencephalogr. Clin. Neurophysiol. Evoked Potentials Section **108**(2), 123–130 (1998). https://doi.org/10.1016/S0168-5597(97)00078-6

26. Ελληνικά Ονόματα Ελλήνων και Ελληνίδων, Στατιστική Συχνότητα. https://www. foundalis.com/grk/EllinikaOnomata.html.
27. Henson, R.N.A.: Neuroimaging studies of priming. Prog. Neurobiol. **70**(1), 53–81 (2003). https://doi.org/10.1016/s0301-0082(03)00086-8
28. Jennings, J.M., Webster, L.M., Kleykamp, B.A., Dagenbach, D.: Recollection training and transfer effects in older adults: successful use of a repetition-lag procedure. Neuropsychol. Dev. Cogn. B Aging Neuropsychol. Cogn. **12**(3), 278–298 (2005). https://doi.org/10.1080/138255890968312
29. Mathe, E., Spyrou, E.: Assessment of User Experience with a Commercial BCI Device, September 2019
30. Mathe, E., Spyrou, E.: Connecting a Consumer Brain-Computer Interface to an Internet-of-Things Ecosystem, pp. 1–2, June 2016. https://doi.org/10.1145/2910674.2935844
31. MindWave. https://store.neurosky.com/pages/mindwave
32. app_notes_and_tutorials [NeuroSky Developer - Docs]. https://developer.neurosky.com/docs/doku.php?id=app_notes_and_tutorials
33. Compilers. https://www.mathworks.com/support/requirements/supported-compilers.html.
34. Mijović, B., De Vos, M., Gligorijević, I., Taelman, J., Van Huffel, S.: Source separation from single-channel recordings by combining empirical-mode decomposition and independent component analysis. IEEE Trans. Biomed. Eng. **57**(9), 2188–2196 (2010). https://doi.org/10.1109/TBME.2010.2051440
35. Al-Subari, K., Al-Baddai, S., Tomé, A.M., Goldhacker, M., Faltermeier, R., Lang, E.W.: EMD-LAB: a toolbox for analysis of single-trial EEG dynamics using empirical mode decomposition. J. Neurosci. Methods **253**, 193–205 (2015). https://doi.org/10.1016/j.jneumeth.2015.06.020
36. Pfurtscheller, G., Lopes da Silva, F.H.: Event-related EEG/MEG synchronization and desynchronization: basic principles. Clin. Neurophysiol. **110**(11), 1842–1857 (1999). https://doi.org/10.1016/s1388-2457(99)00141-8
37. Kalcher, J., Pfurtscheller, G.: Discrimination between phase-locked and non-phase-locked event-related EEG activity. Electroencephalogr. Clin. Neurophysiol. **94**(5), 381–384 (1995). https://doi.org/10.1016/0013-4694(95)00040-6
38. Duncan, C.C., et al.: Event-related potentials in clinical research: guidelines for eliciting, recording, and quantifying mismatch negativity, P300, and N400. Clin. Neurophysiol. **120**(11), 1883–1908 (2009). https://doi.org/10.1016/j.clinph.2009.07.045
39. Güntekin, B., Başar, E.: A review of brain oscillations in perception of faces and emotional pictures. Neuropsychologia **58**, 33–51 (2014). https://doi.org/10.1016/j.neuropsychologia.2014.03.014
40. Sakihara, K., Gunji, A., Furushima, W., Inagaki, M.: Event-related oscillations in structural and semantic encoding of faces. Clin. Neurophysiol. **123**(2), 270–277 (2012). https://doi.org/10.1016/j.clinph.2011.06.023
41. Klimesch, W.: Alpha-band oscillations, attention, and controlled access to stored information. Trends Cogn. Sci. **16**(12), 606–617 (2012). https://doi.org/10.1016/j.tics.2012.10.007
42. Jensen, O., Tesche, C.: Frontal theta activity in humans increases with memory load in a working memory task. Eur. J. Neurosc. **15**, 1395–1399 (2002). https://doi.org/10.1046/j.1460-9568.2002.01975.x
43. Weiss, S., Mueller, H.M.: Too many betas do not spoil the broth': the role of beta brain oscillations in language processing. Front Psychol. **3** (2012). https://doi.org/10.3389/fpsyg.2012.00201.
44. Schmidt, R., Ruiz, M.H., Kilavik, B.E., Lundqvist, M., Starr, P.A., Aron, A.R.: Beta oscillations in working memory, executive control of movement and thought, and sensorimotor function. J. Neurosci. **39**(42), 8231–8238 (2019). https://doi.org/10.1523/JNEUROSCI.1163-19.2019

45. Spitzer, B., Haegens, S.: Beyond the status quo: a role for beta oscillations in endogenous content (re)activation. eNeuro **4**(4), (2017). https://doi.org/10.1523/ENEURO.0170-17.2017
46. Dimitriadis, S., Laskaris, N., Tsirka, V., Vourkas, M., Sifis, M.: What does delta band tell us about cognitive processes: a mental calculation study. Neurosci. Lett. **483**, 11–15 (2010). https://doi.org/10.1016/j.neulet.2010.07.034
47. Harmony, T.: The functional significance of delta oscillations in cognitive processing. Front. Integr. Neurosci. **7** (2013). https://doi.org/10.3389/fnint.2013.00083

Towards Mobile-Based Preprocessing Pipeline for Electroencephalography (EEG) Analyses: The Case of Tinnitus

Muntazir Mehdi[1]([✉]), Lukas Hennig[1], Florian Diemer[1], Albi Dode[2],
Rüdiger Pryss[3], Winfried Schlee[4], Manfred Reichert[2], and Franz J. Hauck[1]

[1] Institute of Distributed Systems, Ulm University, Ulm, Germany
{muntazir.mehdi,lukas.hennig,florian.diemer,franz.hauck}@uni-ulm.de
[2] Institute of Databases and Information Systems, Ulm University, Ulm, Germany
[3] Institute of Clinical Epidemiology and Biometry, University of Würzburg, Würzburg, Germany
[4] Clinic and Policlinic for Psychiatry and Psychotherapy, Regensburg, Germany

Abstract. Recent developments in Brain-Computer Interfaces (BCI)—technologies to collect brain imaging data—allow recording of Electroencephalography (EEG) data outside of a laboratory setting by means of mobile EEG systems. Brain imaging has been pivotal in understanding the neurobiological correlates of human behavior in many complex disorders. This is also the case for tinnitus, a disorder that causes phantom noise sensations in the ears in absence of any sound source. As studies have shown that tinnitus is also influenced by complexities in non-auditory brain areas, mobile EEG can be a viable solution in better understanding the influencing factors causing tinnitus. Mobile EEG will become even more useful, if real-time EEG analysis in mobile experimental environments is enabled, e.g., as an immediate feedback to physicians and patients or in undeveloped areas where a laboratory setup is unfeasible. The volume and complexity of brain imaging data have made preprocessing a pertinent step in the process of analysis, e.g., for data cleaning and artifact removal. We introduce the first smartphone-based preprocessing pipeline for real-time EEG analysis. More specifically, we present a mobile app with a rudimentary EEG preprocessing pipeline and evaluate the app and its resource consumption underpinning the feasibility of smartphones for EEG preprocessing. Our proposed approach will allow researchers to collect brain imaging data of tinnitus and other patients in real-world environments and everyday situations, thereby collecting evidence for previously unknown facts about tinnitus and other conditions.

Keywords: Healthcare · Mobile health · Smartphone apps · Mobile apps · Tinnitus · EEG · Brain imaging · Brain Computer Interfaces

© ICST Institute for Computer Sciences, Social Informatics and Telecommunications Engineering 2021
Published by Springer Nature Switzerland AG 2021. All Rights Reserved
J. Ye et al. (Eds.): MobiHealth 2020, LNICST 362, pp. 67–86, 2021.
https://doi.org/10.1007/978-3-030-70569-5_5

1 Introduction

Brain imaging techniques offer different opportunities to examine the neurobiological correlates of human behavior. Among different brain-imaging techniques, for instance, Magnetoencephalography (MEG), Functional Magnetic Resonance Imaging (fMRI), and Positron Emission Tomography (PET), Electroencephalography (EEG) is the most adaptable and multifaceted one. EEG is a non-invasive tool that allows the investigation of the resting-state electrical activity of the brain by means of electrodes positioned on the scalp [8]. This enables the investigation of human brain functions by recording the communication between neurons in the brain network measured in volts. EEG offers high time resolution (high number of snapshots of electrical activity from various electrodes) in comparison to fMRI and PET [25], and is an inexpensive and low maintenance technique compared to MEG. Thus, EEG is not only an inexpensive but a versatile, lightweight, and portable brain-imaging technique, and it is extensively applied in tinnitus research [3,7,11].

Tinnitus is a common disorder responsible for causing the perception of a ringing sound in the ears without presence of any external sound source. The reasons pertaining to causing this phantom sound are yet to be fully discovered, but it has been firmly established that tinnitus is caused by an underlying anomaly in the ear such as damage and loss of cochlear hair cells [14]. Despite the fact that tinnitus is traditionally considered a problem of the inner ear, recent studies using brain imaging have shown that the complexity of tinnitus goes beyond the auditory cortex into non-auditory brain areas [8,13]. Brain imaging techniques like EEG can be pivotal in collecting evidences for further yet unknown facts regarding the neuronal activity of tinnitus.

Current developments in EEG research have progressed significantly to record EEG outside a laboratory setting by means of ambulatory or mobile EEGs [16,17]. Mobile EEG devices are equipped with necessary hardware to be communicated by a wired (USB) or a wireless connection (Bluetooth or WiFi). Generally, an EEG session is primarily recorded and temporarily stored on the mobile EEG device (either on the built-in flash memory or an external SD card). Since brain imaging outside a controlled laboratory setting and in real-world scenario can result in unnecessary noise in data and useless subject-generated artifacts [12], the EEG recordings are therefore transferred to a computer for preprocessing steps like data cleansing, filtering and artifact removal using EEGLab Scripts [6], MATLAB, or FieldTrip [23]. Alternatively, mobile EEG can also be directly connected to a computer to transfer real-time EEG data and perform on-the-run preprocessing [26].

Although the current paradigm of EEG recording and preprocessing is a significant improvement over conventional EEG, including EEG analysis in real-world settings, it is still limited in terms of offering real-time analysis with freedom of movement or mobility. A major shortcoming of the current EEG analysis paradigm is the requirement of additional hardware for EEG data acquisition, preprocessing, and visualization. For example, currently, the overall process of EEG analysis and visualization requires additional steps of transferring EEG data to a computer, thereby hindering the mobility and introduction of requiring specialized software for EEG data preprocessing. A possible alternative solution to this problem can be *Mobile Sensing*—the process of acquiring sensory data of an individual using a smartphone or mobile device while allowing mobility [20]. Smartphones are capable to be used, and some scientific literature has already reported their successful usage [19,30].

Modern smartphones are ubiquitous devices that provide sophisticated communication hardware, exceptional computing power, and reasonable battery. Additionally, smartphones offer APIs for programming new apps. These characteristics plus the fact that smartphones are literally mobile devices make smartphones an ideal candidate for real-time analysis and recording of EEG data in non-conventional, exceptional, and atypical real-world settings such as swimming, running, or hiking etc. However, it is also notable that the smartphones are manufactured as general purpose devices and are not specialized for real-time EEG recording and analysis, therefore, their feasibility and behavior in such cases require efforts. For instance, continuous sampling of the EEG data might result in excessive battery consumption problems [33], or might introduce scarcity of computational power for general user experience [2]. Furthermore, a continuous Bluetooth connection with the mobile EEG device might cause data transmission problems [10], as well as its associated energy consumption problem [32].

Therefore, for addressing the aforementioned challenges, this article proposes a mobile-based preprocessing pipeline for EEG analysis, more specifically (i) the development and design of a smartphone app with a rudimentary EEG preprocessing pipeline, and (ii) an evaluation of the proposed app to show the feasibility of smartphones to perform EEG preprocessing. The proposed work is motivated and driven by the needs of tinnitus research within the context of the European School for Interdisciplinary Tinnitus Research (ESIT) [29]. One core goal of the ESIT project is the development of a generic, robust and flexible middleware for mobile crowdsensing to monitor real-time measurements of tinnitus-related parameters as well as electroencephalographic and physical activities. The proposed approach will improve mobility for EEG data acquisition and analysis using smartphones and enable preprocessing of EEG data without the need of specialized software and hardware. The proposed smartphone app will also allow researchers to collect brain-imaging data of tinnitus patients in a variety of experimental conditions in real-world environment, thereby, to collect evidence for unknown facts regarding tinnitus in brain regions. In particular, the proposed smartphone app will assist researchers in designing and gathering EEG data for large scale longitudinal studies, for example, to investigate oscillatory brain activity of tinnitus patients in a longitudinal design by investigating patients that have moments with high and low tinnitus intensity. Furthermore, the ability to collect and analyze real-time EEG data in real-world experimental situations as well as in places where a laboratory EEG setup is impossible—for instance, in underdeveloped or undeveloped rural areas—will be a significant asset for brain-imaging and neuro-imaging research. The application possibilities are not limited to tinnitus research, but the proposed solution will also support a variety of application domains where brain-imaging is vital.

Section 2 of this paper gives insights into previously reported related work in this field and briefly discusses the existing preprocessing approaches. Section 3 details the overall design and implementation of the proposed work. The subsequent Sect. 4 evaluates the proposed approach by presenting results and data on the feasibility of smartphones for preprocessing EEG data. Finally, we conclude and present brief insights into future work in Sect. 5.

2   Related Work

In terms of specialized software packages for offline and online preprocessing and analysis of EEG data, EEGLAB [6] and FieldTrip [23] are among the most prominent. EEGLAB is an open source (GNU license) toolbox for MATLAB. It is used for processing EEG data, including data filtering and artifact removal, as well as analysis of EEG data using Independent Component Analysis (ICA). Similarly, FieldTrip is also an open source (GNU license) toolbox for MATLAB for analyzing EEG data. In terms of developing BCI applications, OpenViBE (framework for developing BCI applications for neurofeedback and biofeedback) [27], BCILAB (EEGLAB plugin to develop EEG predictive models) [15], and BCI2000 (a C++ framework for developing real-time BCI applications) [28] are some of the popular frameworks. Furthermore, Esch et al. [9] present the MNE software project, which comprises tools required for EEG and MEG data acquisition, preprocessing, analysis, and visualization. Similarly, Tadel et al. [31] present an open-source platform for EEG and MEG data analysis and visualization.

With reference to existing preprocessing pipelines, it is pertinent to notice that there exists no standard method. Usually, the preprocessing of EEG signals is supervised by EEG experts. However, there has been some existing literature reporting on automated preprocessing of EEG data. Usually, most of the pre-existing preprocessing pipelines perform filtering, removal of line noise, and detection of bad channels including interpolation. Among the preexisting preprocessing pipelines, the PREP Pipeline [4] claims to standardize the preprocessing of EEG data. The main idea of PREP is to distinguish externally generated noise, such as electrical interference and patient-generated artifacts via muscular activation. For instance, the line-noise detection and removal is done using a modified implementation of the *CleanLine* plugin from EEGLAB [1,22]. The PREP Pipeline has been reused in other preprocessing implementations, Automagic [24] and the Batch Electroencephalography Automated Processing Platform (BEAPP) [18]. In [5], da Cruz et al. propose a MATLAB-based automated preprocessing pipeline for EEG data called APP. APP uses the CleanLine plugin from EEGLAB for line-noise removal like the PREP pipeline. Furthermore, APP applies a *3rd Order Butterworth filter* 1 Hz in both forward and reverse direction to correct the direct-current (DC) drift caused by changes in the DC value. After removing the line noises, the channel data is re-referenced. Both PREP and the APP preprocessing pipelines extensively use the EEGLAB preprocessing library. Instructions on how to preprocess EEG data using EEGLAB

Table 1. Overview of the preprocessing pipelines

PREP [4]	APP [5]	Makoto [21]	Result
–	3rd order Butter-worth filter	Highpass filter	3rd order Butter-worth filter
Cleanline	CleanLine	CleanLine	Band-stop filter
Signal true mean estimation with bad channels interpolated	Signal true mean estimation with weighted mean	–	Estimate signal true mean with bad channels interpolated
Detect bad channels relative to mean and interpolate	Detect bad channels relative to neighbors and with high dis-persion to mean	–	Detect bad channels relative to mean and interpolate
Detecting noisy or outlier channels	–	–	–
–	Detecting and remove bad epochs	Reject epochs for cleaning	–
–	ICA	ICA	–
–	Detection, removal and interpolation of bad channels in epochs	–	–
–	Outlier detection	–	–

and development of preprocessing pipelines are given by Makoto Miyakoshi from Swartz Center for Computational Neuroscience [21].

The three foremost and commonly used preprocessing pipelines (PREP, APP, Makoto) are delineated in Table 1, along-with a comparison to our proposed approach. We first apply a *3rd Order Butterworth filter* in both forward and reverse directions for signal filtering like the APP preprocessing pipcline. Next, we use a *Band-stop Filter* (also called notch filter) as an alternative to the Cleanline to remove power line interference between 50 and 60 Hz or 50 and 70 Hz. Despite that this can cause significant signal distortion around the band-stop frequency and phase distortion [4], however, our choice of implementing band-stop filter is due to resource scarcity on the smartphones. Currently, we are working on implementing and optimizing the CleanLinc algorithm for the Android platform. Finally, in order to detect bad channels, we have implemented and modified both phases of the PREP's 'Referencing Procedure' for the Android platform.

In general, there exists a plethora of literature reporting on software packages and toolboxes for online and offline analysis of EEG data. Similarly, there exist plenty of literature reporting on automated preprocessing pipelines and standardizing the preprocessing of EEG data. Our literature review did not yield any study that reports on any application of preprocessing EEG data using smartphones. Specifically, we did not find any article that benchmarks the preprocessing of EEG data using smartphones. To the best of our knowledge, the proposed work is the first of its type towards mobile-based preprocessing pipeline for EEG analysis, including visualization of EEG data, as well as to present evidence regarding feasibility of smartphones to perform preprocessing of EEG data.

3   Implementation

The proposed work aims at preprocessing of EEG data for analysis purposes using a smartphone. Therefore, we have developed an Android application. The overall architecture of the proposed app is presented in Fig. 1. The data from electrodes of the EEG cap are transmitted to the EEG Amplifier. In our implementation, we have used the EEG Amplifier by Brain Products called LiveAmp 16[1]. The EEG Amplifier can be coupled with the smartphone using Bluetooth.

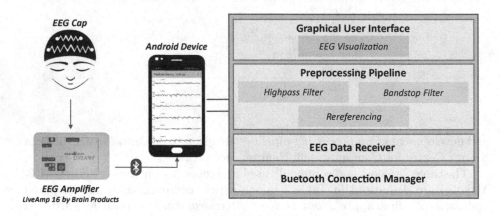

Fig. 1. Architecture

To acquire live EEG data, an EEG cap is connected to LiveAmp 16 using a wired connection. The *Bluetooth Connection Manager* module is responsible for establishing the first connection with LiveAmp 16, and maintaining the

---

[1] https://www.brainproducts.com/productdetails.php?id=63 Accessed: 15/06/2020.

Bluetooth connection for the duration of EEG. The *EEG Data Receiver* module is implemented in Java and included as an external library to the Android application. The EEG data-receiver module is responsible for communicating with the LiveAmp 16 based on the LiveAmp-16's communication protocol, and is assisted by the Bluetooth-connection manager module. All communications between LiveAmp 16 and the Android application are done in a proprietary binary data format using request-response method. Some examples of requests sent to LiveAmp 16 are 'Get Device Information' and 'Get Device Status'. In order to start EEG data acquisition, the EEG data receiver sends a request of type 'Start Data Acquisition' and starts receiving EEG data in binary responses from LiveAmp 16. The data transformation is also managed by the EEG data-receiver module. Once the data has been transformed into an internal Java format, the EEG data is forwarded to the *Preprocessing-Pipeline* module.

3.1   Preprocessing Pipeline

Our current implementation of the preprocessing pipeline offers filtering, removal of line noise, and detection of bad channels including interpolation. As these steps are usually part of any preprocessing pipeline, we identify these steps to be principle components, and therefore we have limited our current implementation to these. Herein, the filtering is offered by `HighPassFilter` with a *3rd Order Butterworth* filter. The line noise removal is carried out by `BandStopFilter`. Finally, the bad-channel detection is done by adopting and implementing both phases of the PREP's 'Referencing Procedure' for Android platform, we refer to as `Rereferencer`. The overall design of our current implementation of the preprocessing pipeline is illustrated in Fig. 2, using a Class Diagram, and the sequential object interactions of the Java classes is given in Fig. 3. The individual classes as well as their relations are briefly discussed below:

Pipeline. The abstract `Pipeline` class defines all the necessary properties and methods, such as the frequencies of filters, and the sampling rate. The `Pipeline` class implements the `Filter` interface, where the `Filter` interface declares the method called `filter()`. To ensure a flexible class design and a uniform filter structure, all filter classes extend the abstract `Pipeline` class (`HighPassFilter`, `Rereferencer`, and `BandStopFilter`). The filter-specific logic is implemented in the overridden `filter()` method of each extending filter class. In addition to other properties, the `Pipeline` class also defines an instance of `EpochBuffer` class. During the filtering process, the `Pipeline` class initializes the buffer with the EEG data values.

EpochBuffer. To work with continuously incoming data, an `EpochBuffer` with a default length of 64 values is used. The `EpochBuffer` implements a `CircularBuffer` and stores the incoming EEG data values. All filters are sequentially applied on the values stored in buffer, thus modifying the EEG data one after the other.

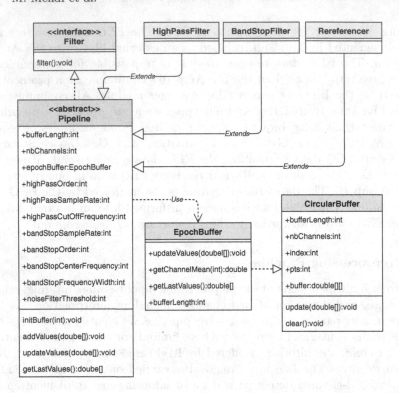

Fig. 2. Class diagram of preprocessing pipeline-related Java classes

HighPassFilter. Class `HighPassFilter` is implemented with the help of an Infinite Impulse Response (IIR) filter library for digital signal processing[2]. The library is integrated into the project using Maven. The library allows application of 3rd Order Butterworth Filter with a default value 1 Hz and a sampling rate 250 Hz to the signal.

Rereferencer. For this filter, both phases of the PREP's re-referencing algorithm presented in [4] was implemented in Java for the Android platform. The `NoiseDetector` from NeuroTechX[3] used in EEG-101 was used to detect noisy channels. The noise detector uses variance thresholding on the data available in `EpochBuffer` to detect and mark noisy channels.

BandStopFilter. The aforementioned IIR library comes with an implementation of the band-stop filter. To remove line noise from the signal, our implementation re-uses the band-stop filter from the IIR library.

---

[2] https://github.com/berndporr/iirj Accessed: 15/06/2020.
[3] https://github.com/NeuroTechX/eeg-101 Accessed: 15/06/2020.

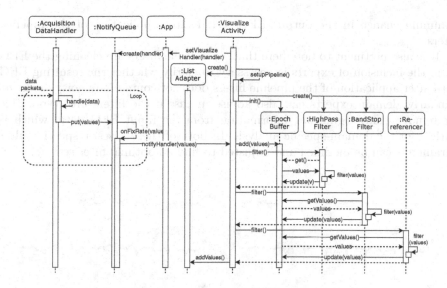

Fig. 3. Sequence diagram of data preprocessing

To better examine the results and behavior of the individual filters, as well as the entire pipeline (all filters applied), a comparison of filter application to the raw EEG data is shown in Fig. 4. In all represented graphs in Fig. 4(a–d), the blue signal represents the raw EEG data without application of any filter, while the blue signal represents the EEG data after application of individual filter. Herein, Fig. 4a shows the comparison of raw EEG data and the high-pass filter, Fig. 4b shows a comparison of the band-stop filter with raw EEG data, and Fig. 4c shows a comparison of raw EEG data and the application of the re-referencer filter. Similarly, Fig. 4d shows a comparison between raw EEG data with all filters applied (high pass, band-stop, re-referencer).

From Fig. 4a, we can observe very minor difference between the two signals, suggesting very little impact on changing the signal. Figure 4b gives a good example of influence of the band-stop filter on the EEG data. Although the signal looks quite similar to the original, but at some points the peaks become more smoother. With the re-referencer filter results shown in Fig. 4c, it can be noticed that the signal peaks remain in their amplitude, but in some places there is a slight upward and downward shift in amplitude of the signal, particularly in the signal comparison of Channel 1. The result of the entire pipeline, depicted in Fig. 4d, shows a mixture of what we experienced at each individual filter.

The exact accuracy of application of individual filters can be questioned, therefore, domain experts can be helpful in validating and improving the filter implementation. Furthermore, please also note that the amount of influence of applying individual filters as well as the entire pipeline on the EEG data is dependent and subjective of the type of raw EEG data used. For instance, a cleaner input EEG signal with minimum noise and noisy artifacts will present minimum change in the output EEG signal after application of the pipeline filters.

It is also pertinent to note here that, even if the filters are cleaning the EEG data, the inclusion of experts is necessary to clarify whether the resulting EEG data after application of the pipeline filters does not contain any noisy artifacts. Similarly, domain experts can also advise in case if the filters are responsible for removing any significant information from the input EEG data, which is critical for the domain-specific analysis. In both of these cases, respective filter parameters can be modified and adjusted to find an optimal filter setting.

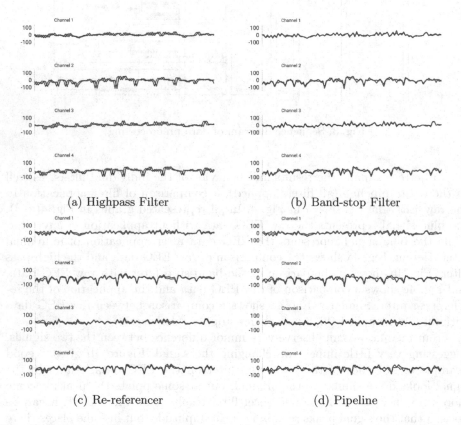

(a) Highpass Filter   (b) Band-stop Filter

(c) Re-referencer   (d) Pipeline

Fig. 4. Comparison between raw simulator data (red) and the filters applied (blue) (Color figure online)

3.2   Graphical User Interface (GUI)

Workspace and Filter Settings

Before running an EEG recording session, the EEG device must be configured properly. The proposed Android application uses workspaces for this task.

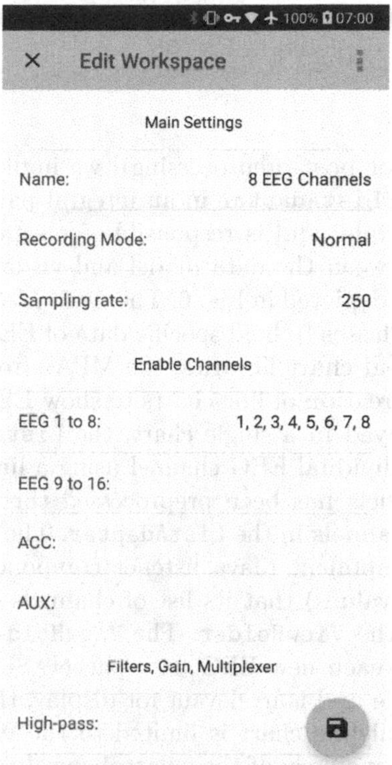

(a) EEG workspace creation

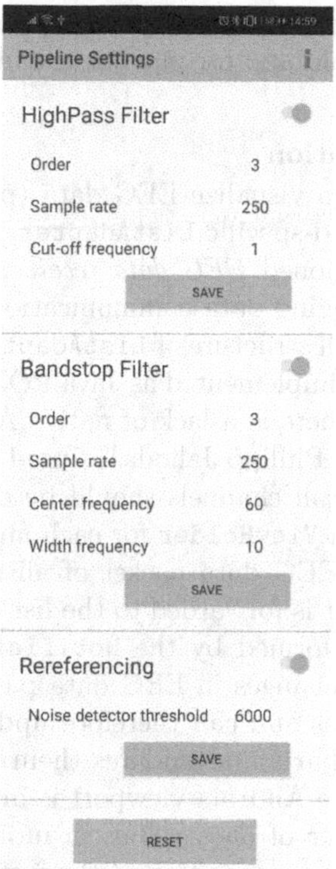

(b) Preprocessing filter settings

Fig. 5. EEG application screenshots

Workspaces are stored and can be edited later. This allows the flexibility to execute multiple EEG sessions with the same workspace configuration. Additionally, changing a single parameter of an existing workspace is also possible. Figure 5a shows the screenshot from the app for the workspace creation. Each workspace consists of several parameter settings like name, recording mode, and sampling rate. Furthermore, the workspace screen also allows enabling and disabling of EEG channels. The workspace configuration can be stored on the Android device and are sent to the EEG amplifier before an EEG session via *EEG Data Receiver* module.

In addition to the workspace configuration, the proposed Android application also allows configuration of filters through a *Pipeline Settings* screen. The pipeline-settings screen allows enabling and disabling of individual pipeline filters as well as configuration of filter parameters. This allows the behavior of individual filters, or different combination of filters on the EEG data to be observed and evaluated. Additionally, changing configuration parameters of individual filters allows optimization of filter application on the EEG signal. A screenshot from the Android app for pipeline settings is depicted in Fig. 5b.

Visualization

In order to visualize EEG data (prior or post-preprocessing), we implemented an Android-specific `ListAdapter`. This `ListAdapter` in an integral part of the aforementioned *EEG data receiver* module, and is responsible for establishing and managing data communication between the data model and visualization. The overall structure of `ListAdapter` is depicted in Fig. 6. The *Data Model* component is implemented as Java POJO Classes to hold specific data of EEG channels. As there is a lack of native Android chart libraries, the MPAndroidChart library by Philipp Jahoda[4] is used for creation of line charts to show EEG data. Since not all channels should be displayed in a single chart, the `ListAdapter` provides a `ViewHolder` for each and individual EEG channel using a line chart. Once an EEG data packet of all channels has been preprocessed through the pipeline, it is forwarded to the list of channels in the `ListAdapter`. The adapter is then informed by the `Notifier` component (Java listener component triggered on changes in EEG data packet values) that its list of channels has new data values and can therefore update the `ViewHolder`. The `ViewHolder` holds the line charts and updates them with each new EEG data packet. Since data outside the Android viewport is invisible and is irrelevant for display, therefore, the number of data values in individual line chart is limited to the viewport, this allows conservation of the working memory of the smartphone. In order to further conserve the smartphone resource, the `RecyclerView` component ensures refreshing of `ViewHolder` based on last used EEG data packets in case the EEG data packet values have not changed.

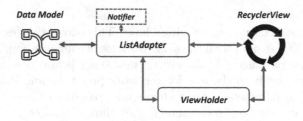

Fig. 6. Structure of the ListAdapter for visualization of EEG data

Figure 7a shows an example visualization of the test signal generated by the EEG amplifier device for Channels 1 to 8. Furthermore, please note the control buttons on the bottom right corner of the screen. The control buttons are divided into three types: 1) The Record button starts recording (storage of EEG data on smartphone and amplifier) of the EEG along with visualization of the EEG

---

[4] https://github.com/PhilJay/MPAndroidChart Accessed: 15/06/2020.

signal on the smartphone, 2) the Monitor button starts visualizing the EEG data without recording, and 3) Start/Stop testing starts respectively stops receiving test signal (sinusoidal wave) generated by the amplifier to test connectivity and data transmission. Figure 7b shows an example visualization of a real EEG data. The pipeline latency on the top of the screen shows the time delay between the preprocessing of two consecutive EEG data packet values. In this example, the latency is shown for all three pipeline filters.

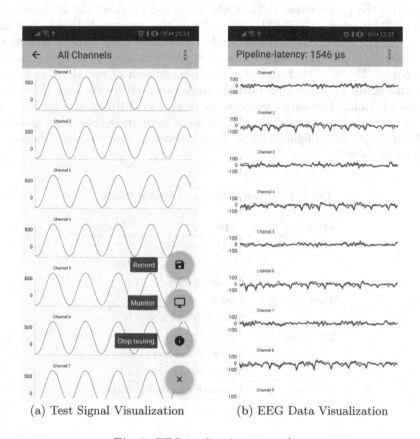

(a) Test Signal Visualization   (b) EEG Data Visualization

Fig. 7. EEG application screenshots

4   Results and Discussions

Since one of the core goals of our proposed work was to test and evaluate the feasibility of smartphones for EEG data preprocessing, in this section we detail the experiments and results examining the performance of the proposed preprocessing pipeline on a mobile device. We have exhaustively tested our proposed approach and run experiments to provide a detailed comparison of resource consumption on the mobile device for acquiring raw EEG data (non-processed EEG data), application of individual filters on the EEG data, and application of all filters on the EEG data. Our experiments focus specifically on mobile resource consumption in terms of CPU usage, working memory usage, and battery consumption.

4.1 Experimental Setup

To measure the performance data of the proposed pipeline and its filters, the Huawei P20 Lite with 4 GB RAM, with an Octacore processor Kirin 659 (4×2.36 GHz + 4×1.7 GHz), and non-removable Li-Po 3000 mAh battery was used[5]. The *Android Profiler* built into Android Studio was used to measure the app performance. The workload and resource consumption of raw data, individual filters and entire preprocessing pipeline were captured by running them for a duration of 5 min. The entire process was repeated 3 times, the performance data was recorded, and the arithmetic mean of 3 separate runs was computed. The EEG amplifier configurations and filter settings used for the experiments are given in Table 2.

Table 2. EEG amplifier and filter settings

Settings	Type	Values
Workspace	EEG channels	1–8
	Data type	Test
	Sampling rate	250
HighPass filter	Order	3
	Cut-off frequency	1
BandStop filter	Order	3
	Center frequency	60
	Width frequency	10
Rereferencing	Variance threshold	4000

4.2 Results

The comparative performance results of the proposed EEG preprocessing pipeline are given in Fig. 8, where Fig. 8a gives performance in terms of CPU usage in percentage, and Fig. 8b shows the amount of working memory used in MB. The battery related results are shown in Fig. 9, where Fig. 9a shows the energy consumption in percentage. Herein, please note that the Android Studio Profiler only distinguishes between three energy levels namely light, medium, and heavy. We divided each of those levels into three equal parts which results

---

[5] https://consumer.huawei.com/de/support/phones/p20-lite/ Accessed: 15/06/2020.

in nine same sized intervals. The introduced nine intervals were used for proper quantization of the energy used by filters and allow better distinction of energy consumption. Figure 9b shows the comparative results of over-all battery run-time duration in hours (hh:mm format). For this purpose, the mobile device was completely charged and the EEG data was continuously sampled, processed, and visualized until the battery was exhausted.

4.3 Discussion

From Fig. 8, in general, we can see minimal usage of critical computing resources of the smartphone. Note that this is suggestive as the regular user experience, including the background services, can not be hindered by the preprocessing and visualization of EEG data. Specifically, from Fig. 8a, the average CPU

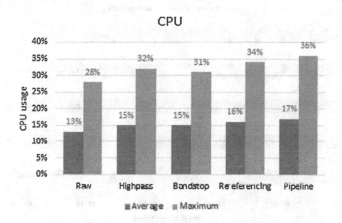

(a) CPU load in percentage

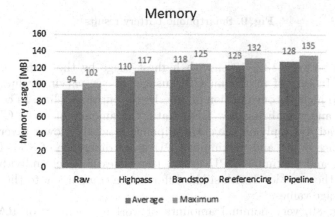

(b) Memory consumption in MB

Fig. 8. Smartphone performance results

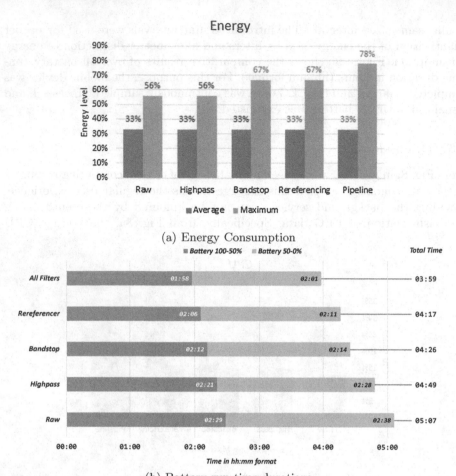

(a) Energy Consumption

(b) Battery run-time durations

Fig. 9. Smartphone battery results

usage ranges between 13%–17%, with highest usage by the entire preprocessing pipeline. In case of maximum CPU usage, we see varying values between 28%–36% and highest consumption of 36% by the entire pipeline. In comparison to acquiring and visualizing raw EEG data, the amount of extra CPU usage (CPU overhead) by applying the entire pipeline is notably lower (average CPU usage difference of 4% and maximum CPU usage difference of 8%). In case of both average and maximum CPU usage, the values for each individual filters remained on the same level with slight difference in comparison to the raw EEG data CPU usage values.

From Fig. 8b, very nominal amounts of working memory or RAM usage can be seen. The average memory usage ranges between 94–128 MB, with most memory usage of 128 MB by the entire preprocessing pipeline. In case of maximum memory usage, a variation of values ranging between 102–135 MB were observed, where the highest memory usage of 135 MB was for the entire pipeline. Comparatively, the amount of additional working memory required for applying the entire pipeline as opposed to acquiring and visualizing raw EEG data is very low (average memory usage difference of 34 MB and maximum memory usage difference of 33 MB).

Apparently, the proposed preprocessing pipeline is resource-intensive in terms of battery and energy consumption (see Fig. 9). A moderate to high requirement for energy consumption was already anticipated due to the involvement of additional resources like Bluetooth and the smartphone screen usage. However, from Fig. 9a, we can conclude an acceptable energy requirement by the app. Specifically, since in case of average energy usage, all filters as well the entire preprocessing pipeline consumed 33% of the smartphone energy, inline with the battery usage for acquiring and visualizing raw EEG data. Conversely, in case of maximum energy usage, we see values ranging from 56% (energy usage to acquire, and visualize raw EEG data) to 78% (energy usage for acquiring, pre-processing with entire pipeline, and visualizing raw EEG data). Herein, we see a notable additional energy usage of 22% by the entire preprocessing pipeline. For HighPass filter, the energy remains same as the raw EEG data acquisition and visualization, but an additional energy usage of 11% for band-stop and referencing (Rereferencer) filters can be seen.

On the other hand, energy usage measure can be subjective in certain scenarios, therefore, an objective measure in terms of overall battery run-time duration is given in Fig. 9b. The overall battery run-time duration represents the amount of time between a full battery charge and empty battery. From Fig. 9b, we see a total of 5 h and 7 min alive time for continuous raw EEG data acquisition and visualization. The overall time duration varied for EEG data acquisition, visualization, and applying individual preprocessing filter. For instance, for Highpass filter the battery lasted for 4 h 49 min, for bandstop filter the battery run-time duration was 4 h 26 min, 4 h 17 min for the Rereferencer, and for the entire pipeline (all filters) the battery lasted for 3 h and 59 min. Herein, we see the lowest battery run-time duration of 3 h and 59 min, which is acceptable since most conventional EEG sessions require maximum of 40 min.

5 Conclusion, Limitations, and Future Work

Portable, ambulatory, or mobile EEG devices allow monitoring of neuronal activities of human brain in real-life scenarios. The mobile EEG devices support the wireless transmission of EEG data over Bluetooth, thus, enabling live EEG data processing and visualization on standard smartphones. In this work, we proposed an elementary mobile-based preprocessing pipeline for EEG analysis and evaluated the feasibility of smartphones for EEG data preprocessing. Our experiments and results show that contemporary smartphones have satisfactory computational capabilities in terms of CPU and working memory to perform EEG data acquisition, preprocessing, and visualization without hindering the user-experience in relation to general smartphone use. Further, our experiments with battery consumption while preprocessing and visualizing EEG data show moderate energy consumption and suggest that the smartphones hold ample battery capacity to allow recording of multiple EEG sessions. The proposed approach was realized within the context of tinnitus research to collect evidence for unknown facts regarding tinnitus using brain imaging techniques. The significant contributions of the proposed approach are to, (i) improve EEG data acquisition, preprocessing, visualization, and analysis, (ii) enable preprocessing of EEG data using smartphones and without the need of specialized software or hardware, (iii) allow researchers the flexibility to gather brain imaging data of tinnitus patients in a variety of experimental conditions in real-world environments. Furthermore, the proposed app serves as an initial step towards smartphone-based automated mobile neurofeedback and biofeedback for tinnitus patients. Nevertheless, our approach can be applied for other domains needing mobile and real-time EEG observations.

Two notable shortcomings of our proposed work are, 1) the number of filters included in the preprocessing pipeline, and 2) our choice of band-stop filter for removal of line noise. For inclusion of additional filters in the preprocessing pipeline, we have ensured the current design is flexible and extendable, and therefore, the pipeline can be easily extended with additional artifact-removing filters. For instance, we are currently implementing the Independent Component Analysis (ICA) algorithm for Android platform. For line interference and noise removal, although, we justify our use of band-stop filter, for future work, we are currently working on an optimized and Android-specific implementation of the CleanLine algorithm. Furthermore, we are running the aforementioned experiments on additional smartphone devices (including old models as well relevantly new models) to observe the behavior of proposed EEG preprocessing pipeline in terms of resource consumption. Finally, for further future work, we intend to apply the proposed smartphone app in the field to acquire and analyze EEG data in real-world experimental settings. This will be specifically done within the context of tinnitus research to gather EEG-related data of tinnitus patients.

Acknowledgment. This publication is a result of research supported by funding from the European Union's Horizon 2020 research and innovation programme under the Marie Skłodowska-Curie grant agreement number 722064 (European School for Interdisciplinary Tinnitus Research, ESIT) [29]. We would also like to acknowledge Brain Products GmbH (https://www.brainproducts.com/ Accessed: 15/06/2020) for their help and support while working with the LiveAmp 16 EEG amplifier.

References

1. Cleanline. https://www.nitrc.org/projects/cleanline. Accessed 04 June 2020
2. Abolfazli, S., Sanaei, Z., Gani, A.: Mobile cloud computing: a review on smartphone augmentation approaches. arXiv preprint arXiv:1205.0451 (2012)
3. Adjamian, P.: The application of electro-and magneto-encephalography in tinnitus research-methods and interpretations. Front. Neurol. **5**, 228 (2014)

4. Bigdely-Shamlo, N., Mullen, T., Kothe, C., Su, K.M., Robbins, K.A.: The prep pipeline: standardized preprocessing for large-scale EEG analysis. Front. Neuroinf. **9**, 16 (2015). https://doi.org/10.3389/fninf.2015.00016, https://www.frontiersin.org/article/10.3389/fninf.2015.00016

5. da Cruz, J.R., Chicherov, V., Herzog, M.H., Figueiredo, P.: An automatic preprocessing pipeline for EEG analysis (APP) based on robust statistics. Clin. Neurophysiol. **129**, 1427–1437 (2018)

6. Delorme, A., Makeig, S.: EEGLAB: an open source toolbox for analysis of single-trial EEG dynamics including independent component analysis. J. Neurosci. Methods **134**(1), 9–21 (2004)

7. Dohrmann, K., Weisz, N., Schlee, W., Hartmann, T., Elbert, T.: Neurofeedback for treating tinnitus. Progress Brain Res. **166**, 473–554 (2007)

8. Elgoyhen, A.B., Langguth, B., De Ridder, D., Vanneste, S.: Tinnitus: perspectives from human neuroimaging. Nature Rev. Neurosci. **16**(10), 632–642 (2015)

9. Esch, L., et al.: MNE: software for acquiring, processing, and visualizing MEG/EEG data. In: Magnetoencephalography: From Signals to Dynamic Cortical Networks, pp. 355–371 (2019)

10. Ganti, R.K., Ye, F., Lei, H.: Mobile crowdsensing: current state and future challenges. IEEE Comm. Mag. **49**(11), 32–39 (2011)

11. Güntensperger, D., Thüring, C., Meyer, M., Neff, P., Kleinjung, T.: Neurofeedback for tinnitus treatment-review and current concepts. Front. Aging Neurosci. **9**, 386 (2017)

12. Hassani, M., Karami, M.R.: Noise estimation in electroencephalogram signal by using Volterra series coefficients. J. Med. Signals Sens. **5**(3), 192 (2015)

13. Jastreboff, P.J.: Phantom auditory perception (Tinnitus): mechanisms of generation and perception. Neurosci. Res. **8**(4), 221–254 (1990)

14. Jastreboff, P.J., Hazell, J.W.: A neurophysiological approach to tinnitus: clinical implications. Br. J. Audiol. **27**(1), 7–17 (1993)

15. Kothe, C.A., Makeig, S.: BCILAB: a platform for brain-computer interface development. J. Neural Eng. **10**(5), 056014 (2013)

16. Kranczioch, C., Zich, C., Schierholz, I., Sterr, A.: Mobile EEG and its potential to promote the theory and application of imagery-based motor rehabilitation. Int. J. Psychophysiol. **91**(1), 10–15 (2014)

17. Lau-Zhu, A., Lau, M.P., McLoughlin, G.: Mobile EEG in research on neurodevelopmental disorders: opportunities and challenges. Develop. Cogn. Neurosci. **36**, 100635 (2019)

18. Levin, A.R., Méndez Leal, A.S., Gabard-Durnam, L.J., O'Leary, H.M.: BEAPP: the batch electroencephalography automated processing platform. Front. Neurosci. **12**, 513 (2018)

19. Lin, Y.P., Wang, Y., Jung, T.P.: Assessing the feasibility of online SSVEP decoding in human walking using a consumer EEG headset. J. Neuroeng. Rehabil. **11**(1), 119 (2014)

20. Mehdi, M.: Smart mobile crowdsensing for tinnitus research: student research abstract. In: Proceedings of the 34th ACM/SIGAPP Symposium on Applied Computing, pp. 1220–1223. ACM (2019)

21. Miyakoshi, M.: Makoto's preprocessing pipeline. Swartz Center for Computational Neuroscience (2018)

22. Mullen, T.: Cleanline EEGLAB plugin. Neuroimaging Informatics Toolsand Resources Clearinghouse (NITRC), San Diego (2012)

23. Oostenveld, R., Fries, P., Maris, E., Schoffelen, J.M.: FieldTrip: open source software for advanced analysis of MEG, EEG, and invasive electrophysiological data. Comput. Intell. Neurosci. **2011**, 156869 (2011)
24. Pedroni, A., Bahreini, A., Langer, N.: Automagic: standardized preprocessing of big EEG data. Neuroimage **200**, 460–473 (2019)
25. Rajkumar, R., et al.: Comparison of EEG microstates with resting state fMRI and FDG-PET measures in the default mode network via simultaneously recorded trimodal (PET/MR/EEG) data. Hum. Brain Mapp. (2018)
26. Reiser, J.E., Wascher, E., Arnau, S.: Recording mobile EEG in an outdoor environment reveals cognitive-motor interference dependent on movement complexity. Sci. Rep. **9**(1), 1–14 (2019)
27. Renard, Y., et al.: Openvibe: an open-source software platform to design, test, and use brain-computer interfaces in real and virtual environments. Presence Teleoper. Virtual Environ. **19**(1), 35–53 (2010)
28. Schalk, G., McFarland, D.J., Hinterberger, T., Birbaumer, N., Wolpaw, J.R.: BCI 2000: a general-purpose brain-computer interface (BCI) system. IEEE Trans. Biomed. Eng. **51**(6), 1034–1043 (2004)
29. Schlee, W., et al.: Innovations in doctoral training and research on tinnitus: the European school on interdisciplinary tinnitus research (ESIT) perspective. Front. Aging Neurosci. **9**, 447 (2018)
30. Stopczynski, A., et al.: Smartphones as pocketable labs: visions for mobile brain imaging and neurofeedback. Int. J. Psychophysiol. **91**(1), 54–66 (2014)
31. Tadel, F., Baillet, S., Mosher, J.C., Pantazis, D., Leahy, R.M.: Brainstorm: a user-friendly application for MEG/EEG analysis. Comput. Intell. Neurosci. **2011**, 879716 (2011)
32. Xiong, H., Zhang, D., Wang, L., Chaouchi, H.: EMC^3: energy-efficient data transfer in mobile crowdsensing under full coverage constraint. IEEE Trans. Mobile Comp. **14**(7), 1355–1368 (2015)
33. Zhuang, Z., Kim, K.H., Singh, J.P.: Improving energy efficiency of location sensing on smartphones. In: Proceedings of the 8th International Conference on Mobile Systems, Applications and Services (MobiSys), pp. 315–330. ACM (2010)

Machine Learning in eHealth Applications

Forecasting Health and Wellbeing for Shift Workers Using Job-Role Based Deep Neural Network

Han Yu[1(✉)], Asami Itoh[2], Ryota Sakamoto[2], Motomu Shimaoka[2],
and Akane Sano[1]

[1] Rice University, Houston, TX 77005, USA
{Han.Yu,akane.sano}@rice.edu
[2] Mie University, Mie 514-8507, Japan
{amasui,sakamoto}@clin.medic.mie-u.ac.jp, shimaoka@doc.medic.mie-u.ac.jp

Abstract. Shift workers who are essential contributors to our society, face high risks of poor health and wellbeing. To help with their problems, we collected and analyzed physiological and behavioral wearable sensor data from shift working nurses and doctors, as well as their behavioral questionnaire data and their self-reported daily health and wellbeing labels, including alertness, happiness, energy, health, and stress. We found the similarities and differences between the responses of nurses and doctors. According to the differences in self-reported health and wellbeing labels between nurses and doctors, and the correlations among their labels, we proposed a job-role based multitask and multilabel deep learning model, where we modeled physiological and behavioral data for nurses and doctors simultaneously to predict participants' next day's multidimensional self-reported health and wellbeing status. Our model showed significantly better performances than baseline models and previous state-of-the-art models in the evaluations of binary/3-class classification and regression prediction tasks. We also found features related to heart rate, sleep, and work shift contributed to shift workers' health and wellbeing.

Keywords: Shift workers · Health · Wellbeing · Wearables · Mobile sensor · Deep learning

1 Introduction

Around 20% of the workforce in the world involves in shift work [48]. Their irregular shift work brings a high risk of poor health and wellbeing. For example, shift work disrupts workers' circadian rhythms and causes problems such as sleep

Supported by National Science Foundation # 1840167 and Japan Agency for Medical Research and Development.

© ICST Institute for Computer Sciences, Social Informatics and Telecommunications Engineering 2021
Published by Springer Nature Switzerland AG 2021. All Rights Reserved
J. Ye et al. (Eds.): MobiHealth 2020, LNICST 362, pp. 89–103, 2021.
https://doi.org/10.1007/978-3-030-70569-5_6

disorder and insomnia [10]. In addition to the sleep issues, decreased alertness levels were found in healthy shift workers [9], which could lead to occupational errors and accidents. Previous studies also showed the potential associations between shift work and pathological disorders such as fatigue, gastrointestinal malfunction [19], and an increased risk of colorectal cancer in night shift nurses [38]. Moreover, more adverse mental health outcomes, emotional exhaustion, and burnout were observed in shift workers compared to daytime workers [5,15,40, 43,46]. In health care domain, physician burnout is estimated to cost 4.6 billion USD per year [13].

To support shift worker's health and wellbeing, monitoring and predicting their day-to-day health and wellbeing trajectories and providing aids to help them prepare for challenging situations might be useful. Besides, mobile devices, such as smartphones and wearable sensors, have become parts of people's daily life, and have been used to detect and predict self-reported health and wellbeing with the help of machine learning models [2,16,21,41,42,49]. These previous works targeted health and wellbeing detection or prediction as binary classification [2,41], 3-class classification [25,49], and regression tasks [1,16,49]. Some of these works developed personalized models by taking participants' demographic information into account [41] or fine-tuning general models to specific users [50]. Correlations among self-reported multi-dimensional labels - including subjective mood, health, and stress- were also used in building multilabel neural network models [41]. In addition, there are some prior works in monitoring shift workers using wearable sensors. Feng *et al.* extracted a behavioral consistency feature from shift worker wearable data and estimated anxiety levels with an accuracy of 57.8% in binary classification. Mulhall *et al.* used sensors integrated in the vehicles to monitor shift workers' eye blinking as a marker of alertness [27] while driving. Actigraphy has been also used widely for studying sleep for shift work nurses [11,17].

Although these previous works have achieved promising results, there is no work to thoroughly monitor and analyze different job types of shift workers' multidimensional wellbeing and forecast them using machine learning. Furthermore, the models developed previously considered the heterogeneity among participants and correlation among wellbeing labels separately; however, since these two characteristics ubiquitously co-exist, modeling them simultaneously for different job types of shift workers might improve prediction model performance.

In this work, we collected physiological and behavioral data from hospital shift workers, then we developed machine learning models to predict their next day's wellbeing in binary/3-class classifications and regression tasks. We also verified the rationale of leveraging job role information and multi wellbeing labels simultaneously in the models by analyzing the data. Then, we proposed a multitask multilabel deep learning model that leveraged job role information and correlations among self-reported health and wellbeing labels.

Our contributions can be summarized as: (i) we collected physiological and behavioral data from hospital shift workers, including nurses and doctors, (ii) we analyzed their physiological and behavioral patterns and found similarities and differences, (iii) we developed a multitask multilabel deep learning model to predict participants' near future wellbeing using wearable sensor, surveys, their job role information, and correlations among wellbeing labels. The details of our proposed model structure, implementation and hyper-parameter information are shared on: https://github.com/comp-well-org/multitask-multilabel-wellbeing-prediction.

2 Related Work

There are numerous studies on shift workers' health and wellbeing. Heath *et al.* collected survey data from shift work nurses, and applied statistical analysis in exploring the association among their work shift types, sleep, mood, and diet [14]. They showed that shift work was significantly negatively related to shit workers' diet, sleep efficiency, and stress levels. Similarly, Books *et al.* analyzed questionnaire data from shift-working nurses and showed an increased risk of sleep deprivation, family stressors, and mood changes due to the night work shift [3].

In addition, with the rapid development of mobile devices and mobile applications, objective data from wearables and smartphones have been used for studying shift workers. For example, Pereira *et al.* collected wearable accelerometer data from hospital shift workers and detected 4 levels of their physical activity intensity with an 83% accuracy score [31]. Feng *et al.* used wearable devices to collect physiological data from shift work nurses for ten weeks and applied a clustering method for extracting behavioral consistency, which intuitively captures unique behavioral patterns between different groups of nurses [7]. They further found that behavioral consistency can help predict self-reported work behaviors and anxiety levels. In another work, Feng *et al.* analyzed physiological and indoor location data from nurses with Fitbit wrist-wearable devices and Bluetooth hubs [6]. They extracted mutual information features and demonstrated the dependency between an individual's movement patterns and physiological responses.

Machine learning models have been designed for detecting or predicting health and wellbeing using mobile and sensor data. For example, Bogomolov *et al.* developed daily stress detection algorithms based on five-month-long weather, mobile phone data (e.g., calls, SMS, and screen usage), and personality survey data from 117 participants [2]. They obtained stress detection accuracy up to 72% in binary classification tasks. In Moodscope paper, mood (1: negative to 5: positive) was detected with the best mean squared error of 0.229 using the data from the mobile phone and a personalized linear regression model [21]. Similarly, Asselbergs *et al.* detected the current mood using mobile phone data with a mean squared error of 0.15 out of -2 to 2 mood scale [1]. For further improving the model performance, Taylor *et al.* developed a multitask machine learning model to predict high/low self-reported stress, mood, and health and separately used (i) the demographic information such as gender and personalities of participants and (ii) correlations among labels [41]. This work also inspired us to use the combination of job role information and label correlations. In this work, we study the differences in daily self-reported health and wellbeing, physiology, and behavior between nurses and doctors, and focus on estimating shift workers' health and wellbeing using the data from mobile sensors and surveys and job-role based deep learning models.

3 Methods

3.1 Data Collection

Two hundred and forty-one days of multi-modal data were collected from 14 shift workers, including 10 nurses (one male) and 4 doctors (all males) in a hospital in Japan. The average age of all participants was 31.4 years old, with a standard deviation (SD) of 4.2. For each study day, participants wore a Fitbit wristwatch (Fitbit Charge 3) for monitoring their physiological and behavioral activities such as heart rate, sleep, and step counts. The data sampled every 1 min was downloaded from the Fitbit server for data analysis and modeling. In addition, participants filled out daily morning and evening questionnaires to record their behavioral activities, including sleep, work schedule, and caffeinated drinks, alcohol & drug intake.

Self-reported health and wellbeing labels - including alertness, happiness, energy, health, and stress - were also collected in the morning questionnaire using 0 to 100 scales, with 0 to the most negative and 100 being the most positive (sleepy-alert, sad-happy, sluggish-energetic, sick-healthy, stressed-calm).

3.2 Features

We calculated the following features from the Fitbit data and daily questionnaires:

Heart Rate. Heart rate and heart rate variability are related to work stress [44] and mood [39]. Based on heart rate collected from Fitbit sensor every 1 min, we computed features including daily mean, standard deviation (SD), and entropy of heart rates. We computed sample entropy of heart rate, which represented the self-similarity of a sequence and has been used in physiological time-series data analysis [34]. To calculate the sample entropy, we first need to set an embedding dimension m. Using the given m, our sequence X with length N can be divided into $N - m + 1$ sliding windows $\{X_1,...,X_{N-m+1}\}$, where $X_i = \{x_i, x_{i+1}, ..., x_{i+m-1}\}$. The equation of sample entropy is:

$$SampEn = -\log \frac{U^m}{U^{m+1}} \tag{1}$$

where

$$U^m = -\frac{1}{N-m} \sum_{i=1}^{N-m} U_i^m \tag{2}$$

$$U_i^m = \frac{[\# \ of \ j \ |d(X_i, X_j) < r]}{N - m - 1} \tag{3}$$

In our case, the distance d is:

$$d(X_i, X_j) = \max |X_i - X_j| = \max_{k=1,\dots,m} |x_{i+k-1} - x_{j+k-1}| \tag{4}$$

Generally, $m = 2$ and $r = [0.2 * (SD \ of \ X)]$.

Sleep. From Fitbit sensors, we obtained sleep duration and sleep efficiency. Then, we calculated the mean and SD values of sleep duration and sleep efficiency across the previous 7, 5, and 3 days. Moreover, using sleep data in one-minute resolution, we calculated sleep regularity with sliding windows across 7 days of participants' data. Sleep regularity is a value of 0–1 based on the likelihood of sleep/wake state being the same time-points 24 h apart, and is associated with health, wellbeing, and academic performance in college students [8,32,37]. From daily surveys, we obtained a daily feature of the time taken to fall asleep in minutes. Participants also reported how they woke up in the morning: waking up naturally, being awakened by the alarm, or other than alarm. Naps have been shown a positive impact on shift workers' performance, alertness [33], and wellbeing [20]. From participants' questionnaires, we summarized the times and total duration of naps across a day.

Steps. Total daily number of steps and minute by minute number of steps were recorded in the Fitbit dataset. To measure the variability of participants' physical activities, we computed the mean and SD to indicate step variability across the previous 7, 5, and 3 days. Excluding the sleep time, we counted the minutes of: (i) duration of segments without steps (stationary segments) and (ii) duration of segments with continuous steps (active segments) in 1-min bins. We used the following information entropy equation to calculate the entropy of the two types of physical activity based stationary and active segments:

$$En = -\sum_i p_i \log p_i \tag{5}$$

where p_i represents the probability that the i_{th} item was observed.

Work. Work schedules and work hours are directly related to symptoms such as sleep disorders and chronic fatigue [4]. Also, excessive work hours are harmful to workers' health and wellbeing [12]. We engineered work related features such as daily work shifts, total work duration per day, and overwork duration in minutes according to participants' answers in the questionnaires. There were three different work shifts, and each shift was for eight hours (1: 8:30-16:30, 2: 16:30-0:30, 3:0:30-8:30). Total work duration was actual work time, and the overwork duration was the difference between the actual work hours and the scheduled hours.

Caffeine, Alcohol and Drug Use. Considering caffeine, alcohol, and drug intake affects workers' alertness [29,35], we computed features related to the intake of caffeinated drinks, drug, and alcohol based on the participants' reports: the number of caffeinated drinks per day, and a binary feature for indicating whether the participant had drug or alcohol each day.

3.3 Statistical Analysis of Physiological and Behavioral Features Between Nurses and Doctors

We applied statistical tests to analyze the differences of physiological and behavioral features between two groups, nurses and doctors. Seventy-seven days of data were in the group of doctors, and 164 days of data were in the nurses' group. Between 2 groups, we compared the numeric features such as daily average heart rate, steps, and overwork time using Mann-Whitney U test (non-normally distributed features) [23] and Welch's t-test (normally distributed features) [45], whereas the categorical features such as awakening types and working shifts were compared with chi-square test [30].

3.4 Job-Role Based Multitask Multilabel Neural Network

Neural networks have been widely used in various areas, including face detection [36], mood, health, and stress prediction [41]. These previous outstanding works showed that the design of neural network structure needs the consideration of unique characteristics of data sets used in different applications. As discussed briefly in Sect. 1, in this work, we considered two important aspects: (1) different distributions in health and wellbeing labels based on our participants' demographic information and (2) correlations among health and wellbeing labels. We observed differences in the distributions of self-reported health and wellbeing labels from two job roles, nurses and doctors. Also, there are correlations among the five labels. The details of the data statistics will be discussed in Sect. 5.1.

To learn different representations corresponding to participant job roles, we applied a multitask learning method, which divided tasks according to participants' job roles. Furthermore, as another form of multitask learning, we used multilabel learning for considering different health and wellbeing labels as tasks. In this way, the model would also fit the correlation among labels. In this work, we designed a job-role based multitask and multilabel neural network model that leveraged user demographic information and correlations among labels at the same time. Figure 1 shows a simplified version of our model. When training the model, there might be redundant features in our input data that would not help health and wellbeing prediction. In contrast, some non-linear combinations of features might improve our model performance. Thus, we applied a one-dimension convolutional neural network (CNN) layer to extract auto-features from our inputs. As shown in Fig. 1, we designed convolutional kernels to learn higher-level features across every day feature vectors: 32 row-wise convolutional kernels embedded 32 channels of new features. Then, the CNN extracted features were fed into the multitask neural network. The shared layers in the network learn the representation from all participant data, and the divided branches of the network structure learn the representation independently from participants in different job roles, nurses and doctors. When doctors' data are fed into the model for training, the weights of loss and optimizer of the nurse branch will be set to 0, and vice verse. Furthermore, each branch of the network outputs all five labels (alertness, happiness, energy, health, and stress) from the shared network layers. Therefore, the outputs of our model simultaneously provide the prediction of all five labels for nurses and doctors. The batch loss function of our model can be represented as:

$$L = \sum_{nurse} L_{ml} + \sum_{doctor} L_{ml} \tag{6}$$

$$L_{ml} = \sum_{l=\{alert,happy,energy,health,stress\}} loss(x, y_l) \tag{7}$$

Where x and y represent the input data and the expected output target, respectively. $loss$ is mean squared error loss in regression tasks and cross-entropy loss in the classification tasks.

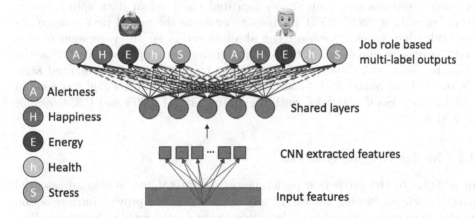

Fig. 1. A simplified version of our job-role based multitask multilabel neural network. Convolutional neural network kernels are applied for extracting high-level features. Our health and wellbeing prediction is designed for nurses and doctors using a portion of the network trained only using data from either nurses or doctors. Shared layers learn representation from all participants. The final output layers provide the prediction of all five labels simultaneously.

4   Experiments

Our tasks are formulated in two ways for evaluation: regression and classification tasks. The regression task is to predict the next day's health and wellbeing scores, each in the range of 0–100, whereas the classification task is to predict next day's high/low (binary classification, defined as 100-51, 50-0) or high/mid/low health and wellbeing levels, and high/ mid/low (3-class classification, defined as 100-67, 66-34, or 33-0). Our models use the wearable and survey data up to and including the current day for predicting nurses' and doctors' next day health and wellbeing labels.

We compared our job-role based multitask multilabel model (MTML-NN) with following approaches to evaluate the benefits of using demographic information and the correlation among labels: (1) random forest (RF), (2) RBF kernel based support vector machine (SVM), (3) multitask neural network (MT-NN) that used clusters of participants and achieved state-of-the-art performance in a previous study [41], (4) multitask neural network with labels as tasks (ML-NN). In addition to applying ML-NN to all participants (ML-NN (all)), we also calculated the prediction results for nurses (ML-NN(N)) and doctors (ML-NN(D)) separately.

For training and testing our models, we randomly split the dataset into training and testing data in a ratio of 80% to 20%. We applied 10-fold cross-validation and grid search to finalize the hyperparameters for all models mentioned above in the training set. Then, we tested models in the testing set. To make the evaluation process more robust, we repeated the random data split strategy (training/testing : 80%/20%) 10 times to evaluate the model performance. As the evaluating metrics, we use mean absolute errors for the regression models and f1-scores for classification tasks. Furthermore, we adopt focal loss[22] as the objective function in the classification tasks to mitigate the unbalanced sample size in both binary and 3-class tasks. The Adam optimizer [18] was used in training the neural networks, with a learning rate of 0.005 and 0.9, 0.999 for β_1 and β_2.

4.1 Model Weights Analysis

In addition to the prediction performance, interpretability is also an essential part of machine learning models. Ideally, we would like to provide our prediction results along with reasonable explanations to our participants or health/medical stakeholders. First, from the weights in the RF model, we analyzed the importance of input features. Then, in our deep learning MTML-NN model, we analyzed the importance of the features by examining the parameters in the first CNN layer before the non-linear activation function. Since the CNN kernel we designed is in one-dimension with a size of the number of features, and parameters in the CNN kernel would correspond to the input features. We calculated the average value of each feature on all channels to check the importance of the features. Also, we computed the correlations between the output of the CNN layer and the input features. Features that have higher correlations with the CNN outputs would also be considered important features.

5 Results and Discussion

5.1 Data Statistics

As shown in Table 1, the average score of alertness label was the lowest among all five labels; while the stress label (0: pressure-1: calm) showed the highest average score. Compared with other labels, the SD of happiness score was lower. Moreover, the distribution of health and wellbeing labels for nurses and doctors were different. For example, doctors generally had higher subjective alertness and energy than nurses in the morning. In addition, we computed correlations among the five health and wellbeing labels. Figure 2 shows the correlation coefficients matrix of all labels, and there are different degrees of correlation among the labels. The Pearson test [26] showed that all five labels were significantly correlated. The linear fitting coefficient of determination (r^2) values [28] between the alert label and other labels ranged from 0.19 to 0.28, while the r^2 values among the happy, energy, health and stress labels were all higher than 0.55, with the highest value being 0.70 (happy and stress).

We also compared feature distributions between nurses and doctors (Table 2). We found that the mean heart rate of doctors was significantly higher than that of nurses; whereas the variability of heart rate, defined as SD and sample entropy, was higher in nurses than doctors. In terms of sleep, we found that doctors showed higher sleep efficiency and lower sleep irregularity than nurses. Further, We found statistical differences between nurses and doctors in movement features, including mean and SD of daily steps across the previous 7 days, and the entropy for stationary/active segments. We did not observe any statistical differences between nurses and doctors in working shifts and total work hours among shift work features. However, we found that overwork was more common among doctors.

Table 1. Mean (SD) of daily wellbeing & P-values from Welch's t-test

	Nurse	Doctor	p-value
Alertness	38.5 (22.9)	52.8 (23.5)	<0.05
Happiness	57.2 (20.9)	59.2 (17.1)	0.38
Energy	54.0 (22.9)	60.5 (22.4)	<0.05
Health	63.3 (22.1)	63.9 (22.4)	0.83
Stress	63.5 (23.4)	65.6 (17.5)	0.39

5.2 Wellbeing Prediction

The classification and regression performance using different models is shown in Table 3. Our proposed job-role based MTML-NN performed the best for four labels in binary classification and all wellbeing labels in 3-class classification and regression (ANOVA, Tukey, p < 0.05). Our results showed the benefits of our proposed simultaneous job role and correlated label modeling, especially in

Table 2. List of main features and the statistics of nurses and doctors. The statistics of numeric features are shown in mean (SD) values, and the differences are tested with Mann-Whitney U-test (non-normally distributed features) and Welch's t-test (normally distributed features, indicated with ⋆); whereas we use percentages to reveal the statistics of categorical features and apply the chi-square test to check their statistical differences.

Source	Daily Features	Nurses (N = 10)	Doctors (N = 4)	P-value
Fitbit	Heart Rate (HR) - Mean ⋆	78.5 (7.1)	70.6 (6.8)	<0.05
	Heart Rate(HR) - SD	13.5 (3.5)	12.3 (3.2)	< 0.05
	Heart Rate(HR) - Entropy ⋆	0.64 (0.23)	0.69 (0.20)	<0.05
	Sleep Duration (mins)	374.3 (134.0)	363.1 (106.3)	0.36
	Sleep Efficiency (0–100)	93.1 (4.9)	95.5 (2.9)	<0.05
	Sleep Regularity ⋆	0.31 (0.25)	0.26 (0.19)	<0.05
	Sleep Duration - Mean across previous 7 days	370.5 (74.4)	359.0 (46.1)	0.21
	Sleep Efficiency - Mean across previous 7 days	94.8 (3.3)	93.2 (3.6)	<0.05
	Sleep Duration - SD across previous 7 days	106.8 (39.1)	88.4 (37.8)	<0.05
	Sleep Efficiency - SD across previous 7 days	2.19 (1.31)	2.20 (1.02)	0.21
	Steps ⋆	8931.2 (4030.3)	8139.9 (3350.8)	0.21
	Steps - Mean across previous 7 days ⋆	8684.8 (2372.8)	9063.4 (2236.9)	<0.05
	Steps - SD across previous 7 days ⋆	3099.5 (1017.8)	2582.5 (849.7)	<0.05
	Entropy (stationary segments)	2.17 (0.53)	2.61 (0.24)	<0.05
	Entropy (active segments)	1.67 (0.45)	1.65 (0.19)	<0.05
Survey	Number of Naps	0.55 (0.68)	0.37 (0.66)	<0.05
	Duration of Naps (mins)	31.1 (68.4)	19.1 (49.4)	0.12
	# of Cups of Caffeinated Drinks	0.47 (0.73)	0.45 (0.62)	0.45
	Wake-up Type	-	-	<0.05
	- Natural	35.5%	35.6%	
	- Alarm	60.9%	46.5%	
	- Other than alarm	3.6%	17.8%	
	Time to Fall Asleep (mins)	-	-	<0.05
	- 0-5	34.0%	40.6%	
	- 6–15	31.4%	41.6%	
	- 16-30	17.3%	11.9%	
	- 31-45	6.6%	3.0%	
	- 45-60	3.6%	3.0%	
	- 60+	7.1%	0%	
	Work Shifts	-	-	0.12
	- Shift 1	53.8%	64.3%	
	- Shift 2	30.4%	19.8%	
	- Shift 3	15.7%	15.8%	
	Work Time (hours)	8.0 (0.0)	8.4 (1.7)	0.08
	Overwork Time (mins)	11.0 (41.8)	202.6 (320.1)	<0.05

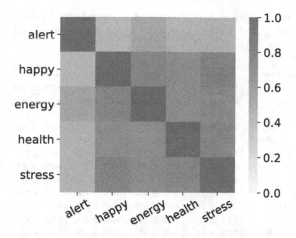

Fig. 2. Correlation coefficients matrix of wellbeing labels

3-class classification and regression. However, according to the performance in 3-class classification, we found poor classification performance for some classes. For example, in the 3-class alertness classification, the high-alertness class precision and recall values were only 0.16 and 0.27 in respectively; and our low-energy class prediction was also relatively low with a precision of 0.33 and a recall of 0.24. These errors might come from the data imbalance problem. In the 3-class classification tasks, the high alertness labels accounted for only 20% of all labels, and the low energy labels accounted for 15% of all labels.

Furthermore, we also found the benefits of using job role information or multiple labels separately. For example, in the alertness prediction, job-role based MT-NN showed significant improvement from NN for both binary and 3-class classification. Besides the overall f1-score, we observed some improvements revealed in each class. For example, in the 3-class alertness classification tasks, MT-NN model provided significantly higher recall and precision scores in low and middle alertness classification compared to NN model (Welch's t-test, $p < 0.05$). We did not observe any significant improvement in the regression tasks. However, the average prediction MAE of MT-NN was lower than that of NN. Significant improvements were observed in ML-NN compared to NN in almost all tasks. For example, in the regression tasks, the ML-NN (all) performed statistically significantly better than NN in predicting alertness, happiness, energy, and stress labels.

5.3   Weight Analysis

From the RF model, for both the binary and 3-class classification happiness prediction tasks, we found features including mean heart rate and heart rate sample entropy across the day, sleep duration, sleep regularity, and the SD of sleep efficiency across the previous seven days, were the most important. In the alertness prediction tasks, work shifts, stationary segment entropy, mean step,

Table 3. Prediction performance (f1-score for classification; mean absolute error (MAE) for regression) of different algorithms. Bold entries represent statistically significantly better results over the other models.

Tasks	Algorithms	Alertness	Happiness	Energy	Health	Stress
Binary	RF	50% ± 7%	78% ± 4%	65% ± 4%	**84% ± 3%**	82% ± 3%
	SVM	52% ± 4%	69% ± 4%	62% ± 6%	80% ± 4%	77% ± 5%
	NN	55% ± 4%	71% ± 5%	65% ± 3%	82% ± 3%	80% ± 3%
	MT-NN	60% ± 4%	76% ± 3%	69% ± 5%	**83% ± 4%**	**83% ± 4%**
	ML-NN (all)	55% ± 7%	74% ± 7%	68% ± 4%	80% ± 4%	**83% ± 3%**
	ML-NN (N)	55% ± 9%	69% ± 5%	64% ± 6%	79% ± 7%	79% ± 7%
	ML-NN (D)	59% ± 8%	75% ± 5%	67% ± 7%	**85% ± 5%**	85% ± 7%
	MTML-NN	**64% ± 7%**	**79% ± 3%**	**71% ± 4%**	81% ± 3%	**84% ± 3%**
3-class	RF	53% ± 5%	39% ± 5%	46% ± 6%	49% ± 7%	44% ± 5%
	SVM	47% ± 7%	40% ± 5%	43% ± 5%	49% ± 7%	46% ± 4%
	NN	51% ± 5%	45% ± 6%	45% ± 5%	53% ± 6%	51% ± 4%
	MT-NN	57% ± 6%	46% ± 5%	48% ± 6%	53% ± 5%	50% ± 5%
	ML-NN (all)	52% ± 8%	**53% ± 7%**	48% ± 7%	55% ± 3%	54% ± 4%
	ML-NN (N)	45% ± 7%	**54% ± 5%**	49% ± 5%	56% ± 2%	53% ± 5%
	ML-NN (D)	54% ± 5%	51% ± 7%	45% ± 6%	54% ± 3%	52% ± 7%
	MTML-NN	**59% ± 5%**	52% ± 4%	51% ± 4%	**58% ± 7%**	57% ± 5%
Regression	SVR	20.6 ± 2.9	19.7 ± 2.5	21.3 ± 2.4	18.9 ± 1.8	21.7 ± 2.1
	NN	19.9 ± 1.8	19.0 ± 1.9	20.3 ± 2.2	19.5 ± 1.9	20.4 ± 1.9
	MT-NN	19.4 ± 2.1	18.8 ± 2.3	20.7 ± 1.6	19.3 ± 2.0	20.3 ± 1.7
	ML-NN (all)	18.6 ± 1.3	16.9 ± 3.1	18.6 ± 2.0	18.7 ± 2.6	19.4 ± 2.6
	ML-NN (N)	18.0 ± 1.1	15.9 ± 1.9	17.3 ± 1.7	15.6 ± 1.7	17.7 ± 1.3
	ML-NN (D)	20.4 ± 2.1	16.0 ± 2.0	19.3 ± 2.0	17.4 ± 2.0	19.4 ± 3.1
	MTML-NN	**17.4 ± 1.4**	**15.1± 1.6**	**17.7 ± 1.2**	**15.4 ± 1.5**	**15.6 ± 1.9**

and mean sleep duration across the previous 7, 5 days played important roles. The analysis of the parameters in the CNN layer in the MTML-NN model and the correlations between the CNN output and input features indicated that features including heart rate sample entropy, sleep regularity, sleep efficiency, work shifts, steps, and active segment entropy - contributed to health and wellbeing prediction. For example, from the correlation analysis, we found that the sleep efficiency, sleep regularity, and daytime work shift were positively related to the wellbeing (Pearson test, p-value $< 0.05/(\#$ of features)); whereas the step and the entropy of active segments were negatively related to the wellbeing (Pearson test, p-value $< 0.05/(\#$ of features)). Our findings were consistent with some prior results. For example, according to the previous works, sleep influences physical and psychological health [47], and stress [24]; sleep regularity is associated with mood [37]. Previous studies also indicated the association between work shifts and stress levels [46].

6   Conclusion

In this work, we collected physiological and behavioral wearable sensor data as well as survey data from shift-work nurses and doctors, and compared their physiology and behaviors between two job roles. Then, we proposed a job-role based multitask and multilabel learning model structure to predict shift workers' health and wellbeing for next day using sensor and questionnaire data. The proposed model outperformed the benchmark models, including RF and SVM as well as the previous state-of-the-art models. The analysis of model weights showed that health rate, work shifts, sleep parameters such as sleep regularity and sleep efficiency contributed to shift workers' health and wellbeing labels. As future work, we will collect more data from shift workers and design a system to improve shift workers' health and wellbeing.

References

1. Asselbergs, J., Ruwaard, J., Ejdys, M., Schrader, N., Sijbrandij, M., Riper, H.: Mobile phone-based unobtrusive ecological momentary assessment of day-to-day mood: an explorative study. J. Med. Internet Res. **18**(3), e72 (2016)
2. Bogomolov, A., Lepri, B., Ferron, M., Pianesi, F., et al.: Daily stress recognition from mobile phone data, weather conditions and individual traits. In: Proceedings of the 22nd ACM International Conference on Multimedia, pp. 477–486 (2014)
3. Books, C., Coody, L.C., Kauffman, R., Abraham, S.: Night shift work and its health effects on nurses. Health Care Manager **36**(4), 347–353 (2017)
4. Bourdouxhe, M., Quéinnec, Y., Guertin, S.: The interaction between work schedule and workload: case study of 12-hour shifts in a Canadian refinery. In: Shiftwork International Newsletter, p. 19 (2000)
5. Courtney, J.A., Francis, A.J., Paxton, S.J.: Caring for the carers: fatigue, sleep, and mental health in Australian paramedic shiftworkers. Aust. J. Organisational Psychol. **3**, 32–41 (2010)
6. Feng, T., Booth, B.M., Narayanan, S.S.: Modeling behavior as mutual dependency between physiological signals and indoor location in large-scale wearable sensor study. In: ICASSP 2020 IEEE International Conference on Acoustics, Speech and Signal Processing (ICASSP), pp. 1016–1020. IEEE (2020)
7. Feng, T., Narayanan, S.S.: Modeling behavioral consistency in large-scale wearable recordings of human bio-behavioral signals. In: ICASSP 2020 IEEE International Conference on Acoustics, Speech and Signal Processing (ICASSP), pp. 1011–1015. IEEE (2020)
8. Fischer, D., et al.: Irregular sleep and event schedules are associated with poorer self-reported well-being in us college students. Sleep **43**(6), zsz300 (2020)
9. Ganesan, S., et al.: The impact of shift work on sleep, alertness and performance in healthcare workers. Sci. Rep. **9**(1), 1–13 (2019)
10. Garbarino, S., et al.: Sleepiness and sleep disorders in shift workers: a study on a group of Italian police officers. Sleep **25**(6), 642–647 (2002)
11. Geiger-Brown, J., Rogers, V.E., Trinkoff, A.M., Kane, R.L., Bausell, R.B., Scharf, S.M.: Sleep, sleepiness, fatigue, and performance of 12-hour-shift nurses. Chronobiol. Int. **29**(2), 211–219 (2012)
12. Golden, L., Wiens-Tuers, B.: Overtime work and wellbeing at home. Rev. Soc. Econ. **66**(1), 25–49 (2008)
13. Han, S., et al.: Estimating the attributable cost of physician burnout in the United States. Ann. Intern.Med. **170**(11), 784–790 (2019)
14. Heath, G., Dorrian, J., Coates, A.: Associations between shift type, sleep, mood, and diet in a group of shift working nurses. Scand. J. Work Environ. Health **45**(4), 402–412 (2019)

15. Jamal, M.: Burnout, stress and health of employees on non-standard work schedules: a study of Canadian workers. Stress Health: J. Int. Soc. Invest. Stress **20**(3), 113–119 (2004)
16. Jaques, N., Taylor, S., Sano, A., Picard, R., et al.: Predicting tomorrow's mood, health, and stress level using personalized multitask learning and domain adaptation. In: IJCAI 2017 Workshop on Artificial Intelligence in Affective Computing, pp. 17–33 (2017)
17. Kato, C., Shimada, J., Hayashi, K.: Sleepiness during shift work in Japanese nurses: a comparison study using JESS, SSS, and actigraphy. Sleep Biol. Rhythms **10**(2), 109–117 (2012)
18. Kingma, D.P., Ba, J.: Adam: a method for stochastic optimization. arXiv preprint arXiv:1412.6980 (2014)
19. Knutsson, A.: Health disorders of shift workers. Occup. Med. **53**(2), 103–108 (2003)
20. Li, H., et al.: Napping on night-shifts among nursing staff: a mixed-methods systematic review. J. Adv. Nurs. **75**(2), 291–312 (2019)
21. LiKamWa, R., Liu, Y., Lane, N.D., Zhong, L.: MoodScope: building a mood sensor from smartphone usage patterns. In: Proceeding of the 11th Annual International Conference on Mobile Systems, Applications, and Services, pp. 389–402 (2013)
22. Lin, T.Y., Goyal, P., Girshick, R., He, K., Dollár, P.: Focal loss for dense object detection. In: Proceedings of the IEEE International Conference on Computer Vision, pp. 2980–2988 (2017)
23. Mann, H.B., Whitney, D.R.: On a test of whether one of two random variables is stochastically larger than the other. Ann. Math. Stat. 50–60 (1947)
24. Mezick, E.J., et al.: Intra-individual variability in sleep duration and fragmentation: associations with stress. Psychoneuroendocrinology **34**(9), 1346–1354 (2009)
25. Muaremi, A., Arnrich, B., Tröster, G.: Towards measuring stress with smartphones and wearable devices during workday and sleep. BioNanoScience **3**(2), 172–183 (2013). https://doi.org/10.1007/s12668-013-0089-2
26. Mukaka, M.M.: A guide to appropriate use of correlation coefficient in medical research. Malawi Med. J. **24**(3), 69–71 (2012)
27. Mulhall, M.D., et al.: A pre-drive ocular assessment predicts alertness and driving impairment: a naturalistic driving study in shift workers. Accid. Anal. Prev. **135**, 105386 (2020)
28. Nagelkerke, N.J., et al.: A note on a general definition of the coefficient of determination. Biometrika **78**(3), 691–692 (1991)
29. Pasman, W.J., Boessen, R., Donner, Y., Clabbers, N., Boorsma, A.: Effect of caffeine on attention and alertness measured in a home-setting, using web-based cognition tests. JMIR Res. Protoc. **6**(9), e169 (2017)
30. Pearson, K.: X. on the criterion that a given system of deviations from the probable in the case of a correlated system of variables is such that it can be reasonably supposed to have arisen from random sampling. Lond. Edinb. Dublin Philos. Mag. J. Sci. **50**(302), 157–175 (1900)
31. Pereira, A., Nunes, F.: Physical activity intensity monitoring of hospital workers using a wearable sensor. In: 12th EAI International Conference on Pervasive Computing Technologies for Healthcare-Demos, Posters, Doctoral Colloquium. European Alliance for Innovation (EAI) (2018)
32. Phillips, A.J., et al.: Irregular sleep/wake patterns are associated with poorer academic performance and delayed circadian and sleep/wake timing. Sci. Rep. **7**(1), 1–13 (2017)

33. Purnell, M., Feyer, A.M., Herbison, G.: The impact of a nap opportunity during the night shift on the performance and alertness of 12-h shift workers. J. Sleep Res. **11**(3), 219–227 (2002)
34. Richman, J.S., Moorman, J.R.: Physiological time-series analysis using approximate entropy and sample entropy. Am. J. Physiol. Heart Circulatory Physiol. **278**(6), H2039–H2049 (2000)
35. Roehrs, T., Roth, T.: Sleep, sleepiness, and alcohol use. Alcohol Res. Health: J. Nat. Inst. Alcohol Abuse Alcoholism **25**(2), 101–109 (2001)
36. Rowley, H.A., Baluja, S., Kanade, T.: Neural network-based face detection. IEEE Trans. Pattern Anal. Mach. Intell. **20**(1), 23–38 (1998)
37. Sano, A.: Measuring college students' sleep, stress. Mental Health and Wellbeing with Wearable Sensors and Mobile Phones. Ph.D. thesis, MIT (2015)
38. Schernhammer, E.S., et al.: Night-shift work and risk of colorectal cancer in the nurses' health study. J. Nat. Cancer Inst. **95**(11), 825–828 (2003)
39. Shapiro, D., Jamner, L.D., Goldstein, I.B., Delfino, R.J.: Striking a chord: moods, blood pressure, and heart rate in everyday life. Psychophysiology **38**(2), 197–204 (2001)
40. Srivastava, U.R.: Shift work related to stress, health and mood states: a study of dairy workers. J. Health Manag. **12**(2), 173–200 (2010)
41. Taylor, S.A., Jaques, N., Nosakhare, E., Sano, A., Picard, R.: Personalized multitask learning for predicting tomorrow's mood, stress, and health. IEEE Trans. Affective Comput. **11**, 200 (2017)
42. Umematsu, T., Sano, A., Taylor, S., Picard, R.W.: Improving students' daily life stress forecasting using LSTM neural networks. In: 2019 IEEE EMBS International Conference on Biomedical and Health Informatics (BHI), pp. 1–4. IEEE (2019)
43. Vogel, M., Braungardt, T., Meyer, W., Schneider, W.: The effects of shift work on physical and mental health. J. Neural Transm. **119**(10), 1121–1132 (2012)
44. Vrijkotte, T.G., Van Doornen, L.J., De Geus, E.J.: Effects of work stress on ambulatory blood pressure, heart rate, and heart rate variability. Hypertension **35**(4), 880–886 (2000)
45. Welch, B.L.: The generalization of student's' problem when several different population variances are involved. Biometrika **34**(1/2), 28–35 (1947)
46. Wisetborisut, A., Angkurawaranon, C., Jiraporncharoen, W., Uaphanthasath, R., Wiwatanadate, P.: Shift work and burnout among health care workers. Occup. Med. **64**(4), 279–286 (2014)
47. Wong, M.L., Lau, E.Y.Y., Wan, J.H.Y., Cheung, S.F., Hui, C.H., Mok, D.S.Y.: The interplay between sleep and mood in predicting academic functioning, physical health and psychological health: a longitudinal study. J. Psychosomatic Res. **74**(4), 271–277 (2013)
48. Wright Jr., K.P., Bogan, R.K., Wyatt, J.K.: Shift work and the assessment and management of shift work disorder (SWD). Sleep Med. Rev. **17**(1), 41–54 (2013)
49. Yu, H., Klerman, E.B., Picard, R.W., Sano, A.: Personalized wellbeing prediction using behavioral, physiological and weather data. In: 2019 IEEE EMBS International Conference on Biomedical and Health Informatics (BHI), pp. 1–4. IEEE (2019)
50. Yu, H., Sano, A.: Passive sensor data based future mood, health, and stress prediction: User adaptation using deep learning. In: 2020 42nd Annual International Conference of the IEEE Engineering in Medicine and Biology Society (EMBC), pp. 5884–5887. IEEE (2020)

A Deep Learning Model for Exercise-Based Rehabilitation Using Multi-channel Time-Series Data from a Single Wearable Sensor

Ghanashyama Prabhu[1,2,4]([✉]) [iD], Noel E. O'Connor[1,2] [iD], and Kieran Moran[1,3] [iD]

[1] Insight SFI Research Centre for Data Analytics, Dublin City University, Dublin, Ireland
ghanashyama.prabhu2@mail.dcu.ie, gs.prabhu@manipal.edu
[2] School of Electronic Engineering, Dublin City University, Dublin, Ireland
[3] School of Health and Human Performance, Dublin City University, Dublin, Ireland
[4] Department of Information and Communication Technology, Manipal Institute of Technology, Manipal Academy of Higher Education, Manipal, India
https://www.insight-centre.org/

Abstract. The ability to accurately and automatically recognize and count the repetitions of exercises using a single sensor is essential for technology-assisted exercise-based rehabilitation. In this paper, we present a single deep learning architecture to undertake both of these tasks based on multi-channel time-series data. The models are constructed and tested using the INSIGHT-LME [1] exercise dataset which consists of ten local muscular endurance (LME) exercises. For exercise recognition, we achieved an overall F1-score measure of 96% and for repetition counting, we were correct within an error of ± 1 repetitions in 88% of the observed exercise sets. To the best of our knowledge, our approach of using the same deep learning model for both tasks using raw time-series sensor data information is novel.

Keywords: INSIGHT-LME dataset · CNN · Wearable sensor · Exercise-based rehabilitation · Multi-channel time-series

1 Introduction

Community-based or home-based exercising are approaches commonly adopted for rehabilitation. Exercise-based rehabilitation often needs to be long-term. Unfortunately, for a variety of reasons (including travel distances, organized classes not being schedule-friendly and some people not wanting to exercise in front of others) adherence to organised programmes tend to be very low [2,3]. Alternatively, if people could exercise anywhere convenient to them, at any time,

Supported by Insight SFI Research Centre for Data Analytics.

it may act to motivate the uptake and adherence to exercise-based rehabilitation. Such an approach would be facilitated if information on the type and amount of exercise was automatically detected for real-time and summary feedback, which has been shown to be a motivating factor rehabilitating patients. Technology advances in wearable sensors have resulted in cost-effective devices capable of recording human movements effectively [4,5]. Human activity recognition (HAR) is an increasingly important research topic where human movements and associated activities are studied using advanced artificial intelligence algorithms, e.g. machine learning and deep learning models, applied to sensor data from wearables. In recent years, the use of a single wearable sensor has gained prominence in different areas of HAR such as: day-to-day activity(e.g. jogging, running, walking, drinking, sitting) [6–9], gym activity [10] and exercise [11–14] recognition and in repetition counting [11,15,16]. Studies have shown that elderly rehabilitation patients (about 68%) have indicated their interest in using a single sensor (inertial measurement unit) within exercise-based rehabilitation [2].

The increased interest in using deep learning models in the field of HAR and especially exercise [1,11,17] has resulted in various models being used for exercise recognition and repetition counting. However, it appears that no studies have used a single deep CNN model architecture using multi-channel time-series data for exercise recognition and repetition counting. Using a single model architecture for both tasks simplifies implementation and training. This is an important consideration if the AI-based technique were ultimately to be implemented as an embedded function of the wearable sensing platform. As such, this study aims to demonstrate how a single CNN model architecture can be used for automatic exercise recognition and repetition counting using multi-channel time-series data obtained from a single inertial measurement unit.

2 Proposed Framework

Figure 1 represents the end-to-end pipeline framework used for the exercise recognition and repetition counting. This framework consists of a data processing unit, two CNN models and an output processing component. The data processing unit processes the INSIGHT-LME dataset [1] into 6D time-series arrays. Two CNN models were constructed using a single architecture for both the exercise recognition and the repetition counting tasks. The output processor consists of two fully connected layers, the first one is used at the output of the CNN model for exercise recognition and the second one is used at the output of the CNN model for repetition counting.

3 Methodology

3.1 Data Set

We have used the INSIGHT-LME dataset, a data set recently made publicly available (https://bit.ly/30UCsmR), consisting of eleven classes of movements with first ten classes corresponding to ten LME exercises commonly used in

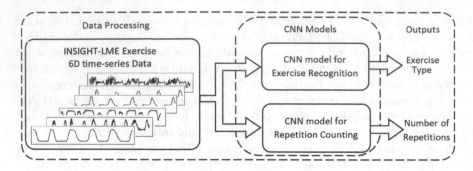

Fig. 1. End-to-End pipeline for exercise recognition and repetition counting.

exercise-based cardiovascular disease (CVD) rehabilitation and the eleventh class corresponding to movements commonly observed between exercises. The ten LME exercises consists of six upper-body LMEs (*Bicep Curls* (BC), *Frontal Raise* (FR), *Lateral Raise* (LR), *Triceps Extension Right arm* (TER), *Pec Dec* (PD) and *Trunk Twist* (TT)), and four lower-body LMEs (*Squats* (SQ), *Lunges* (L), *Leg Lateral Raise* (LLR) and *Standing Bicycle Crunches* (SBC)). The dataset consists of raw time-series data from a 3D accelerometer and a 3D gyroscope using a single inertial measurement unit (IMU) mounted on the right-wrist and was collected from 76 healthy and able bodied participants. The IMUa used in the dataset was Shimmer3 IMUs which were light-weight wearable sensor units from Shimmer[1]. Each IMU used in the data collection process was calibrated using Shimmer's 9DoF calibration application[2] and a sampling rate 512 Hz was used. Exercise data were collected in two sets from the participants under constrained and unconstrained environments. 6D time-series data (3D accelerometer and 3D gyroscope) were further used in the data processing. As an illustrative example, Fig. 2 represents 25 s segmented time-series sensor signal plots of 3D accelerometer and 3D gyroscope for the *Frontal Raise* exercise.

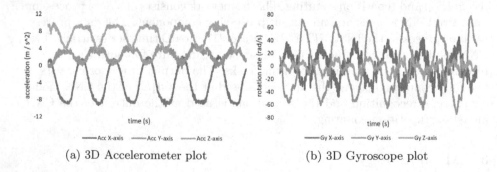

(a) 3D Accelerometer plot   (b) 3D Gyroscope plot

Fig. 2. 25 s segmented plots of Frontal Raise exercise

---

[1] http://www.shimmersensing.com/products/shimmer3.
[2] https://www.shimmersensing.com/products/shimmer-9dof-calibration.

3.2   Data Processing

Data processing was performed on the INSIGHT-LME dataset to have 6D time-series array information with two target labels. The new 6D time-series information was generated from data segmentation process using a sliding window method. A window-length of 4 s and an overlap of 0.5 s was used in data segmentation process. From every 4 s segment of exercise data, a 6D time-series data array was formed and was computed for all exercise data. The processed data, from 76 participants, was divided into three subsets. A training set was formed with data from 46 participants. Additionally, from the remaining participants a test set and a validation set were formed with data from 15 participants each.

The two class labels were generated for the new 6D time-series information. First target labels were used for the exercise recognition task and the second target labels were used in the repetition counting task. The first target labels were for the exercise recognition task and were the eleven class label information of the exercise movements. However, for the repetition counting task, a new binary class label was added on each 4 s segmented array data using a 50% grid method. Ground truth with the newer binary class information was generated using dominant signal information for each exercise [1,16,18]. If the dominant signal peak lay at the left half of the grid then a label information "Peak" (or "1") was added, otherwise "No Peak" (or "0") label information was added.

3.3   A Deep CNN Architecture for Recognition and Repetition Counting

HAR recognition, especially in the field of exercise recognition and repetition counting, few recent studies [1,11,17] have used different deep CNN structures. A single CNN architecture was used by [11] which uses one model for exercise recognition but uses ten different models for repetition counting. However, in our previous study [1] we have successfully demonstrated building two models using the state of the art AlexNET architecture, one for all the exercise recognition and the other for repetition counting from all the exercises in contrast to Soro et al. [11]. However, it appears that no studies have used a single deep CNN model architecture using multi-channel time-series data for exercise recognition and repetition counting.

We designed and built deep CNN models from scratch using the same base structure (Fig. 3), one for the exercise recognition and other for the repetition counting. The architecture consists of seven 2D convolutional layers (*ConvLayer*) in addition to an input layer, two fully connected layers and a dropout layer. The number of filters used in seven convolution layers were 16, 16, 32, 32, 64, 64 and 96 respectively. The selection of the number of convolutional layers and the number of filters in each layer of the CNN_Model2 architecture were arrived after the initial few trials with different configurations. Output of each *ConvLayer* was batch normalized [19] and rectified linear units (ReLU) [20] were used along with MaxPooling. The output of the seventh *ConvLayer* was flattened and a fully connected layer was used. A drop out rate of 0.5 was used in the fully

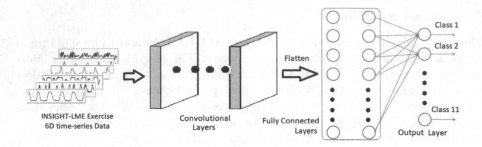

Fig. 3. CNN_Model Architecture for exercise recognition

connected layer to prevent overfitting of the data. The LME exercise recognition task was an 11 class classification problem and hence we used a fully-connected output layer with a softmax activation function capable of classifying output into 11 classes. Table 1 lists the complete list of the parameters of the CNN architecture.

The same single CNN architecture 1 was used as a binary classifier for the repetition counting task. We used a fully-connected output layer with a sigmoid activation function capable of classifying binary class. The binary class label information associated with the input was used for output prediction in the fully connected output layer. This single CNN model for repetition counting works parallel to the exercise recognition task and the predicted output are used along with exercise-type information from the exercise recognition model. Finally, a counting function was used to count the total number of repetitions using the transition information associated with the binary predicted output (Fig. 4).

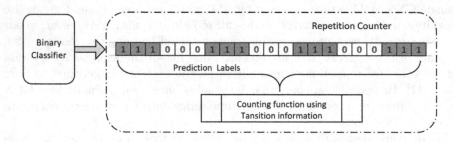

Fig. 4. Repetition Counter

The optimum model was evaluated for individual class performance based on statistical measures such as precision, recall and F1-score using Eqs. (1)–(3) respectively, where TP represents the number of times the model correctly predicts the given exercise class, FP represents the number of times the model incorrectly predicts the given exercise class and FN represents the number of times the model incorrectly predicts other than the given exercise class.

$$Precision = \frac{TP}{TP + FP} \tag{1}$$

Table 1. All architecture parameters for CNN_Model2. CL: Convolution Layer and DL: Dense Layer

Layer	Value	Parameters
Input layer	2048 × 1 × 6	0
Convolution filters CL1	16	304
Kernel size CL1	(3, 1)	–
Strides CL1	(1, 1)	–
Convolution filters CL2	16	784
Kernel size CL2	(3, 1)	–
Strides CL2	(1, 1)	–
Convolution filters CL3	32	1568
Kernel size CL3	(3, 1)	–
Strides CL3	(1, 1)	–
Convolution filters CL4	32	3104
Kernel size CL4	(3, 1)	–
Strides CL4	(1, 1)	–
Convolution filters CL5	64	6208
Kernel size CL5	(3, 1)	–
Strides CL5	(1, 1)	–
Convolution filters CL6	64	12352
Kernel size CL6	(3, 1)	–
Strides CL6	(1, 1)	–
Convolution filters CL7	96	18528
Kernel size CL7	(3, 1)	–
Strides CL7	(1, 1)	–
Batch normalization CL1, CL2, CL3, CL4, CL5, CL6, CL7	Yes	64 + 64 + 128 + 128 + 256 + 256 + 384
Activation function CL1, CL2, CL3, CL4, CL5, CL6, CL7	ReLU	0
Dense Layer DL1	128	25165952
Dropout DL1	0.25	0
Dense Layer DL2	11	1419
Activation function DL2	softmax	0
Total parameters	:	**25,211,499**
Trainable parameters	:	**25,210,859**
Non-trainable parameters	:	**640**

$$Recall = \frac{TP}{TP + FN} \qquad (2)$$

$$F1 = \frac{2 * Precision * Recall}{Precision + Recall} \qquad (3)$$

4 Experimental Results

The CNN models for both tasks were constructed using Keras API [21] with the TensorFlow [22] back end with the choice of optimizer function among stochastic gradient descent (SGD) [23], Adam [24], and RMSprop [25]. The best learning rate was selected by training the model over a range of 1e−03 to 1e−10 with a decay of 1e−01. The multi-class classification model for exercise recognition was optimized using the loss functions such as categorical cross-entropy (CCE) [26] and Kullback–Leibler divergence (KLD) [27] to have lower losses. However, the binary-class model for repetition counting was optimized using binary cross-entropy loss function. We used early stopping during model building by monitoring the validation loss. A learning rate scheduler was used effectively using the "ReduceOnPlateau" function from Keras. Data augmentations like shearing, resizing, flipping, rotation were not performed on the time-series data. Models were trained using the training set and validated using the validation set. A model with a minimum validation loss and with the best validation accuracy was selected as the optimum CNN model in both tasks and was further tested using the test set.

4.1   Exercise Recognition Using CNN Model

A CNN model with an Adam optimizer having a learning rate 1e-7 and a KLD loss function was found to be the best model. The model recorded an overall training score of 96.89% and a validation score of 88.97%. For the test set, the model recorded an overall test accuracy of 95.61% and an overall F1-score measure of 96% and an overall loss of 0.1288. Figure 5(a) and Fig. 5(b) shows the learning curves in terms of training and validation accuracies as well as training and validation losses.

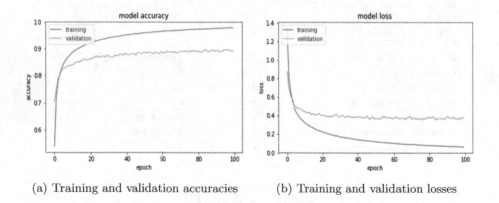

(a) Training and validation accuracies   (b) Training and validation losses

Fig. 5. Learning curves

The performance of the CNN model, in terms of statistical parameter measurements such as precision, recall and F1-score, for individual exercise are tabulated in Table 2. The model recorded an overall precision of 96.52%, overall recall rate of 97.13% and an overall F1-score of 96.80% for the upper-body LME exercises. The overall performance for the lower body LME in terms of precision, recall rate and F1-score measures were 95.99%, 97.08% and 96.5% respectively.

Table 2. Performance evaluation measures of the CNN model

Exercise type		Precision	Recall	F1-score	Support
Upper-body LME exercises	Bicep Curls	0.9952	0.9713	0.9831	1290
	Frontal Raise	0.8917	0.9574	0.9234	1290
	Lateral Raise	0.9389	0.9178	0.9283	1290
	Triceps Extension	0.9985	1.0000	0.9992	1290
	Pec Dec	0.9953	0.9837	0.9895	1290
	Trunk Twist	0.9721	0.9977	0.9847	1290
Lower-body LME exercises	Standing Bicycle	0.9834	0.9651	0.9742	1290
	Squats	0.9874	0.9698	0.9785	1290
	Leg Lateral Raise	0.9771	0.9907	0.9838	1290
	Lunges	0.8917	0.9574	0.9234	1290
Common movements	Others	0.8975	0.8389	0.8672	1440
Micro average		0.96	0.96	0.96	14340
Macro average		0.96	0.96	0.96	14340
Weighted average		0.96	0.96	0.96	14340

4.2   Repetition Counting Using the CNN Model

The optimum model was selected based on the validation score and incorporated an Adam optimizer and had a learning rate of 1e-06. The optimum model was further tested with the test data set to count the repetitions. The test data set consisted of 30 exercise data from each exercise type corresponding to the fifteen participants performing each exercise twice and 6 to 7 repetitions over 25 s of data segment.

Table 3. Number of error counts in the repetition using CNN model

Exercise type	Acronym	Total subjects	Error count			
			$e|0|$	$e|1|$	$e|2|$	$e > |2|$
Upper-body LME exercises	BC	30	28	1	0	1
	FR	30	25	4	0	1
	LR	30	30	0	0	0
	TER	30	29	1	0	0
	PD	30	29	1	0	0
	TT	30	27	3	0	0
Lower-body LME exercises	SBC	30	18	7	4	1
	SQ	30	15	9	4	2
	LLR	30	23	5	2	0
	L	30	6	4	4	16

Table 3 shows the results of repetition counting for individual LME exercise in terms of the number of absolute errors. The total number of subjects used in the test set for testing each exercise is also indicated in the table. The repetition error counts are indicated by the columns "Error Count" or "$e|X|$", where "$e|X|$" indicates the number of exercise sets with '$|X|$' repetition error count. '$|X|$' represents the absolute error count in terms of 0, 1, 2, or more than 2 errors. The repetition counting method performed better for upper-body exercises like BC, FR, LR and TER in comparison to the repetition counting of the lower-body exercises. For example, from Table 3, for the upper-body LME exercises, zero errors in repetition counting were reported in 168 instances among 180 observed sets.

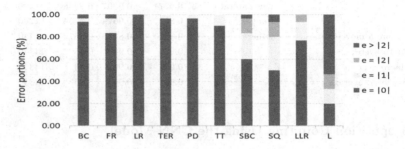

Fig. 6. Number of errors of the repetition counting using the CNN model (Color figure online)

A significant amount of error count for the upper-body LME exercises was with one count error. We could achieve 100% correct counting only in the case of LR exercise trials. Repetition counting performance for Lunges, a lower-body exercise, was very poor. Performance of the model can be evaluated with a tolerance of one repetition count error (i.e. blue + yellow, Fig. 6). The repetition counting from the model was within an error of ±1 repetitions in 88% of the observed exercise sets.

5   Discussion

In this paper, we studied a deep CNN model architecture on the INSIGHT-LME dataset for automatic recognition and repetition counting in LME exercises. The dataset used was based on the data from single wrist-worn inertial measurement unit from the exercises used in CVD rehabilitation program. We found that the deep CNN model constructed on the time-series data was an efficient model for exercise recognition and repetition counting in terms of accuracy measure. In addition, we demonstrated a novel method of using a single model based on multi-channel time-series data for the repetition counting from all the ten exercises.

We would like to discuss the outcome of our study with the findings of recent relevant studies in the area of exercise-based rehabilitation using wearables. First, this study of ours was an extension of findings from our work [1], where a comparative approach was adopted in LME exercise recognition and repetition counting using different supervised machine learning models and a deep CNN model using AlexNet architecture. In addition, using the earlier study [1] we had made the INSIGHT-LME dataset publicly available. The CNN model using AlexNet architecture was the best approach, however, requires the input data in terms of 2D images. However, this study of exercise recognition and repetition counting uses the multi-channel raw time-series data and achieves the overall same result.

Second, Soro et al. [11], a recent work on exercise recognition and repetition counting on ten Cross-Fit exercises using deep CNN models uses two sensors one on a foot and one on hand. The study makes use of a single deep CNN model for the exercise recognition task but uses ten different models for the repetition counting. 9D data from accelerometer, gyroscope and orientation sensor was used and reports an overall accuracy measure of 97% in exercise recognition with only exercise data. In contrast, our model for the exercise recognition uses 6D data and the recognition task considers an additional eleventh class ("Others"), with non-exercise movement data along with the ten exercise class data. We built a single CNN model for repetition counting in contrast to the ten individual models.

While our studies and those of Soro et al. [11] were on different exercises and different data-sets, the main aim was to address exercise-based rehabilitation using deep learning models. The current study using multi-channel information with a deep CNN appear also shows that it is possible to use a single model to count exercise repetition, with very little loss in accuracy. This may be beneficial in reducing the dependency on the total number of resources required in repetition computation in the case of multiple exercise evaluation.

6   Conclusion

We studied a single deep CNN architecture based model on the exercises used in an exercise-based CVD rehabilitation program. The automatic recognition and repetition counting of the exercises was achieved using multi-channel (6D) time-series data obtained from a single wearable sensor. We achieved an overall F1-score measure of 96% in the exercise recognition task and the repetition counting was within an error of ± 1 count among 88% of the observed exercise sets. Our study also showed that it is possible to use a single CNN model for repetition count with very little loss in accuracy.

Acknowledgement. This publication has emanated from research supported by INSIGHT SFI Research Centre for Data Analytics and Science Foundation Ireland (SFI) under Grant Number SFI/12/RC/2289_P2, co-funded by the European Regional Development Fund.

References

1. Prabhu, G., O'Connor, N.E., Moran, K.: Recognition and repetition counting for local muscular endurance exercises in exercise-based rehabilitation: a comparative study using artificial intelligence models. Sensors **20**(17), 4791 (2020)
2. Buys, R., et al.: Cardiac patients show high interest in technology enabled cardiovascular rehabilitation. BMC Med. Inform. Decis. Mak. **16**(1), 95 (2016)
3. Dalal, H.M., Zawada, A., Jolly, K., Moxham, T., Taylor, R.S.: Home based versus centre based cardiac rehabilitation: cochrane systematic review and meta-analysis. BMJ **340**, b5631 (2010)
4. Foerster, F., Smeja, M., Fahrenberg, J.: Detection of posture and motion by accelerometry: a validation study in ambulatory monitoring. Comput. Hum. Behav. **15**(5), 571–583 (1999)
5. Lara, O.D., Labrador, M.A.: A survey on human activity recognition using wearable sensors. IEEE Commun. Surv. Tutor. **15**(3), 1192–1209 (2012)
6. Weiss, G.M., Timko, J.L., Gallagher, C.M., Yoneda, K., Schreiber, A.J.: Smartwatch-based activity recognition: a machine learning approach. In: 2016 IEEE-EMBS International Conference on Biomedical and Health Informatics (BHI), pp. 426–429. IEEE (2016)
7. Sarcevic, P., Pletl, S., Kincses, Z.: Comparison of time-and frequency-domain features for movement classification using data from wrist-worn sensors. In: 2017 IEEE 15th International Symposium on Intelligent Systems and Informatics (SISY), pp. 000261–000266. IEEE (2017)
8. Chernbumroong, S., Atkins, A.S., Yu, H.: Activity classification using a single wrist-worn accelerometer. In: 2011 5th International Conference on Software, Knowledge Information, Industrial Management and Applications (SKIMA) Proceedings, pp. 1–6. IEEE (2011)
9. Zhu, C., Sheng, W.: Recognizing human daily activity using a single inertial sensor. In: 2010 8th World Congress on Intelligent Control and Automation, pp. 282–287. IEEE (2010)
10. Crema, C., Depari, A., Flammini, A., Sisinni, E., Haslwanter, T., Salzmann, S.: IMU-based solution for automatic detection and classification of exercises in the fitness scenario. In: 2017 IEEE Sensors Applications Symposium (SAS), pp. 1–6. IEEE (2017)
11. Soro, A., Brunner, G., Tanner, S., Wattenhofer, R.: Recognition and repetition counting for complex physical exercises with deep learning. Sensors **19**(3), 714 (2019)
12. Um, T.T., Babakeshizadeh, V., Kulić, D.: Exercise motion classification from large-scale wearable sensor data using convolutional neural networks. In: 2017 IEEE/RSJ International Conference on Intelligent Robots and Systems (IROS), pp. 2385–2390. IEEE (2017)
13. O'Reilly, M.A., Whelan, D.F., Ward, T.E., Delahunt, E., Caulfield, B.: Classification of lunge biomechanics with multiple and individual inertial measurement units. Sports Biomech. **16**(3), 342–360 (2017)
14. Whelan, D., O'Reilly, M., Ward, T., Delahunt, E., Caulfield, B.: Evaluating performance of the single leg squat exercise with a single inertial measurement unit. In: Proceedings of the 3rd 2015 Workshop on ICTs for Improving Patients Rehabilitation Research Techniques, pp. 144–147 (2015)
15. Morris, D., Saponas, T.S., Guillory, A., Kelner, I.: RecoFit: using a wearable sensor to find, recognize, and count repetitive exercises. In: Proceedings of the SIGCHI Conference on Human Factors in Computing Systems, pp. 3225–3234 (2014)

16. Mortazavi, B.J., Pourhomayoun, M., Alsheikh, G., Alshurafa, N., Lee, S.I., Sarrafzadeh, M.: Determining the single best axis for exercise repetition recognition and counting on smartwatches. In: 2014 11th International Conference on Wearable and Implantable Body Sensor Networks, pp. 33–38. IEEE (2014)

17. Whelan, D., O'Reilly, M., Ward, T., Delahunt, E., Caulfield, B.: Evaluating performance of the lunge exercise with multiple and individual inertial measurement units. In: Pervasive Health 2016: 10th EAI International Conference on Pervasive Computing Technologies for Healthcare, Cancun, Mexico, 16–19 May 2016. ACM (2016)

18. Prabhu, G., Ahmadi, A., O'Connor, N.E., Moran, K.: Activity recognition of local muscular endurance (LME) exercises using an inertial sensor. In: Lames, M., Saupe, D., Wiemeyer, J. (eds.) IACSS 2017. AISC, vol. 663, pp. 35–47. Springer, Cham (2018). https://doi.org/10.1007/978-3-319-67846-7_4

19. Ioffe, S., Szegedy, C.: Batch normalization: accelerating deep network training by reducing internal covariate shift. arXiv preprint arXiv:1502.03167 (2015)

20. Nair, V., Hinton, G.E.: Rectified linear units improve restricted Boltzmann machines. In: ICML (2010)

21. Chollet, F., et al.: Keras (2015). https://github.com/fchollet/keras

22. Abadi, M., et al.: TensorFlow: large-scale machine learning on heterogeneous systems (2015). https://www.tensorflow.org/. Software available from tensorflow.org

23. Kiefer, J., Wolfowitz, J., et al.: Stochastic estimation of the maximum of a regression function. Ann. Math. Stat. **23**(3), 462–466 (1952)

24. Kingma, D.P., Ba, J.: Adam: a method for stochastic optimization. arXiv preprint arXiv:1412.6980 (2014)

25. Tieleman, T., Hinton, G.: Lecture 6.5–RmsProp: divide the gradient by a running average of its recent magnitude. COURSERA Neural Netw. Mach. Learn. 4, 26–31 (2012)

26. Rubinstein, R.Y., Kroese, D.P.: The Cross-Entropy Method: A Unified Approach to Combinatorial Optimization, Monte-Carlo Simulation and Machine Learning. Springer, New York (2004). https://doi.org/10.1007/978-1-4757-4321-0

27. Joyce, J.M.: Kullback-Leibler divergence (2011)

Bayesian Inference Federated Learning for Heart Rate Prediction

Lei Fang[1]([✉]), Xiaoli Liu[2], Xiang Su[2,3], Juan Ye[1], Simon Dobson[1], Pan Hui[2,4], and Sasu Tarkoma[2]

[1] University of St Andrews, St Andrews KY16 9SX, UK
lf28@st-andrews.ac.uk
[2] University of Helsinki, 00014 Helsinki, Finland
[3] University of Oulu, 90014 Oulu, Finland
[4] The Hong Kong University of Science and Technology,
Clear Water Bay, Hong Kong

Abstract. The advances of sensing and computing technologies pave the way to develop novel applications and services for wearable devices. For example, wearable devices measure heart rate, which accurately reflects the intensity of physical exercise. Therefore, heart rate prediction from wearable devices benefits users with optimization of the training process. Conventionally, Cloud collects user data from wearable devices and conducts inference. However, this paradigm introduces significant privacy concerns. Federated learning is an emerging paradigm that enhances user privacy by remaining the majority of personal data on users' devices. In this paper, we propose a statistically sound, Bayesian inference federated learning for heart rate prediction with autoregression with exogenous variable (ARX) model. The proposed privacy-preserving method achieves accurate and robust heart rate prediction. To validate our method, we conduct extensive experiments with real-world outdoor running exercise data collected from wearable devices.

Keywords: Federated learning · Bayesian inference · Wearable computing · Heart rate prediction

1 Introduction

Cardiovascular diseases (CVD) are the number one cause of death globally. According to the world health organization report, 17.9 million people die from CVD each year, an estimated 31% of all deaths worldwide [1]. Many factors can trigger these diseases, including tobacco use, unhealthy diet, physical inactivity, and harmful use of alcohol. Preventing CVD is becoming an urgent task. It is well-known that exercising has a proven therapeutic effect on the cardiovascular system. Hence, predicting and controlling heart rates during the exercise is important to avoid overstrain and prevent sudden heart rate break.

Wearable devices enable intelligent human-computer interactions. The wearable fitness, sport technologies, and service business are expected to grow

© ICST Institute for Computer Sciences, Social Informatics and Telecommunications Engineering 2021
Published by Springer Nature Switzerland AG 2021. All Rights Reserved
J. Ye et al. (Eds.): MobiHealth 2020, LNICST 362, pp. 116–130, 2021.
https://doi.org/10.1007/978-3-030-70569-5_8

exponentially in the near future. Users of wearable devices are expecting the service that can guide their smart exercise coaching, rather than only tracking their activities. Heart rate based training is a well-known technique to improve the effectiveness of training and prevent over-exercising. Designing an optimal exercise training plan to avoid overstrain is crucial. Ignoring the limits of the physical activities will not only nullify the effect of the exercise but also cause harmful effect on the cardiovascular system. The first step of designing the optimal exercise training plan is predicting heart rate from the exercise, which will be then used for the training control. The designed recommendation and control systems can be adopted in the mobile phone or smart watches. Subjects can use the control system in those smart devices to guide their exercise in order to reach the desired heart rate response and avoid overtraining, which will benefit the users' health. However, most existing research work related to heart rate prediction focuses on indoor exercises. For outdoor physical exercise, it is not possible to automatically regulate the workload intensity due to the dependence on environmental conditions. Hence, it's typical for an outdoor exerciser to continuously check heart rate and increase or decrease the speed accordingly for regulating his or her heart rate.

Machine learning has demonstrated its promising performance in providing the users with recommendations regarding to physical activity and physiological response [2,3]. Machine learning algorithms typically learn from centralized data in order to train a powerful model. However, pooling data from many users to the Cloud introduces significant privacy concern; for example, leaking sensitive health information of users. Recently, EU General Data Protection Regulation (GDPR) [4] states the need for trust to be built into personal data services and allows users to control their own data, including data their devices generate. Based on GDPR, collecting a massive amount of user data from wearables is not allowed. Federated learning has been regarded as a promising architecture, allowing learning from a large volume of distributed local data without pooling users' private data to the Cloud [5]. Federated learning preserves the users' privacy by training the model in a decentralized manner where multiple local models are synthesized to a global model which is used for future applications.

In this paper, we propose a Bayesian inference based federated learning for heart rate prediction. Bayesian inference provides a statistically sound way to combine local models; and at the same time achieves robust predictions even when data are unevenly distributed among the peripheral nodes, which is common in real world applications. Our work is the first Bayesian inference federated learning approach for heart rate prediction with autoregression with exogenous variable model (ARX) and this framework can be extended to other ARX prediction problems.

Our contributions are threefold:

- We propose two Bayesian federated learning methods, namely Federated Learning based on Sequential Bayesian method (*FD Seq Bayes*) and the Empirical Bayes based Hierarchical Bayesian method (*FD HBayes-EB*), for heart rate prediction without pooling data to the Cloud for privacy

preservation. The former model *FD Seq Bayes* is proposed to provide a statistically sound way of integrating local models; whereas the latter model, *FD HBayes-EB*, provides an alternative but more scalable way from a Bayesian hierarchical model perspective.
- We have conducted extensive evaluation on real-world data from wearable devices. Compared to various state-of-the-art baseline models, our proposed methods have demonstrated their strength in achieving higher prediction accuracy on unseen, new users with lower computation cost.
- Our proposed Bayesian federated learning methods can be easily extended to address other ARX regression problems taking consideration of user privacy preservation and achieving good performance.

The remainder of this paper is organized as follows. Section 2 describes the background and related work. Section 3 presents the proposed Bayesian inference federated learning methods. We present experimentation setup and results in Sect. 4 and summarize our insights and conclude the paper in Sect. 5.

2   Related Work

In this section, we review the state-of-the-art techniques in heart rate prediction and federated learning.

2.1   Heart Rate Prediction

Heart rate modelling and prediction have been extensively studied. Existing approaches to model and predict the heart rate response to running exercises can be divided into two categories: (1) Physiological models, which are usually described by deterministic mathematical formulas and used in specific biological systems; and (2) machine learning approaches, which do not encode any prior information but will learn and generalize the response model in the learning process. While approaches in the first category gain its appeal from its analytical closed-form notation, the approaches in the second category are more attractive, because they allow accounting for environmental parameters and other relevant information that is not represented in the analytic equations.

An ordinary differential equation (ODE) model had been proposed by Cheng et al. [6] to describe the dynamical changes of heart rate from resting heart rate by taking consideration of exercise speed and heart rate effects from hormonal system. Levenberg-Marquardt algorithm is used for estimating the optimized parameters. The proposed ODE model is designed for speed control in the treadmill for heart rate regulation. In order to use those models, the subject's resting heart rate need to be known beforehand and special test need to be performed in order to get subject's resting heart rate.

A nonparametric hammerstein model decoupled the linear and nonlinear parts using pseudorandom binary sequences is proposed by Su et al. [7] for heart rate regulation. Support vector regression is adopted to estimate the parameters of the model. Mohammad et al. [8] have used takagi-sugeno fuzzy model for controlling the heart rate in cycling exercises. They build a takagi-sugeno fuzzy model for each subject based on that subject's own observed data. Subjects did not share their data nor model parameters.

Machine learning methods, such as time series linear regression, support vector regression, feedforward artificial neural network, and long short-term memory (LSTM) [2] have also been used in modelling and predicting the heart rate in exercise. Ni et al. [3] propose an LSTM-based context-aware sequential model to capture the heart rate and the personalized patterns of fitness data. Ludwig et al. [9] summarize most of the recent models related to predicting and controlling heart rate response to exercise.

Current research work related to heart rate modeling and prediction for wearable devices mainly develop general models on the Cloud by sharing subjects' data or developing the personal model with using each subject's own data without sharing other subjects' data. Less attention has been paid on building a general model that can be used for all subjects while keeping data isolated for privacy preservation.

2.2   Federated Learning

Kairouz et al. [10] define federated learning as a machine learning setting where multiple entities (clients) collaborate in solving a machine learning problem, under the coordination of a central server or service provider. Each client's raw data is stored locally and not exchanged or transferred; instead, focused updates intended for immediate aggregation are used to achieve the learning objective [10]. Federated learning was firstly proposed by Google [5], aiming to keep the training data on the device while collaboratively learning a shared model by coveraging the parameters changes learned from local models. Privacy and communication efficiency are most important concerns in federated learning.

Recently, federated learning has attracted widespread attention and made considerable success in many applications [11]. McMahan et al. [12] have introduced the Federate Averaging (FedAvg) algorithm, which learns the federated global model based on averaging of local learner parameters trained using stochastic gradient descent. Smith et al. [13] treat federated learning as a multi-task learning problem and develop MOCHA method to solve the statistical challenges in federated setting. More significant research work on distributed deep learning can refer to [14,15]. Chen et al. [16] develop a federated transfer learning framework, named FedHealth, for wearable healthcare. Their proposed approaches combine transfer learning and federated learning using the FedAvg algorithm, which requires to share the same random initialization and is not applicable for combing pre-trained models. Here, we look into a Bayesian model for integrating local models.

Yurochkin et al. [17] propose a Bayesian federated learning framework to aggregate pre-trained neural networks, each being trained locally in parallel with its own specific dataset. The parameters of these local neural networks will be matched to a global model, which is governed by the posterior of a Bayesian nonparametric model. Different from existing work, we focus on learning time-series data with ARX model and we propose two variants of Bayesian methods.

3 Proposed Approach

This section presents the problem statement on federated learning for heart rate prediction and introduces two Bayesian-based techniques: sequential and hierarchical models.

3.1 Problem Definition

The objective of heart rate prediction is to predict the heart rate y_t given the historic readings of the previous heart rates and other useful inputs like speed:

$$y_t = f(y_{1:t-1}, x_{1:t}) + e_t,$$

where e_t is the error term and f can be any parametric function, say a linear function or neural network. The objective of federated learning is to learn such a parametric model f in the server without sending each user's raw data. In particular, given data from n different users stored at each distributed node, and denote the reading from user i as $\mathcal{D}_i$, the learning outcome is a trained global model in the server with datasets $\{\mathcal{D}_i\}_{i=1}^n$; and the global learning should only involve model parameters rather than raw user data. For later prediction, the trained model at the server can then be directly used for predictions of future users with personalization if possible.

3.2 Autoregression with Exogenous Variable Model

As the heart rate data is a time series with serial correlations, a suitable model for such data sets is ARX. An ARX model with p autoregression components and $q + 1$ lagged inputs can be formally written as:

$$y_t = \theta_0 + \sum_{i=1}^p \theta_i y_{t-i} + \sum_{j=0}^q \omega_j z_{t-j} + e_t$$

where $e_t \sim N(0, \sigma^2)$ is white noise with variance σ^2, y_t, z_t are heart rate and speed measurements at time t. By defining β, x as the vectors concatenating the model parameters and covariates, the model can be succinctly written as

$$y_t = x^T \beta + e_t,$$

where $\beta^T = [\theta_0, \theta_1, \ldots, \theta_p, \omega_0, \ldots, \omega_q]$ and $x^T = [1, y_{t-1}, \ldots, y_{t-p}, x_t, \ldots, x_{t-q}]$.

3.3 Federated Learning with Sequential Bayesian Inference

Bayesian inference provides a natural solution to the federated learning problem, where the inference is on the posterior distribution of model parameters. By making conditional independent assumption of the data at different nodes given the model parameter, the posterior distribution of the model parameter can be learnt in a sequential manner. Denoting $\mathcal{D}_i = \{\boldsymbol{X}_i, \boldsymbol{y}_i\}$ as the dataset at node i where $\boldsymbol{y}_i = [y_{i,1}, \ldots, y_{i,n_i}]^T$ and $\boldsymbol{X}_i = [\boldsymbol{x}_{i,1}, \ldots, \boldsymbol{x}_{i,n_i}]^T$, and n_i is the number of time instances for user i; then the posterior distribution is

$$p(\boldsymbol{\beta}, \sigma^2 | \mathcal{D}_1, \mathcal{D}_2, \ldots \mathcal{D}_n) \propto p(\boldsymbol{\beta}, \sigma^2) p(\mathcal{D}_1, \mathcal{D}_2, \ldots \mathcal{D}_n | \boldsymbol{\beta}, \sigma^2) \tag{1}$$

$$= p(\boldsymbol{\beta}, \sigma^2) \prod_{i=1}^{n} p(\mathcal{D}_i | \boldsymbol{\beta}, \sigma^2) \propto p(\boldsymbol{\beta}, \sigma^2 | \mathcal{D}_1, \mathcal{D}_2, \ldots \mathcal{D}_{n-1}) p(\mathcal{D}_n | \boldsymbol{\beta}, \sigma^2), \tag{2}$$

where the second equation has used the conditional independence assumption and the last equation shows that the posterior can be recursively learnt by updating the posterior of the previous $n-1$ sites.

For an ARX model with fixed p, q terms, the model parameters are $\boldsymbol{\beta}$ and σ^2. A conjugate prior for the unknown parameters are Normal-Inverse Gamma distribution, *i.e.*

$$p(\boldsymbol{\beta}, \sigma^2) = \mathrm{NIG}(\boldsymbol{\beta}, \sigma^2; \boldsymbol{m}_0, \boldsymbol{\Lambda}_0, a_0, b_0) \tag{3a}$$

$$= \mathrm{N}(\boldsymbol{\beta}; \boldsymbol{m}_0, \sigma^2 \boldsymbol{\Lambda}_0^{-1}) \mathrm{Inv\text{-}Gamma}(\sigma^2; a_0, b_0), \tag{3b}$$

where $\mathrm{N}(\boldsymbol{\mu}, \boldsymbol{\Sigma})$ denotes a Gaussian distribution with mean and variance $\boldsymbol{\mu}$ and $\boldsymbol{\Sigma}$; and $\mathrm{Inv\text{-}Gamma}(a, b)$ denotes a inverse Gamma distribution with shape and rate parameter a, b respectively.

It can be shown that the posterior distribution can be obtained recursively in a closed form by updating the prior parameters, $\{\boldsymbol{m}_0, \boldsymbol{\Lambda}_0, a_0, b_0\}$, and the inference result is summarized in Theorem 1. According to the update procedure in Eq. (5a), instead of averaging all the model parameters learnt at different sites, the Bayesian method essentially provides an alternative weighted average procedure that takes into account of the model uncertainties as well as the parameters themselves. That is, the weights depend on the variance $\boldsymbol{\Lambda}_n^{-1}$, indicating the uncertainty of the parameter.

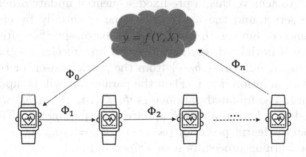

Fig. 1. Federated learning with sequential Bayesian inference

Theorem 1 (Sequential Bayesian inference). *Adopt the NIG prior for* $\boldsymbol{\beta}, \sigma^2 | \emptyset$ *as defined in Eq. (3) for some pre-determined parameters* $\boldsymbol{m}_0, \boldsymbol{\Lambda}_0, a_0, b_0$;

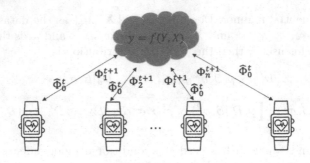

Fig. 2. Federated learning with hierarchical Bayesian inference and empirical Bayes method

for user datasets $\{\mathcal{D}_i\}_{i=1}^n$, the posterior distribution can be learnt sequentially, i.e. for $n > 0$:

$$p(\boldsymbol{\beta}, \sigma^2 | \mathcal{D}_1, \dots, \mathcal{D}_n) = NIG(\boldsymbol{\beta}, \sigma^2; m_n, \boldsymbol{\Lambda}_n, a_n, b_n), \tag{4}$$

where,

$$m_n = (\boldsymbol{\Lambda}_n)^{-1}(\boldsymbol{\Lambda}_{n-1}m_{n-1} + \boldsymbol{X}_n^T \boldsymbol{y}_n) \tag{5a}$$

$$\boldsymbol{\Lambda}_n = \boldsymbol{X}_n^T \boldsymbol{X}_n + \boldsymbol{\Lambda}_{n-1} \tag{5b}$$

$$a_n = a_{n-1} + \frac{N_n}{2} \tag{5c}$$

$$b_n = b_{n-1} + \frac{1}{2}(\boldsymbol{y}_n^T \boldsymbol{y}_n + m_{n-1}^T \boldsymbol{\Lambda}_{n-1} m_{n-1} - m_n^T \boldsymbol{\Lambda}_n m_n) \tag{5d}$$

and N_n is the number of data points at site n.

To protect the privacy of the user, instead of sending all the raw data $\{\mathcal{D}_i\}$ to the server, we carry out the inference locally in a sequential manner. Each node will learn the posterior sequentially, where the posterior parameters are communicated. To achieve this, a pre-fixed sequential update order needs to be decided at the server and the learning is done essentially by circulating the posterior parameters among the sites. To be more specific, after an update sequential order is initialized, each node i will first receive the model parameters $\boldsymbol{\Phi}_{i-1} = \{m_{i-1}, \boldsymbol{\Lambda}_{i-1}, a_{i-1}, b_{i-1}\}$ from the previous user, or the server if it is the first update iteration, $i = 1$. Then the parameters will be updated according to Theorem 1. The updated parameters $\boldsymbol{\Phi}_i = \{m_i, \boldsymbol{\Lambda}_i, a_i, b_i\}$ will be relayed to the next node $i + 1$ until all sites update their parameters. The server will receive and keep the learnt posterior parameter $\boldsymbol{\Phi}_n = \{m_n, \boldsymbol{\Lambda}_n, a_n, b_n\}$ for later prediction. The learning procedure is described in Fig. 1.

3.4 Federated Learning with Hierarchical Bayesian Inference

The sequential processing algorithm clearly does not scale well when the number of users/nodes increases. A distributed inference algorithm that allows parallel processing therefore is more appealing. To achieve this, hierarchical Bayesian model is proposed, where hyper-priors over the prior parameters are introduced and the model parameters at each individual site become conditionally independent. By using a hierarchical model, we also achieve a principled way of learning hyperparameters, $\{m_0, \Lambda_0, a_0, b_0\}$.

Formally, a hierarchical Bayesian linear regression model can be formulated as follows

$$y_i|\beta_i, \sigma_i^2, X_i \sim N(X_i\beta_i, \sigma_i^2 I)$$
$$\beta_i, \sigma_i^2|m_0, \Lambda_0, a_0, b_0 \sim \text{NIG}(m_0, \Lambda_0, a_0, b_0)$$
$$m_0, \Lambda_0, a_0, b_0|\Psi \sim P(.),$$

where each user/node has its own model parameter $\{\beta_i, \sigma_i^2\}$. A common Normal-InvGamma prior is imposed on the model parameters and the model parameters become conditionally independent or exchangeable given the hyperparameters $\Phi_0 = \{m_0, \Lambda_0, a_0, b_0\}$. A further hierarchical hyper-prior P of appropriate form is imposed on the hyperparameters Φ_0. For example, Gaussian is for m_0, Inverse-Wishart is for Λ_0, and Gamma is for a_0 and b_0. Usually vague uninformative hyper-priors are used for the second tier distributions [18].

Empirical Bayes. The inference for the hierarchical model cannot be solved in closed form any more. Usually computationally expensive inference procedures like Markov Chain Monte Carlo (MCMC) has to be used. An alternative is Empirical Bayes (EB) method where hyperparameters $\Phi_0 = \{m_0, \Lambda_0, a_0, b_0\}$ are not sampled but directly maximised against the model evidence

$$\hat{\Phi}_0 = \underset{\Phi_0}{\operatorname{argmax}}\, P(\mathcal{D}_1, \mathcal{D}_2 \ldots \mathcal{D}_n|m_0, \Lambda_0, a_0, b_0).$$

By treating the model parameters $\{\beta_i, \sigma_i^2\}_{i=1}^n$ as missing data, an EM algorithm can be derived to find the optimal hyperparameters. The detailed derivation and the EM algorithm is listed in the appendix.

The EB-based federated learning becomes an iterative procedure to accommodate the learning of the hyperparameters Φ_0. The learning procedure iterates between the following two steps:

1. Update the hyperparameter at the server given $P(\{\beta_i, \sigma_i^2\}_{i=1}^n|\{\mathcal{D}_i\}_{i=1}^n, \hat{\Phi}_0^{t-1})$ by an EM procedure listed Eq. (9):

$$\hat{\Phi}_0^t = \underset{\Phi_0}{\operatorname{argmax}}\, P(\mathcal{D}_1, \mathcal{D}_2 \ldots \mathcal{D}_n|m_0, \Lambda_0, a_0, b_0).$$

2. At each site i, update the local posterior given $\hat{\Phi}_0^t = \{\hat{m}_0, \hat{\Lambda}_0, \hat{a}_0, \hat{b}_0\}$ in parallel:

$$P(\beta_i, \sigma_i^2|\hat{\Phi}_0^t, \mathcal{D}_i) = \text{NIG}(m_i, \Lambda_i, a_i, b_i), \quad \text{where} \tag{6a}$$

Table 1. Physical characteristics of the subjects.

	Age (yr)	Height (cm)	Weight (kg)	BMI (kg/m^2)
Mean	30.4	175.2	70.8	23.05
Standard deviation	2.5	7.5	9.2	1.6
Range	(27, 34)	(162, 187)	(55, 87)	(19.9, 24.8)

$$m_i = (\Lambda_i)^{-1}(\hat{\Lambda}_0 \hat{m}_0 + X_n^T y_n)$$
$$\Lambda_i = X_i^T X_i + \hat{\Lambda}_0$$
$$a_i = \hat{a}_0 + \frac{N_i}{2}$$
$$b_i = \hat{b}_0 + \frac{1}{2}(y_i^T y_i + \hat{m}_0^T \hat{\Lambda}_0 \hat{m}_0 - m_i^T \Lambda_i m_i) \tag{6b}$$

To be more specific, at each iteration $t \geq 1$, the server will propagate the current hyperparameter $\hat{\boldsymbol{\Phi}}_0^{t-1}$ to the clients (some initial non-informative piror's parameters are used for the first iteration), each node then updates their posterior distributions of the local parameters according to a variant of Theorem 1 and sends back the learnt posterior parameters $\boldsymbol{\Phi}_i^t = \{m_i, \Lambda_i, a_i, b_i\}$ to the server. The server will then optimize the hyperparameter $\hat{\boldsymbol{\Phi}}_0^t$ based on the received posterior distributions by the EM algorithm. Figure 2 summarizes the learning procedure at iteration t. Note that the local learning in Eq. (6) is still in closed form hence computationally cheap. Thanks to this conjugacy, we find that only two to three iterations are usually good enough for the EB method to work in practice.

4   Evaluation and Results

This section illustrates our evaluation methodology, including the dataset and comparison techniques, and then present the results.

4.1   Dataset

We analyze the performance of proposed Bayesian inference federated learning with collecting real-world outdoor running exercise data from 10 subjects wearing Polar smart watches. Exercise time, running speed, and heart rate are recorded in each exercise. The physical characteristics of subjects are listed in Table 1. The duration of one exercise ranges from 30 min to 90 min and heart rate ranges from 60 bpm to 200 bpm. Outliers are removed based on the interquartile range criteria and missing values are imputed with linear interpolation. The ten subjects are regarded as isolated to each other and cannot share their data due to the privacy concern during the federated learning process.

4.2   Evaluation Methods

We evaluate the two proposed Bayesian Federated learning, *FD Seq Bayes* and *FD HBayes-EB*, with two baseline solutions.

- FedAvg: a simple average based federated learning method where the local regression models are trained by the least squared error method. A simple average of the learnt parameters is used for future testing and prediction.
- HBayes-MCMC: It refers to hierarchical Bayesian model inferred by Markov Chain Monte Carlo (MCMC) method [18]. Note that this method does not belong to federated learning realm as the training data from all the users is aggregated and stored in the server.

4.3   Experiment Procedure

To evaluate the effects of the proposed methods thoroughly, we firstly randomly select nine out of ten users as the existing users, leaving one user's data for testing as new users. For the nine chosen users, a random subset of each user's K_i exercises data is selected for model training: the selected exercises data is further split into training and testing. The following three types of errors are compared, including training error, testing error, and new exercise error (on the left-out user's and the unselected exercises' data). We assume that the training and testing data are drawn from the same population, and thus the training and testing errors are used to assess the learning capability of the model. The new exercise error represents the model performance on new users and new exercises from selected users (which might have different distributions from the training and testing data), indicating the generalization of the model. Squared errors are used for evaluating the performance of the models. The errors are further decomposed as by time-instance error and by-user error. The definitions of these two errors are as follows.

$$\text{error}_{\text{time}} = \frac{\sum_{i=1}^{n} \sum_{t=1}^{n_i} (y_{i,t} - \hat{y}_{,it})^2}{\sum_{i=1}^{n} n_i},$$

$$\text{error}_{\text{user}} = \frac{\sum_{i=1}^{n} (\sum_{t=1}^{n_i} (y_{i,t} - \hat{y}_{i,t})^2 / n_i)}{n},$$

where n is the total number of users (10 users in our case) and n_i is the number of data records of user i's data.

4.4   Results

Table 2 and Fig. 3 report the experiment results of $K_i = 10$ for 100 repeated experiments. Table 2 reports the means of squared errors and standard deviations of means. As we can see that the proposed two federated learning methods, i.e. FD Seq Bayes and FD HBayes-EB outperform the simple FedAvg by significant margins in all six types of errors; *e.g.*, FD Seq Bayes and FD HBayes-EB reduce

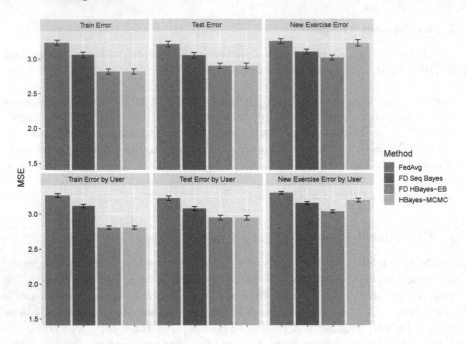

Fig. 3. Experiment results on the four methods; where $K_i = 10$ exercises data are used for training; where the error bars are the standard error

Table 2. Experiment results of by user error on the four methods; where $K_i = 10$ exercises data are used for training. The mean and the standard deviations (in brackets) are reported.

	Train error by user	Test error by user	New Ex error by user
FedAvg	3.27 (0.27)	3.23 (0.31)	3.3 (0.18)
FD Seq Bayes	3.11 (0.26)	3.08 (0.28)	3.16 (0.19)
FD HBayes-EB	2.81 (0.23)	2.95 (0.33)	3.04 (0.19)
HBayes-MCMC	2.81 (0.23)	2.95 (0.33)	3.2 (0.26)

0.16 and 0.46 on the mean of train error and 0.15 and 0.28 on the mean of test error from FedAvg.

The hierarchical Bayesian method achieves better result compared to the sequential method. The empirical Bayes method also achieves very similar results compared to the more computation intensive MCMC-based method in both training and testing errors and outperforms its counterpart in the new exercise error. Our results show that Bayesian based federated learning methods provide a more sound model synthesis (smaller testing error) and also new user personalization performance (new exercise error).

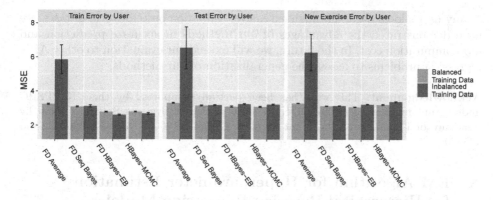

Fig. 4. Experiments on imbalanced training data scenario

Effects of Varied Training Datasets. To further demonstrate the effects of the Bayesian inference federated learning method, we deliberately make the training data imbalanced to better simulate the real world scenario. To be more specific, a random selection ratio $(0.01\%, 25\%, 50\%, 75\%, 100\%)$ is applied to each user's training data to make the training data imbalanced among the users. We assume different amounts of data from users might have a negative impact on federated learning; for example, the prediction might be biased towards the users whose data takes the majority. The results of 100 random experiments are listed in Fig. 4. It is obvious that all Bayesian based methods, both federated and traditional learning, outperform the likelihood based average method. When imbalanced training data is used, the average methods fail in all three error categories, and their large standard error also signifies the instability of the methods. The Bayesian methods however are all more robust, i.e. the performance deteriorates to a much less degree. We can also observe that the sequential Bayesian method achieves slightly better results than the hierarchical model, as the sequential method essentially pools the data together by integrating all local parameters with weights but at the price of scalability.

5   Conclusion

When users perform physical exercises, one important goal is to optimize the training process. Heart rate has been used as a most important indicator for monitoring the training strain. Therefore, predicting heart rate during physical exercise is crucial for tracking physiological responses and improving the effect of the exercise. The majority of the existing research focuses on pooling together a large amount of users' data for building a robust model, which often has incurred much privacy concern. To tackle this issue, we leverage a statistically sound model – Bayesian inference and propose two Bayesian-based federated learning methods, i.e. *FD Seq Bayes* and *FD HBayes-EB*. They enable collaborative model training under the orchestration of a central server, while not accessing to any user's local data. Through extensive evaluation on real-world dataset, we have demonstrated the advantages of our methods in accurate prediction and low computation cost. In the future, we will extend our evaluation to other ARX regression problems to assess the generalization of our methods.

Acknowledgement. This work has been partially supported by the UK EPSRC under grant number EP/N007565/1, "Science of Sensor Systems Software", and by Academy of Finland projects, grant number 325774, 3196669, 319670, 326305, and 325570.

A   EM Algorithm for Hyperparameter Estimation for Hierarchical Bayesian Regression Model

E step: The complete data log likelihood is

$$
\begin{aligned}
L(\boldsymbol{\Phi}_0) &= \log P(\{\boldsymbol{\beta}_i, \sigma_i^2\}_1^n, \{\mathcal{D}_i\}_i^n | \boldsymbol{\Phi}_0) \\
&= \log(P(\{\mathcal{D}_i\}_i^n | \{\boldsymbol{\beta}_i, \sigma_i^2\}_1^n, \boldsymbol{\Phi}_0) P(\{\boldsymbol{\beta}_i, \sigma_i^2\}_1^n | \boldsymbol{\Phi}_0)) \\
&= \log \left(\prod_{i=1}^n \mathrm{N}(\boldsymbol{y}_i; \boldsymbol{X}_i \boldsymbol{\beta}_i, \sigma_i^2 \boldsymbol{I}) \mathrm{NIG}\left(\{\boldsymbol{\beta}_i, \sigma_i^2\}; \boldsymbol{\Phi}_0\right) \right) \\
&= \sum_{i=1}^n \log \left(\mathrm{NIG}\left(\{\boldsymbol{\beta}_i, \sigma_i^2\}; \boldsymbol{\Phi}_0\right) \right) + C,
\end{aligned}
$$

where C contains all the terms that are independent of $\boldsymbol{\Phi}_0$. The conditional expected complete data likelihood is:

$$
\begin{aligned}
Q(\boldsymbol{\Phi}_0 | \boldsymbol{\Phi}_0^{t-1}) &= E_{\{\boldsymbol{\beta}_i, \sigma_i^2\}_1^n | \boldsymbol{\Phi}_0^{t-1}, \{\mathcal{D}_i\}_i^n}[L(\boldsymbol{\Phi}_0)] \\
&\approx \frac{1}{nL} \sum_{m=1}^L \sum_{i=1}^n \log(\mathrm{NIG}(\{\boldsymbol{\beta}_i, \sigma_i^2\}^{(m)}; \boldsymbol{\Phi}_0)
\end{aligned}
$$

where $\{\boldsymbol{\beta}_i, \sigma_i^2\}^{(m)}$ denotes the m-th i.i.d. sample from $P(\boldsymbol{\beta}_i, \sigma_i^2 | \mathcal{D}_i, \boldsymbol{\Phi}_0^{t-1})$, which are NIG distributed. Sampling from a NIG distribution is straightforward by a standard two step procedure by firstly sampling σ^2 from Inv-Gamma(a_i, b_i) then sampling from $\boldsymbol{\beta}$ from $\mathrm{N}(\boldsymbol{m}_i, \sigma^2 \boldsymbol{\Lambda}_i^{-1})$. Essentially, we are approximating the conditional expectation with a Monte Carlo estimator with L samples from the posterior $P(\{\boldsymbol{\beta}_i, \sigma_i^2\}_1^n | \{\mathcal{D}_i\}_1^n, \boldsymbol{\Phi}_0^{t-1})$. The EM algorithm degenerates to a Monte Carlo Expectation Maximization (MCEM) [19].

M step: the objective here is to maximize the conditional expectation, namely

$$
\hat{\boldsymbol{\Phi}}_0 = \operatorname*{argmax}_{\boldsymbol{\Phi}_0} Q(\boldsymbol{\Phi}_0 | \boldsymbol{\Phi}_0^{t-1}) \tag{7}
$$

$$
= \operatorname*{argmax}_{\boldsymbol{\Phi}_0} \frac{1}{nL} \sum_{m=1}^L \sum_{i=1}^n \log(\mathrm{N}(\boldsymbol{\beta}_i^{(m)}; \boldsymbol{m}_0, \sigma_i^{2(m)} \boldsymbol{\Lambda}_0^{-1})) + \log\left(\mathrm{G}\left(\sigma_i^{-2(m)}; a_0, b_0\right)\right) \tag{8}
$$

where we have used the property that if $x \sim$ Inv-Gamma(a, b), then $1/x$ is Gamma distributed with shape and rate parameters a, b, denoted as $G(a, b)$. It is easy to see that the optimal $\hat{a}_0, \hat{b}_0$ w.r.t Q are just the maximum likelihood estimator of a Gamma distribution with dataset $\{\sigma_i^{2(m)}\}_{i,m=1}^{n,L}$ (the second term of Eq. (8)). An iterative generalized Newton's method can be used to find the ML estimator of Gamma as follows [20].

$$\frac{1}{a_0} = \frac{1}{a_0} + \frac{\overline{\log \sigma^{-2}} - \log(\overline{\sigma^{-2}}) + \log a_0 - \Psi(a_0)}{a_0^2(1/a_0 - \Psi'(a_0))} \tag{9a}$$

$$b_0 = \frac{\overline{\sigma^{-2}}}{a_0}, \tag{9b}$$

where

$$\overline{\sigma^{-2}} = \frac{\sum_{m=1}^{L} \sum_{i=1}^{n} 1/\sigma_i^{2(m)}}{nL}, \quad \overline{\log \sigma^{-2}} = \frac{\sum_{m=1}^{L} \sum_{i=1}^{n} \log(1/\sigma_i^{2(m)})}{nL}.$$

Take the derivative of the Gaussian term in Eq. (8) w.r.t m_0, Λ_0 and set them to zero, we can find the estimators for m_0, Λ_0:

$$m_0 - \frac{\sum_{m=1}^{L} \sum_{i=1}^{n} \frac{1}{\sigma_i^{2(m)}} \beta_i^{(m)}}{\sum_{m=1}^{L} \sum_{i=1}^{n} \frac{1}{\sigma_i^{2(m)}}} \tag{9c}$$

$$\Lambda_0^{-1} = \frac{1}{nL} \sum_{m=1}^{L} \sum_{i=1}^{n} \frac{1}{\sigma_i^{2(m)}} (\beta_i^{(m)} - m_0)(\beta_i^{(m)} - m_0)^T \tag{9d}$$

References

1. Cardiovascular diseases. https://www.who.int/health-topics/cardiovascular-diseases/#tab=tab_1. Accessed 22 Aug 2020
2. Hilmkil, A., Ivarsson, O., Johansson, M., Kuylenstierna, D., Erp, T.V.: Towards machine learning on data from professional cyclists. In: 12th World Congress on Performance Analysis of Sports, Opatija, Croatia (2018)
3. Ni, J.M., Muhlstein, L., McAuley, J.: Modeling heart rate and activity data for personalized fitness. In: WWW 2019, 13–17 May 2019, San Francisco, CA, USA (2019)
4. EU: Regulation (EU) 2016/679 of the European Parliament and of the Council of 27 April 2016 on the protection of natural persons with regard to the processing of personal data and on the free movement of such data, and repealing directive 95/46/EC (general data protection regulation). Off. J. Eur. Union L119, 1–88 (2016). http://eur-lex.europa.eu/legal-content/EN/TXT/?uri=OJ:L:2016:119:TOC
5. Konečný, J., McMahan, H.B., Ramage, D., Richtárik, P.: Federated optimization: distributed machine learning for on-device intelligence. arXiv:1610.02527 (2016)
6. Cheng, T.M., Savkin, A.V., Celler, B.G., Su, S.W., Wang, L.: Nonlinear modeling and control of human heart rate response during exercise with various work load intensities. IEEE Trans. Biomed. Eng. 55(11), 2499–2508 (2008)

7. Su, S.W., Wang, L., Celler, B.G., Savkin, A.V., Guo, Y.: Identification and control for heart rate regulation during treadmill exercise. IEEE Trans. Biomed. Eng. **54**(7), 1238–1246 (2007b)
8. Mohammad, S., Guerra, T.M., Grobois, J.M., Hecquet, B.: Heart rate control during cycling exercise using Takagi-Sugeno models. In: 8th IFAC World Congress, Milano, Italy, pp. 12783–12788 (2011)
9. Ludwig, M., Hoffmann, K., Endler, S., Asteroth, A., Wiemeyer, J.: Measurement, prediction, and control of individual heart rate responses to exercise-basics and options for wearable devices. Front. Physiol. (2018). https://doi.org/10.3389/fphys.2018.00778
10. Kairouz, P., et al.: Advances and open problems in federated learning. arXiv:1912.04977 (2019)
11. Xu, D.L., et al.: Edge intelligence: architectures, challenges, and applications. arXiv:2003.12172 (2020)
12. McMahan, B., Moore, E., Ramage, D., Hampson, S., Arcas, B.A.: Communication-efficient learning of deep networks from decentralized data. In: Proceedings of the 20th International Conference on Artificial Intelligence and Statistics, pp. 1273–1282 (2017)
13. Smith, V., Chiang, C.K., Sanjabi, M., Talwalkar, A.S.: Federated multi-task learning. In: NIPS 2017, Long Beach, CA, USA, pp. 4424–4434 (2017)
14. Lian, X., Zhang, C., Zhang, H., Hsieh, C.J., Zhang, W., Liu, J.: Can decentralized algorithms outperform centralized algorithms? A case study for decentralized parallel stochastic gradient descent. In: Advances in Neural Information Processing Systems, vol. 30, pp. 5330–5340 (2017)
15. Dean, J., et al.: Large scale distributed deep networks. In: Advances in Neural Information Processing Systems, vol. 25, pp. 1223–1231 (2012)
16. Chen, Y., Qin, X., Wang, J., Yu, C., Gao, W.: FedHealth: a federated transfer learning framework for wearable healthcare. IEEE Intell. Syst. **35**(4), 83–93 (2020)
17. Yurochkin, M., Agarwal, M., Ghosh, S., Greenewald, K., Hoang, N., Khazaeni, Y.: Bayesian nonparametric federated learning of neural networks. In: PMLR, vol. 97, pp. 7252–7261 (2019)
18. Gelman, A., Carlin, J.B., Stern, H.S., Dunson, D.B., Vehtari, A., Rubin, D.B.: Bayesian Data Analysis. CRC Press, Boca Raton (2013)
19. Wei, G.C., Tanner, M.A.: A Monte Carlo implementation of the EM algorithm and the poor man's data augmentation algorithms. J. Am. Stat. Assoc. **85**(411), 699–704 (1990)
20. Minka, T.P.: Estimating a gamma distribution. Technical report, Microsoft Research, Cambridge, UK (2002)

Health Telemetry and Platforms

A Home-Based Self-administered Assessment of Neck Proprioception

Angelo Basteris(✉) ⓘ, Charlotte Egeskov Tornbjerg, Fredcrikke Birkeholm Leth, and Uffe Kock Wiil ⓘ

Health Informatics and Technology Center, SDU HIT, Mærsk McKinney Møllier Institute, Faculty of Engineering, University of Southern Denmark, 5230 Odense, Denmark
angelobasteris@gmail.com

Abstract. Proprioception is fundamental for maintaining balance and moving-hence for daily living. As proprioception deficits may occur with aging, neurological and musculoskeletal (especially cervical) conditions, assessment of proprioception can be relevant for a very large cohort of individuals.

We designed a web page that allows measuring the neck joint position sense while sitting in front of a standard webcam. The web page tracks the subjects' head movement and instructs them on how to perform a head repositioning accuracy protocol. We performed a test retest analysis of this tool in order to assess its feasibility and reliability. Eleven healthy subjects participated in two sessions over consecutive days, at their homes. We calculated average errors across four directions Bland-Altman level of agreement between the measurements on the two sessions.

All participants could complete the test in approximately six minutes. The average absolute error did not differ between the two sessions, showing close to zero bias and a 95% limit of agreement of 1.676°. These values changed significantly across directions, suggesting that the performance of the head tracking software for neck flexion movements may be limited.

By comparing our results with normative values, we suggest that the narrow limit of agreement we observed makes the web page potentially capable of distinguishing healthy subjects from subjects with proprioceptive deficit in the neck joint.

Keywords: eHealth · Movement analysis · Proprioception

1 Introduction

Neck pain is a highly prevalent condition, as it is estimated that 37% of people worldwide will experience neck pain at least once a year [1]. Not only it already is very common, but due to population growth and aging it is expected to become even more relevant in the next future [2]. The burden of neck pain worldwide is heavy both in terms of disability [3] and economically [4].

© ICST Institute for Computer Sciences, Social Informatics and Telecommunications Engineering 2021
Published by Springer Nature Switzerland AG 2021. All Rights Reserved
J. Ye et al. (Eds.): MobiHealth 2020, LNICST 362, pp. 133–144, 2021.
https://doi.org/10.1007/978-3-030-70569-5_9

A coarse classification of neck pain can be made based on whether it is of known (specific) or unknown (idiopathic) non-traumatic origin, or it is trauma-induced [5].

Regardless of the cause of neck pain, loss of proprioception (*"the sense of one's own body"*) is a symptom frequently associated with conditions which affect the neck joint. Also, aging is frequently associated with a progressive loss for vestibular function [6].

As proprioceptive deficits significantly impact quality of living, it is not surprising that several methods have been developed for assessment of cervical Joint Position Sense (JPS). The standard to measure JPS in clinical practice is to place a headband with a laser pointer on top of the person's head, in order to observe the errors–as distance of the laser dot from the center of a target placed in front of the person – when he/she moves the head back to the central position [7] after an either passive or active movement of the neck. However, this simple method is time-consuming as it requires a trained person to administer the test.

Technology has come into help for measuring JPS with systems which have so far been used mostly in research facilities. Proprioceptive assessment can be done with electrogoniometers [8], electromagnetic trackers [9] and optoelectronic systems [10]. Unsurprisingly, a more recent technology like VR head mounted displays have been used to monitor head stability [11]. Notably, all these systems require dedicated hardware, and this may limit accessibility to these methods. Moreover, all of these systems also require the subject to wear some equipment – with consequent burdens in terms of comfort and hygiene.

We previously proposed the use of webcam-based head tracking to measure JPS [12]. Our method showed that results in neurologically intact individuals who participated in a lab-based session under the supervision of a researcher were comparable to normative values described in literature. In this work, we aim at evaluating the feasibility and the reliability of remote unsupervised measurement of neck JPS.

2 Methods

2.1 Task

The task consisted in an active-active neck joint position sense test. The participant was asked to sit still and look straight ahead. Each repetition consisted of five phases. Transition between phases occurred based on subject's movement or actions (click).

1) *Initial.* The neutral, starting position acquired when the participant clicks, at the beginning of the session, is acquired as the reference (target) position with respect to which errors are calculated.
2) *Outward movement.* Once the target position is set by clicking, the participant is asked to close the eyes (so that the task relies only on his/her proprioception, and no visual information is used) and to move the head, as far as possible, in one of four possible neck movement directions (extension, flexion, right and left rotation)
3) *Matching.* The subject moves the head to return to the neutral position, trying to match it as accurately as possible. He/she confirms the response (*final position*) by clicking.

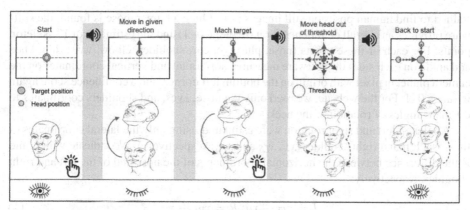

Fig. 1. Each repetition of a JPS measurement articulates in 5 phases: initial, outward movement, matching, distraction and return to center

4) *Distraction.* Once the final position was confirmed, the participants was asked to move the head for an amplitude of at least approximately 5°, still with the eyes closed; in this way, no feedback was provided before
5) *Return to center.* The subject can open the eyes and return to the target position (by aligning a cursor showing the head angles on the screen) in preparation for the next repetition.

2.2 Experimental Protocol

A convenience sample of eleven neurologically intact volunteers (5M/6F, age: 23 ± 1) participated in this study. A restricted access web page was set up, and participants were recruited through referral among peers. Information about this study, including instructions on how to take part in the experiment, and informed consent were provided and acquired through the same website.

Participants accessed the website without any supervision, from their homes and using their laptops. They were requested to place the camera at eye level in front of their eyes and they were instructed to repeat the test on two consecutive days, at the same time of the day. On each day, each participant performed a total of 28 repetitions (7 in each of the 4 directions) in a pseudo-randomized order. For each day, the first four repetitions (one per direction) were considered as familiarization and discarded from further analysis. Participants did not receive any feedback about their performance upon completion of the first session, while a graph showing the final positions on day 2 was display at the end of the second session.

2.3 Head Tracking Software

While the standard, responsive webpage was created using standard HTML and JavaScript code, the core of the functionality for proprioceptive assessment (i.e. movement analysis) was implemented using PoseNet [13]. PoseNet is a community supported library for markerless skeleton tracking. The library is built on top of TensorFlow models trained to find human poses on still images [14]. Once a human pose is found, the software provides an overall confidence for it (in range 0–1) and the estimates of 17 skeleton points. For each of these points (nose, plus eye, ear, shoulder, elbow, wrist, hip, knee and ankle on each side) the software measures horizontal and vertical coordinates on the camera plane, in pixel with origin on the bottom left corner, and a confidence score again in range 0–1. For the website, we used only the nose, eyes, and shoulders coordinates to estimate angles of rotation of the neck.

Angles of left and right rotation were estimated using only the lateral coordinates of the nose, left and right shoulder (x_N, x_{LS} and x_{RS}, respectively). We indicate with L and R the difference between the horizontal coordinates of the nose and of the left and right shoulder, respectively:

$$L = x_{LS} - x_N; R = x_{RS} - x_N \qquad (1)$$

Assuming that the subject is facing the camera and looking straight at it, these distances will be equal and opposite in sign ($L = -R$). Leftwards rotation causes L to decrease and R to increase, while rightward rotation provokes an opposite increase in L and decrease in R. We thus estimated angle of lateral rotation of the head as

$$\theta_L = +45 - \arctan\frac{L}{R} \qquad (2)$$

causing $\theta_L = 0°$ in the reference position and $\theta_L > 0$ for rightward rotations.

We estimated neck flexion/extension movements by using the nose, left and right shoulders vertical coordinates (y_N, y_{LS} and y_{RS}, respectively). Let E be the vertical coordinate of the midpoint between the eyes:

$$E = \frac{y_{LE} + y_{RE}}{2} \qquad (3)$$

and D_0 the value of E when the subject is facing the camera, in the initial position. As the subject turns the head downwards, the value of E decreases (that is, the projection of the eyes on the camera plane appear closer to the projection of the nose than in the initial position), while upwards rotation likewise cause an increase of E. We thus estimated angle of vertical rotation of the head as

$$\theta_V = -45 - \arctan\frac{y_N - E}{D_0} \qquad (4)$$

causing $\theta_V = 0°$ in the reference target position and $\theta_V > 0$ for neck extension.

2.4 Data Analysis

For each repetition, the software measured the absolute error and the constant error (absolute value and value of the difference between final and target position). We retained only the angle θ_L after lateral rotations and only θ_V after vertical movements, so that movements off the main movement axis were not accounted for in the error amplitude. We calculated the absolute error for each subject, direction and session as median value of the six repetitions, and the average of the four values as an indication of subject's accuracy. We compared the time taken to complete the experiment and the absolute error for each day by a paired samples t-test.

We also performed a Bland-Altman analysis to establish the bias and the level of agreement for the head tracking software across the two days [15]. The Bland-Altman method reveals systematic differences between two measurements and the limit of agreement represent the 95% confidence interval due to random fluctuations of the measurement method. We repeated the same Bland-Altman analysis were repeated on the median values in each of the four directions, in order to understand whether reliability of the proposed software method differed across movement direction.

3 Results

3.1 Test Duration

Figure 2 displays the duration of the test for each subject on both days. On the first day, subjects could complete the test in an average of 400 s (range: 312–520 s). On the second day, it took all subjects a lower time to perform the same test (p < .001), with an average duration of 312 s (range: 240–366 s).

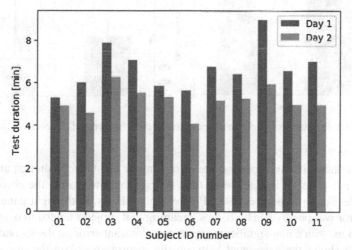

Fig. 2. Time taken to complete the full test (28 repetitions) by each subject on two consecutive days

3.2 Absolute Error – All Directions

Figure 3 shows the average error for each subject on both days. Subject 11 showed errors higher than the average of the other participants (three to four times higher) and his data were than excluded from further analysis.

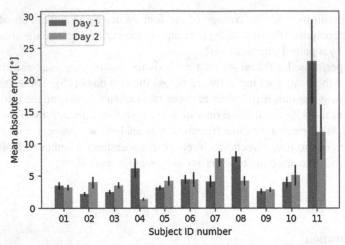

Fig. 3. Mean absolute error for each subject, on both days. The mean value was calculated among the four median values (one per direction) among six repetitions. Errorbars represent the standard error of the mean.

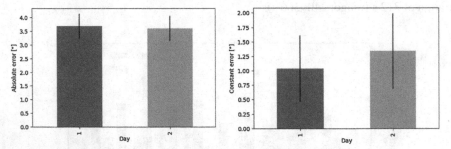

Fig. 4. Average absolute error (left panel) and constant error (right panel) for each day, all subjects.

Figure 4 shows the average absolute error (among all subjects) on first and second day, in the left panel. It is noteworthy that, despite the lower time, the absolute error did not differ across days (p = 0.95). Figure 4 also shows, in the right panel, that the constant error was positive on both days, meaning that subjects tended to overshoot the target position, with a non-significant increase in constant error on the second day.

Figure 5 shows the agreement between the measurements on the two days. The method was proven to have very low bias (0.079°) and a 95% level of agreement interval of 1.676° (range between −1.597° and 1.755°).

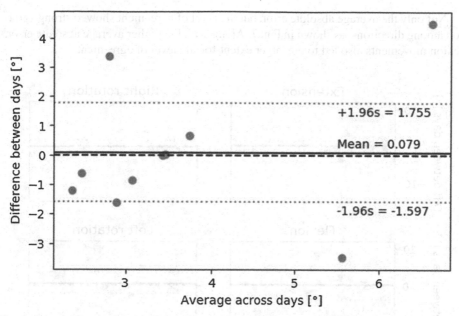

Fig. 5. Bland-Altman plot showing 95% level of agreement between repeated measures of neck JPS

3.3 Effect of Movement Direction on Absolute Error

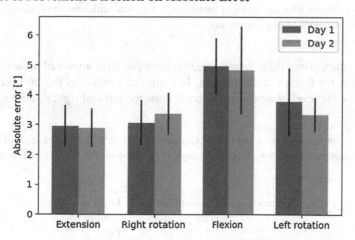

Fig. 6. Average error for all subjects after each of the four movement directions.

Errorbars represent the standard error of the mean.

Figure 6 shows the average error on both days, for each direction. While no significant changes were observed among days, our results show higher error when trying to match the target position after returning from flexion movement. Also, it is noteworthy left rotation movements led to slightly higher error than right rotation.

Not only the average absolute error, but the level of agreement showed strong variation among directions, as shown in Fig. 7. Along with the higher average absolute error, flexion movements also led to the larger extent for the level of agreement.

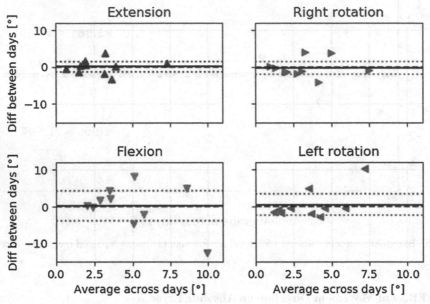

Fig. 7. Bland-Altman plot for repeated measures across four different directions, all subjects. Dashed lines mark 95% level of agreement.

Table 1 summarizes these results: the bias between days appeared higher for lateral rotations than for flexion and extension. In a similar fashion as the average absolute error, also the the level of agreement differed between left and right rotations.

Table 1. Average absolute error and Bland-Altman bias and 95% confidence level of agreement between measurements on two consecutive days after movement in each of the four different directions.

Direction	Absolute error [°]	Bias [°]	Level of agreement [°]
Extension	2.91	0.057	1.387
Flexion	4.89	0.135	4.14
Right rotation	3.21	−0.301	1.791
Left rotation	3.55	0.427	2.877

4 Discussion

4.1 Feasibility of Self Administered Assessment of Neck Proprioception.

Our results prove the feasibility of a home-based, self-administered assessment of the neck joint position sense. Previous work using hardware compatible with a home environment included gaming devices like the WiiMote [16], and it was also suggested that a 3D camera could be used for postural assessment [17]. Unfortunately, these devices are not available to many users. A more inclusive solution is the use of smartphone for vestibular rehabilitation [18]. However, our solution only relies on the availability of a webcam, and it is thus potentially available to any user of a standard laptop or smartphone. Also, the same solution can be easily adapted to measure proprioception of the other body joints (i.e. shoulder, elbow, knee) already tracked by the skeleton tracking software used in this study.

The subjects participated in tests from their homes, without any live interaction with the researchers. They only received an email with the information sheet and instructions about their participation, and they were then guided by the website by means of voice guidance provided through speech synthesis, during the test. This potentially saves work hours from the healthcare professionals, who can then dedicate their time to treat patients, and resources for unnecessary travels for the patients. Of the 11 subjects who participated in this study, only one (subject 11) showed abnormal values on both days. It is possible that the instructions were somehow not clear to this participant, but as no information about the participants', other than the results of their tests was recorded, it is no possible to ascertain the reason for this exceptionally high values.

The test proven to be quick to be performed, as all the subjects could complete it in less than 9 min, with an average of 400 s on the first day. The fact that on the second day all participants could perform within a smaller duration suggests that there is some familiarization with the test. However, the similarity of results across the two days, also considering that no feedback was provided, reduces the concerns raised by this familiarization.

4.2 Test-Retest Reliability of the Proposed Method and Implications for Diagnostic Value

The average absolute error across the two days was $3.64 \pm 2.62°$, with a small change $(0.08°)$ between the two days, and a 95% level of agreement of $1.676°$. The average value is comparable with the values reported by other studies which used conventional methods for using the neck JPS. There are indeed two other studies reporting $3.6°$ as the average absolute error for healthy subjects [19, 20]. Armstrong et al. reported $3.25 \pm 2.32°$ as absolute error for healthy subjects [8] when averaging all movement directions, while Revel et al. had previously suggested $3.50 \pm 0.82°$ for lateral rotations and $3.37 \pm 0.73°$.

A review about evidence of impaired proprioception in chronic idiopathic neck pain considered 10 studies, indicating a absolute difference in error between people with chronic neck pain and healthy controls ranging from 0.1 to 3.0 [21]. As the extent of our level of agreement falls within this range, our test may be reliable enough to distinguish between people with chronic neck pain and healthy individuals, with potential diagnostic value – that needs however to be assessed in a specific study.

4.3 Effect of Direction on Average Error and Test-Retest Reliability

Our system performed differently along movement directions. It is important to stress that our system estimated the rotation angles based on the method described in Sect. 2.3 (Eq. 2 and 4). Concerning lateral rotations, there was a small difference between left and right rotations. However, the amplitude of such difference is compatible with those reported by a number of other studies (e.g. 0.3 [10]) and may be affected as an instance by subjects' handedness [22]. The high difference in level of agreement between the two lateral directions may be a consequence of the low number of subjects who participated in this study.

We found a high difference between errors after flexion and extension movement, with higher errors after flexion. Also, the level of agreement for the former was approximately three times higher than for the latter. These results may be a consequence by factors that we could not control for, in particular, the camera positioning. If the camera was placed below the participants' head, the misalignment between the camera optics and the head's rotation axis would have caused errors in the vertical angle estimation. We rely that this may have been the case, especially if subjects performed the test using a standard laptop and did not follow the instructions of facing the camera directly. Further studies may use the position of the shoulders– as it was successfully done for the lateral angle - also for estimating the vertical angle.

4.4 Limitations of This Study

This study involved only young healthy individuals (average age 23 years). A population with higher age range may show a significantly higher absolute error, and possibly altering the level of agreement. Also, the head tracking system is not yet validated against a gold standard, which would provide estimates of its precision in tracking the head movement.

5 Conclusions

Our results prove that a webcam-based face tracking system can be used for a remote, unsupervised assessment of proprioception. This will allow people with neck pain to monitor their performance in proprioceptive tests at home, without the supervision of a healthcare professional.

The good level of agreement observed in this study between measurements on two consecutive days on healthy individuals suggests that the tool has good reliability, especially after extension, left and right rotation movements – while results after flexion movements require further testing.

The level of agreement found in this study - lower than differences in JPS error between healthy individuals and people with neck pain reported in literature – supports future studies aimed at establishing the diagnostic value of this tool by comparing results in populations with and without proprioceptive impairment.

References

1. Haldeman, S., Carroll, L., Cassidy, J.D.: Findings from the bone and joint decade 2000 to 2010 task force on neck pain and its associated disorders. J. Occup. Environ. Med. **52**(4), 424–427 (2010). https://doi.org/10.1097/JOM.0b013e3181d44f3b
2. Hoy, D., et al.: The global burden of neck pain: estimates from the global burden of Disease 2010 study. Ann. Rheum. Dis. **73**, 1309–1315 (2014). https://doi.org/10.1136/annrheumdis-2013-204431
3. Vos, T., et al.: Years lived with disability (YLDs) for 1160 sequelae of 289 diseases and injuries 1990–2010: a systematic analysis for the global burden of Disease Study 2010. Lancet **380**, 2163–2196 (2012). https://doi.org/10.1016/S0140-6736(12)61729-2
4. Childs, J.D. et al.: Neck pain: clinical practice guidelines linked to the international classification of functioning, disability, and health from the orthopaedic section of the American physical therapy association. J. Orthop. Sports Phys. Therapy. **38**(9), A1–A34 (2008) https://pubmed.ncbi.nlm.nih.gov/18758050/. https://doi.org/10.2519/jospt.2008.0303
5. Coppieters, I., et al.: Differences between women with traumatic and idiopathic chronic neck pain and women without neck pain: interrelationships among disability, cognitive deficits, and central sensitization. Phys. Ther. **97**, 338–353 (2017). https://doi.org/10.2522/ptj.20160259
6. Eibling, D.: Balance disorders in older adults. Clin. Geriatr. Med. **34**(2), 175–181 (2018) https://pubmed.ncbi.nlm.nih.gov/29661330/. https://doi.org/10.1016/j.cger.2018.01.002.
7. Clark, N.C., Röijezon, U., Treleaven, J.: Proprioception in musculoskeletal rehabilitation. Part 2: clinical assessment and intervention. Man. Ther. **20**, 378–387 (2015). https://doi.org/10.1016/j.math.2015.01.009
8. Armstrong, B.S., McNair, P.J., Williams, M.: Head and neck position sense in whiplash patients and healthy individuals and the effect of the cranio-cervical flexion action. Clin. Biomech. **20**, 675–684 (2005). https://doi.org/10.1016/j.clinbiomech.2005.03.009
9. Cheng, C.H., Wang, J.L., Lin, J.J., Wang, S.F., Lin, K.H.: Position accuracy and electromyographic responses during head reposition in young adults with chronic neck pain. J. Electromyogr. Kinesiol. **20**, 1014–1020 (2010). https://doi.org/10.1016/j.jelekin.2009.11.002
10. Grip, H., Sundelin, G., Gerdle, B., Karlsson, J.S.: Variations in the axis of motion during head repositioning–a comparison of subjects with whiplash-associated disorders or non-specific neck pain and healthy controls. Clin. Biomech. **22**, 865–873 (2007). https://doi.org/10.1016/j.clinbiomech.2007.05.008
11. Lubetzky, A.V., Hujsak, B.D.: A virtual reality head stability test for patients with vestibular dysfunction. J. Vestib. Res. Equilib. Orientat. **28**, 393–400 (2019). https://doi.org/10.3233/VES-190650
12. Basteris, A., Pedler, A., Sterling, M.: Evaluating the neck joint position sense error with a standard computer and a webcam. Manual Therapy **26**, 231–234 (2016). https://doi.org/10.1016/j.math.2016.04.008
13. Clark, R.A., Mentiplay, B.F., Hough, E., Pua, Y.H.: Three-dimensional cameras and skeleton pose tracking for physical function assessment: a review of uses, validity, current developments and Kinect alternatives. Gait Posture. **68**, 193–200 (2019). https://doi.org/10.1016/j.gaitpost.2018.11.029
14. Smilkov, D., et al.: TensorFlow.js: machine learning for the web and beyond (2019)
15. Bland, J.M., Altman, D.G.: Statistical methods for assessing agreement between two methods of clinical measurement. Lancet **1**, 307–310 (1986)
16. Chen, P.Y., Hsieh, W.L., Wei, S.H., Kao, C.L.: Interactive wiimote gaze stabilization exercise training system for patients with vestibular hypofunction. J. Neuroeng. Rehabil. **9**(1), 1–10 (2012). https://doi.org/10.1186/1743-0003-9-77

17. Placidi, G., et al.: A low-cost real time virtual system for postural stability assessment at home. Comput. Methods Programs Biomed. **117**, 322–333 (2014). https://doi.org/10.1016/j.cmpb.2014.06.020
18. Nehrujee, A., Vasanthan, L., Lepcha, A., Balasubramanian, S.: A Smartphone-based gaming system for vestibular rehabilitation: a usability study. J. Vestib. Res. Equilib. Orientat. **29**, 147–160 (2019). https://doi.org/10.3233/VES-190660
19. Palmgren, P.J., Andreasson, D., Eriksson, M., Hägglund, A.: Cervicocephalic kinesthetic sensibility and postural balance in patients with nontraumatic chronic neck pain - a pilot study. Chiropr. Osteopat. **17**, 6 (2009). https://doi.org/10.1186/1746-1340-17-6
20. Uthaikhup, S., Jull, G., Sungkarat, S., Treleaven, J.: The influence of neck pain on sensorimotor function in the elderly. Arch. Gerontol. Geriatr. **55**, 667–672 (2012). https://doi.org/10.1016/j.archger.2012.01.013
21. Stanton, T.R., Leake, H.B., Chalmers, K.J., Moseley, G.L.: Evidence of impaired proprioception in chronic, idiopathic neck pain: systematic review and meta-analysis. Phys. Ther. **96**, 876–887 (2016). https://doi.org/10.2522/ptj.20150241
22. Dempsey-Jones, H., Kritikos, A.: Handedness modulates proprioceptive drift in the rubber hand illusion. Exp. Brain Res. **237**(2), 351–361 (2018). https://doi.org/10.1007/s00221-018-5391-3

Health Telescope: System Design for Longitudinal Data Collection Using Mobile Applications

Bas Willemse[1,2,3](✉), Maurits Kaptein[1,2,3], Nikolaos Batalas[3,4], and Fleur Hasaart[5]

[1] Jheronimus Academy of Data Science, 's-Hertogenbosch, The Netherlands
[2] Eindhoven University, Eindhoven, The Netherlands
[3] Tilburg University, Tilburg, The Netherlands
{b.j.p.c.willemse,m.c.kaptein}@tilburguniversity.edu,
nikolaos.batalas@gmail.com
[4] RoboticBit, Eindhoven, The Netherlands
[5] CZ Zorgverzekeraars, Tilburg, The Netherlands
fleur.hasaart@cz.nl

Abstract. This paper describes the process of developing the technical infrastructure of the Health Telescope: an interventional panel study designed to measure the long term effects of eHealth usage. We describe the design and implementation of both the Health Telescope application—an Android application that allows us to interact with participants and obtain measurements—and the researcher authoring client—a web-based application that allows us to flexibly submit experience sampling tasks to participants. This paper serves as a blueprint for those wanting to study long-term behavioral change in the wild. The paper furthermore describes a pilot study that was conducted to evaluate the research software. We conclude with design guidelines aimed at those aiming to undertake a similar endeavor that are vital when developing similar software; this paper aims to highlight both the importance and challenges of measuring the effects of eHealth applications longitudinally.

Keywords: eHealth · mHealth · Longitudinal data collection · Interventional panel study · Wearable research · Technical guidelines

1 Introduction

Physical activity has decreased globally over the last 50 years [14]. In parallel, the last 50 years have brought forth a lot of research on health and physical activity. Given the developments in recent years, with new technological advances such as smartphones, wearable bands, smart scales, and many other examples entering the consumer market, we can now analyze health behaviors at an unprecedented level by generating high amounts of data on activity and physical health.

© ICST Institute for Computer Sciences, Social Informatics and Telecommunications Engineering 2021
Published by Springer Nature Switzerland AG 2021. All Rights Reserved
J. Ye et al. (Eds.): MobiHealth 2020, LNICST 362, pp. 145–165, 2021.
https://doi.org/10.1007/978-3-030-70569-5_10

However, research utilizing modern technology like cellphones and activity trackers still has some challenges: for one, long-term engagement with this technology has proven challenging [8,24]. The accuracy of devices is often inconsistent [6] and not validated [15]. Measuring the effects of usage may stretch beyond simply measuring step count for some period of time, and changes in health behaviors are made in different ways. These factors, among others, make it hard to conduct large-scale longitudinal research using activity trackers to measure participant physical activity. Furthermore, developing the technical infrastructure for such research can be challenging, as the technologies used are complex.

This paper describes the development of the system design and technical implementation of the Health Telescope, an interventional longitudinal study investigating the effects of eHealth app usage. With this paper, we aim to show the process through which the technical infrastructure for the Health Telescope project was developed. The paper covers the thoughts going into building the system, the details of the architecture, the evaluation process, done through a pilot study, followed by the improvements made after receiving feedback. These details on the development process may be interesting for readers trying to set up longitudinal research using mobile phones to generate data, or to communicate to participants. It can also be informative for researchers interested in using data generated in the project.

In the Health Telescope study, we measure the activity and mood of $N = 450$ participants for a minimum of four months. During this time, participants will be monitored and recommended to download existing applications for health behavior change. This study is significant for the field of eHealth for the following three reasons: (i) carrying out intensive longitudinal research contributes to helping the general understanding of the effects of eHealth application usage, as well as health behavior change; (ii) uncertainty exists regarding how to fully capture the effects of eHealth apps, in this study a broad range of information such as daily activity, sleep, mood, and phone usage is collected, allowing a unique, detailed look into the effects of usage of the apps distributed in the study; (iii) different approaches for health behavior change can help different users. In the study, we will experiment with personalization of eHealth app allocation: by prescribing different applications to different users, we aim to learn if an eHealth app is more effective for users with certain characteristics (i.e. "elderly women", "20-year olds that wake up at 6 am", "participants that make intense use of their smartphone"). We can then test these hypotheses by recommending the applications to users with similar characteristics. The study objectives are further detailed in Sect. 2. A detailed setup for the study can be found in [26].

The remainder of this paper is structured as follows: the paper starts by introducing the background, objectives and architecture of the Health Telescope Project (Sect. 2); then, the implementation of the system created for the study is described (Sect. 3). Next, we show how the system usage allows us to accomplish use cases (Sect. 4). We furthermore expand on a pilot that was used to evaluate and improve the system (Sect. 5) and close off by discussing improvements and related work, as well as describing a set of guidelines following our development process (Sect. 6).

2 The Health Telescope Software

The infrastructure described in the paper was created as part of the Health Telescope project. The project goals inspired us to build an infrastructure that can communicate with study participants' cellphones, and capture behavioral data like step count and phone usage to investigate the effects of using eHealth applications. In this section, we briefly discuss the Health Telescope project, listing its goals and motivations. We do so to show the rationale behind the development process and infrastructure that we discuss in the remainder of the paper. Additionally, we describe the requirements that implementations will need to satisfy. We first do this through sketching the data flow needed for the project, followed up by use cases that help make the details of the architecture concrete.

2.1 Study Objectives

The system is designed as part of the Health Telescope project, an interventional panel study measuring activity data using wearables. The objectives of this project are as follows:

- O_1. We aim to investigate the effect of using eHealth apps focused on increasing physical activity on activity and mood, for a long period,
- O_2. We want to see if there is a correlated effect between short-term measures and long-term measures after interacting with eHealth apps,
- O_3. We want to test different ways of personalizing eHealth offerings.

To effectively accomplish these objectives, we chose to not simply design or test a single app, but instead investigate how individuals respond to existing eHealth apps that focus on different, distinct persuasive elements. We will recommend study participants different, existing eHealth applications that all focus on improving physical activity, using different behavioral change techniques. For more information on the reasoning and design of the study, we refer to our study protocol [26].

2.2 System Architecture

To enable the goals of the Health Telescope project, we developed a system that allows a researcher to directly communicate to study participants, through a mobile app, as well as have that app transfer data generated by participants to the researcher. The architecture for this system has been largely inspired by a previous application for conducting event and signal contingent experience sampling studies, TEMPEST [11]. Like TEMPEST, the Health Telescope architecture consists of 3 software components:

- A mobile application for the Android OS, available to participants via Google play store, which collects data in the background on app usage and location from the phone, and steps, activity, and heart rate from the wristband. It also receives and renders content as produced by the researchers, such as questionnaires or cloud messages.
- An authoring web application, to be used by the researchers for creating content and managing its distribution to the participants in the study.
- A server that stores content and collected data in a database, and allows information to be shared between the authoring web application and the mobile application.

2.3   Considerations in Developing the System

We intend to create an application that serves as an observer app: that is, it gathers data relevant to the study from a user's phone, and transfers it to the database. The Health Telescope app is meant to a) transfer wearable and phone data to the database, and b) help evaluate existing apps. Importantly, the purpose of the app is not to function as a behavior change app in itself. Instead, we would like to use the app to observe how active users are before, during and after using eHealth apps that will be recommended to them during the study. To accomplish this, focus is put on making sure communication and data transmission happen correctly, not on experimenting with incentivizing activity or ways of engaging participants.

To ensure that the system can perform the tasks required to accomplish the study goals, we used use cases as a measure of internal testing during development [7]. These use cases resemble queries that need to be run during the study. The value of use cases shows in two different stages of development: a concrete, step-by-step plan on how the system should function can help during implementation by showing explicit restrictions that the system will need to uphold. During evaluation, each action in a use case can be tested to effectively isolate and communicate about existing flaws in the software. We expand further on use cases by giving two examples in Sect. 4 as a way of demonstrating the system's flexibility, as well providing detail on our evaluation process.

3   Implementation of the System

In this section, we discuss the framework that was created for the project. Below, we will detail the structure and interactions of the mobile app and authoring client.

3.1   Mobile Application

The goals of the Health Telescope application are:

1. To serve as a tool for users to self-report on their mood;

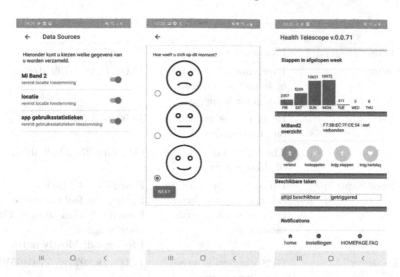

Fig. 1. Screenshots from the Health Telescope application. The first panel shows the privacy configuration for data collection, the second panel shows an example of a questionnaire loaded in the app, and the third panel shows the home screen, displaying the daily step counts, a wearable connection menu, and a notifications bar.

2. To gather GPS and phone usage data;
3. To collect sensor data from the wearable band, visually display this data, and transmit collected data to our servers;
4. To deliver interventions to participants; and
5. To monitor participant engagement.

The Health Telescope application is designed as a tool to observe participant behavior closely, without requiring active effort from participants. The data collection is completely passive, excluding the participant's self-reporting on mood, which is also designed to minimize the strain by making short multiple-choice questions. Figure 1 shows screenshots of different parts of the Health Telescope Application.

Data. The Health Telescope application collects a total of **six** different types of data: step count, heart rate, sleep, experience sampling, GPS location, and phone usage. Examples of these data can be seen in Table 1. We employ Experience Sampling as a tool for participants to self-assess how they are feeling throughout the week. To capture this, we investigated different constructs, such as wellbeing [17], happiness [21], and mood [28]. Out of these options, we chose mood and happiness. Mood is a construct chosen for its day-to-day variance, displaying direct effects of events happening in the life of participants. Different ways of evaluating mood exist, and one commonly used dichotomy fundamentally separates this mood into *valence* (the intrinsic attractiveness or aversiveness of the mood) and *activity/arousal* (expressing the calm or exciting nature of the mood) [5].

Table 1. Summary of data used in the Health Telescope

Data Type	Frequency	Example
Step Count	Every hour, the number of steps taken during that hour is measured	14.00–15.00 - 739 steps
Heart rate	Heart rate is measured on one hour intervals	14.00 - 73 bpm
Sleep Data	The start and end time of sleep are measured	February 23: 23:16–07:12
Experience Sampling	Up to once per day, we ask participants brief questions using push messages	February 23 14:00: I generally feel energetic: Yes I currently feel happy: Completely agree I feel good: Mostly agree
GPS Location	GPS location is saved every four hours	14:00: 38.8977N, 77.0365W
Phone Usage	We measure screen time and usage of applications on participants' mobile phones. Note: We only measure the duration of use, and do not in any way measure what happens within an application	Chrome: 14:03–14:04 Facebook: 14:04–14:17 Messages: 14:23–14:25 Mail: 14:25–14:37

Most existing surveys measuring mood in this way consist of 10–30 questions. Given our setup, it seems infeasible to regularly ask participants this many questions: participant burden is a large factor of dropout in longitudinal studies and questionnaires are lengthy. As a result, we directly ask for the underlying constructs of the questionnaires: one question asks participants about *activity*, one question asks participants about *valence*. A third question measures happiness using a three-point smiley face question, with a face for sad, neutral, and happy.

Technical Implementation. The mobile application is a hybrid of a web-based component and a native android component. The web-based component is an Ionic/Angular app, which renders the User Interface and also renders the questionnaires or other documents created by the researchers. The user interface consists of two major parts; one is a setup guide, for allow participants to log in and manage their system account, provide necessary permissions for data collection and pair their wristband with the phone; the other is the main screen which displays documents available for access, as well as an Inbox screen for notifications received so far. Notifications are Firebase cloud-messages that can consist of a single message body, but can also have documents attached. All documents in this environment can be any HTML/JavaScript content, which gives researchers the freedom to serve rich styling and interactions according to the needs of the study as it develops.

The native android component is tasked with downloading configuration and content created by the researchers, setting alarms for signal-contingent experience sampling, receiving Firebase cloud messages, collecting app usage statistics and location data, and connecting to the wristband via Bluetooth for sampling step count, activity data, and heart rate. Data is stored in the phone's SQLite3 database and is only uploaded to the server at opportune moments, as decided by the android OS's facilities for managing communications and power consumption. Additionally, Firebase cloud messages are not only notifications to be presented to the users but also commands to the application itself. This allows researchers to remotely control functions of the application, such as forcing the downloading of a new configuration, or the uploading of collected data.

3.2 Authoring Client

The authoring client is designed as a tool for researchers to carry out experiments. It accomplishes this goal by providing a simple interface for researchers to a) monitor enrolment and participant engagement; b) conduct experiments by setting up scheduled surveys and alerts; c) communicate to participants. The authoring client groups allow researchers to set up the following:

Participants. The authoring client allows researchers to monitor participants in their activity and engagement with the panel. While participant data can be directly accessed from the database, the authoring client provides a visual interface tracking data transfer and daily activity. The authoring client provides control of participant creation and deletion in the database.

Documents. The authoring client allows researchers to design any kind of content using HTML and JavaScript to create and serve rich styling and interactions as the study progresses. Specifically for questionnaires though, the application allows their creation using custom web components, which can be read in the semantic terms of the questionnaire's content and computational logic rather than the syntactic features of their HTML structure. The motivation and method of the approach for this particular feature can be found in [11]. It provides a live preview of the documents to prepare (see Fig. 2).

Allocation and Rules. The authoring client allows researchers to assign documents to (groups of) participants, using *rules* and *allocations*. Rules specify the conditions under which a document should be available for participants, and allows for researchers to set moments for the phone to trigger. Rules can be "always available", or "time-triggered". We can use the 'always available' setting for documents that users will need to have the ability to fill in whenever they want, as often as they want (tracking water consumption is an application for this rule). Time triggered rules, on the other hand, can be used when users should respond up to once per day. After completion, a document shown with a time-triggered rule will be hidden until the next day.

Allocations are the glue that holds everything together: an allocation is a triplet connecting *rules* specifying a timeframe, to a *document* that will be available for a (group of) *participants*. After an allocation has been created, participants will be able to see a document in their task list to be filled in, as well as receiving a system notification that they have a new task available (see Fig. 4). After completing a task, it disappears from the home screen of the app.

Communication. Furthermore, the authoring app allows researchers to send cloud messages to participants. Cloud messages are flexible: they can be used to "silently" contact the phone or can make notifications appear in the participants' Android notification screen. Cloud messages can contain the following: (i) a simple message, containing a head and body; (ii) a prompt for the participant phone to upload its allocation, forcing a new allocation onto the phone; (iii) a prompt for the phone to sample sensor data (as described in Table 1) to the server; and (iv) a notification that has a document attached to it. Cloud messages that contain notifications are stored and available to view for participants in the Messages tab of the app. In our setup, we use cloud messages to deliver interventions.

Technical Implementation. The authoring web-application was built using the Ionic/Angular framework. The interface components that are available in the authoring client belong to two main categories: lists and editors. Lists correspond to database tables and display the rows for a particular entity, such as participants, documents, rules, etc. Editors allow the researcher to create new such entities or edit existing ones, and they are generally custom UI components that are tailored to the properties of each. Both lists and editors offer options for accessing other related entities, e.g. a group editor can be opened from a participant list because a listed participant might belong in that group.

4   Testing the Software: Use Cases

In this section, we will demonstrate the flexibility and ease of use of the described system, by going over two distinct use cases and displaying step-by-step how these use cases can be implemented in the system. The use cases are as follows:

– **Use case 1 - Questionnaire**: Set up a questionnaire that asks every participant in the panel three questions daily for the next three months between 11:00 and 20:00.
– **Use case 2 - Intervention**: Send out a cloud message containing advice to download an interventional application to participants that walked an average of less than 7000 steps per day for the last 30 days.

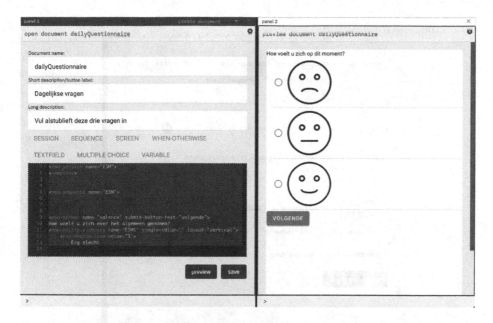

Fig. 2. Document creation interface. There are several pre-made buttons that create blocks of HTML code to create multiple-choice questions, create screen sequences, and more options. We are not limited to these pre-made buttons and could choose to manually insert other HTML. There is a live preview button, that renders the document in a separate pane.

4.1 Use Case 1 - Questionnaire

Here we describe how our system can be used to achieve the following steps:

1. Create a *document* in the authoring client to distribute to participants,
2. Select a *group* containing *participant* that will see the document,
3. Create a *rule* that makes this *document* appear within a time frame, and
4. Tie everything together by creating an *allocation*.

Figure 2 shows how a document can be created in the authoring client's *document creation* interface. On account creation, every new participant is added to the *'allParticipants'* group, containing the full set of participants, as part of the information sent from Google Scripts to the database.

Next, we create a rule that determines when the document is visible for participants. For this use case, we choose the latter, setting up a time-triggered rule. Here, we set the interval for the document to appear to 11:00–20:00, and enable the document for every day in the next three months.

After this, we have created the document we want to distribute, have chosen the time frame during which participants should see it, and have a group of participants that we would like to show the document to. To tie these three parts together, we set up the allocation by navigating to the *allocation creation*

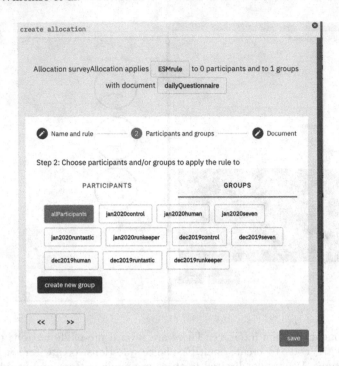

Fig. 3. Allocation creation interface in the authoring client. Researchers can use this to select documents to display for (groups of) users given some rule for when to show the content.

interface in the authoring client. The allocation interface (shown in Fig. 3) allows us to select the rule, participant, and document, which finalizes the use case. After taking these steps, every user will receive a notification, every day at 11:00, asking them to fill out a questionnaire.

4.2 Use Case 2 - Intervention

To complete this use case, we need to:

1. create a *group* of participants that will receive the intervention,
2. create a *document* containing the intervention, and
3. add the document to a *cloud message* that will be sent to the group of selected participants.

Use case 2 requires some work outside of the interface: we want to get to a point where we've identified the group of users that walk an average of fewer than 7000 steps per day, to feed this to the database. After this, we can create a *cloud message* with the advice, to send to this group. The first part of this can be done in any pre-made script, that connects to the database, selects the activity data for all participants for the last 30 days, then averages this out. From the

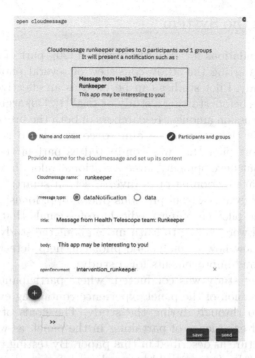

Fig. 4. Cloud message creation. Here, researchers can send notifications to participant cellphones, and specify the content for these notifications. There is a live preview of the notification at the top.

resulting list, select only the participants whose average activity is lower than 7.000 steps. Next, we add the IDs of these users that were insufficiently active to a group and use the database connection to create a new group in the database, containing this list of participants.

After these steps, the database contains the group of participants that will receive the intervention. We use the authoring client to create the cloud message. Cloud messages are messages appearing in the app's message box, that can be read back by users at any time. For this use case, we will attach a document to the notification, containing the intervention. We create this document in the same way we created the questionnaire in use case 1. Figure 4 shows how the message is given a title and body, that will appear to users as a notification, then add the document by selecting the key-value type openDocument, and selecting the earlier created message as our document. Then, we select the group that was created using the pre-made script as the receivers, and finally, we send the message. With this, the second use case has been completed.

5   Evaluating the System

Following recommendations for eHealth design in [20], part of the evaluation of the system before starting the study consisted of several pilot studies, testing elements of the study. Pilot studies can be used as an effective tool for testing experimental setups before starting a study or trial [1]. [30] argues that "There is a need for more discussion amongst researchers of both the process and outcomes of pilot studies". In this section, we aim to contribute to this discussion, by expanding on a short pilot that was conducted as part of the development of the app. Throughout development, three additional pilots have been held: one to test the technical functioning on a diverse set on smartphones; one to test the improved (after feedback from previous pilots) app, focusing mainly on user experience; and one pilot enrolling medical professionals that will be involved in recruitment, and were willing to learn more about the study by conducting a pilot. We aim to show how a small-scale pilot can help detect a wide range of necessary changes and improvements for a study.

A two-week pilot study was conducted, where participants were subjected to an accelerated version of the panel experience containing every element that participants will go through during the study. The goals of the pilot are to investigate the user experience of partaking in the panel, as well as testing the technical infrastructure as described in this paper. By testing the setup through a pilot, the developed software could be used on different phone configurations, and communication channels and data transfer can be validated. Below, we detail the design of the pilot, as well as providing a summary of the findings obtained in interviews that were held with pilot participants.

5.1   Pilot Design

The design for the pilot is as follows:

- **Intro survey.** Participants complete the introductory survey
- **Installation.** Participants download and install the application
- **Set-up.** Participants log into the app, set their data preferences, and set up the connection to the wearable
- **Daily survey.** Every morning, the participants receive a notification to fill in the three-question survey
- **Intervention I.** After three days, the participants receive a cloud message containing an app recommendation for an eHealth app
- **Intervention II.** After ten days, participants that have not installed the application recommended in Intervention I will receive another cloud message, containing a recommendation for a different health app

The pilot concludes with individual, semi-structured interviews with each participant. During this interview, we have specific points on which we would like to gather information. Section 5.2 expands on these points.

Technical Functioning. One of the main objectives of the pilot was to test the technical functioning of the system. The pilot was held briefly after the first version of the software was developed, and while the system was tested on multiple phones during development, the use of Bluetooth, connecting phone and wearable, can function slightly differently for different phones. It is difficult to comprehensively test Bluetooth functionality during the development of an app, as Android Studio's virtual machine can not utilize Bluetooth. As such, connectivity and stability testing during development were limited - increasing the value of a pilot.

There are several specific points that we were interested in seeing during and after the pilot. The general stability of the software on different phone and OS configurations; the quality of the data transfer from phone to database; the functioning of our cloud messages, that should send alerts to users; the content of the data generated being in the desired format; the connectivity and general use of the wearable.

Users install the app through a platform called TestFairy. This platform provides valuable information for testing and developing software, by e.g. providing crash reports that help isolate technical issues.

User Experience. The other main objective of the pilot was to improve the user experience, by having a set of participants undertake the same actions that participants of the study will. While the decreased duration of such an accelerated version of the study may influence the perceived strain of participation, we believe such an accelerated path can be used to effectively find possible issues in user experience.

The interviews conducted after the pilot contained questions regarding the ease of enrolment, the general use of the mobile application, experiences in using the wearable, perceived strain of participation, privacy, and quality of the information provided to participants.

5.2 Pilot Results

This section describes the results of the pilot. We begin by describing the participant set, and split our findings up in two parts: first the technical functioning of the software, which had just finished the first cycle of development; secondly the user experience of participating in the study. We summarize the findings from the interviews and include relevant participant quotes.

Respondents. Recruitment for the pilot happened through one of the largest health-insurance companies in the Netherlands, respondents were all employees of this company. Seven respondents expressed interest in participating in the pilot. Two participants were unable to join due to not having an Android phone. One respondent changed his/her mind and did not participate in the pilot. The final pilot group consisted of four participants, aged 34 on average

(SD = 6.76). All participants were male. The pilot took place in Tilburg, Noord-Brabant, the Netherlands. Participants were given the information letter and informed consent form before participation, as well as a letter explaining the process of the pilot. These documents can be found at https://health-telescope.com/documents/. Participants all used Android phones and were given a Xiaomi MiBand 2.

Technical Functioning. The findings from the pilot and interviews are summarized below:

- **Stability of software.** On the first day of the pilot, two participants reported being unable to open the ESM questionnaires in the app. This issue got resolved within the next day, and participants were able to open the app, connect to the database, and respond to daily questionnaires. One participant noted that they were unable to open a questionnaire from their phone's home screen, but manually opening the app would make the questionnaire show up in his task list. This issue did not exist for the other participants.
- **Data transfer.** All of the data came into the database as expected: for each participant, activity, phone usage, and GPS data are periodically sent from the phone to the database.
- **Cloud messages and documents.** The cloud message functionality of the app showed clear issues: Intervention I was received by three out of four participants. Out of these three participants, two were unable to open the message. Intervention II was not received by any participant. One participant reported a measured step count of over 20.000 steps per day on average. This is likely a result of a malfunctioning wearable.
- **Wearable.** Participants reported that the wearables mostly functioned properly: there was one participant whose wearable reported abnormally high step counts, possibly caused by some malfunction in the band. Aside from this issue, the bands stayed connected and reported activity hourly.

User Experience. Participants noted that the introduction questionnaire that is asked on the website might be confusing, as it was written in English (as opposed to the native language of participants, Dutch). Participants noted that the questionnaire contains personal questions, but understood the significance of the questions asked. Excluding the technical issues that users experienced on the first day of the pilot, participants found the app easy in use. Three out of four participants found the wording used within the app clear and understandable. Participants thought the app UI was functional, but not visually attractive:

> "I normally use a different wearable and am fairly spoiled with the app's dashboards. Because of that, I don't think this app is particularly attractive".

Participants noted the visualization of the heart rate in the app's home screen is nice, but they hoped to see more: distance metrics, a visualization of their questionnaire responses, sleep analysis, and heart rate graphs were all suggested.

Participants found the effort of answering a survey every day to not be a problem, which they stated was because the questionnaires were very short and multiple choice. One participant pointed out that two years of answering the same
daily questions could bore participants, and suggested changing the questions
we asked periodically. Participants found the setup process to be well explained,
but reported not knowing what to do after completing the setup, and trying to
find actions that they were supposed to perform in the app:

> "After the setup, I wanted to get more active, but I couldn't find any tips
> or activities in the app."

When asked if it is realistic to expect panel members to participate for two years,
the pilot participants responded positively.

6   Discussion

This section of the paper discusses the changes made based on the pilot, as well as
listing related work that inspired us. Furthermore, we provide a list of guidelines
that we believe are important to consider during development of longitudinal
studies using electronic devices.

6.1   Lessons Taken from Pilot

The feedback received from the pilot allowed us to make the following changes
to the system:

Technical Functioning. The pilot showed us important technical issues that
needed to be worked out before starting the study. In the weeks following the
pilot, various technical improvements were made that ultimately led to stability
on, as far as we know, every Android phone version 7.0 and up. The pilot showed
that the configuration of data gathering and the transfer was correctly set up.
The issues concerning the allocation of cloud messages to different phones were
traced down and resolved after the pilot. Lastly, one of the take-aways from the
pilot is that while generally the wearable functions just fine, some wearables that
we distribute may malfunction. It is imperative to detect this and replace the
wearable. To allow for this, we now include a specific point on malfunctioning
wearables and replacement in the participant briefing of the study. Participants
can contact us if the wearable reports incorrect step counts, breaks, or gets lost,
to have the wearable replaced.

User Experience. Participants indicated that the amount of effort that participation took was reasonable, and could be done on a longer-term. One participant
described it as following:

"The effort needed to participate is not too high. I think it's reasonable to expect people to participate for longer periods. Also, if I were to enroll in a university study, there'd be some motivating aspect of contributing to science that helps me stay engaged".

After the pilot, we made significant changes to allow for easier understanding of the setup process: texts were clarified and made simpler; and more emphasis was put on the voluntary nature of the introduction survey, to ensure participants are aware they do not need to fill in every question. The pilot also allowed us to proceed with the planned rewards for participation: participants can earn their wearable over time, and we will host guest lectures relevant to the general understanding of eHealth that participants will be able to follow. Feedback from the pilot showed that participants did not fully comprehend the intended purpose for the app: despite information material outlining the interventional apps that are supplied during the study, some participants were under the impression that the Health Telescope app would provide them health advice. After hearing this, we have made significant changes to the briefing, putting more emphasis on the functions of the mobile application and communicating that the eHealth apps recommended during the study are what is being tested. Additionally, the introductory texts that guide participants through the setup now include at multiple points that there are no immediate actions for users after finalizing the setup.

6.2 Related Work

Here, we would like to highlight related research that guided us in this work. As mentioned before, the TEMPEST architecture, which contributed to the Health Telescope system, is described in [12], and the Health Telescope protocol is found at [26].

There exists a large amount of work on tracking physical activity. Before mobile phones became widely spread, these studies often had participants report on their physical activity [16,29]. These studies however often utilize self-reporting and surveys to measure activity/BMI. A possibly more reliable alternative used in longitudinal studies is to actively test their participants' physical condition periodically through exercise tests [18].

The rise of wearable technology may be able to provide researchers with a very direct way to measure activity. Usability and acceptability studies have been done on a wide range of participants and features [13,23,27], which can inform researchers when a target audience or outcome variable is chosen. Research analyzing the attrition rate of wearable use [2,8] should be considered in the design process. Additionally, research investigating the accuracy and reliability of data created by wearable devices [6,10] can help choose an appropriate device for a study, given the important trade-off in features, comfort, and accuracy for different features.

Wearables can be utilized in studies investigating physical activity in several ways: the reported activity can be used as an outcome variable [3,19]; notifications received on a wearable can be used to motivate participants [32], and there is a wide range of studies investigating individual wearables and their effect [25,31,33]. Regarding study design using wearables for physical activity, we advise researchers to use the informative design recommendations in [20]. Additionally, researchers should look into how wearables and their accompanying apps incorporate behavior change [22].

In designing the database and data sharing policies, we drew inspiration from various longitudinal Dutch studies, that we note here for their data sharing policies: the Lifelines cohort study [4] is a large-scale longitudinal study following the physical activity and weight in non-obese people. The Longitudinal Internet Study for the Social Sciences (LISS) panel [9] is a longitudinal study sampling the Dutch population and conducting periodical surveys and experiments. These studies may be interesting for researchers looking for longitudinal datasets.

6.3   Design Guidelines

As part of our findings, we would like to present a set of design guidelines, based on the experiences of developing this technical infrastructure:

Design and Implementation of Infrastructure

- When designing the technical infrastructure of a project, researchers should choose to measure data that is appropriate for the study objectives. As an example, for research regarding activity, step count is generally more accurate and reliable than heart rate, especially at higher intensity activity.
- It is important to consider the details on how data should be collected, transmitted and saved. We recommend regularly gathering the desired data, and periodically, encryptedly transmitting this data to a secure database.
- We recommend careful investigation of factors both in user experience such as comfort and battery life, as well as research done on the accuracy and reliability of the data generated by the instruments (e.g. wearable) considered.
- We strongly encourage researchers to consider privacy and participant rights while designing the study, to ensure the infrastructure is set up in a GDPR-proof manner. As an example, it is necessary for the system to allow for individual participant data excerpts, and full deletion of data belonging to individuals. These rights should be considered in the design.
- Design the setup process of a study or app in a way that informs participants of the purpose of the app, and actions they should take. As an example, we discovered through feedback that users were confused on their next actions after the initial setup, and considerably changed the information provided to users during this setup to inform them of the possible actions within the app.
- When implementing software of this sort, it is important, besides data collection, to collect data on how the client application functions, e.g., when a cloudmessage was received, when something was downloaded from the server, etc. This information can be helpful for isolating technical issues (e.g., if data is missing, is it because the application is not capturing that particular source

of data, or is the device perhaps turned off?). There are ways in which participants use their phones which can account for what data gets collected, which are not necessarily obvious from looking at the data of the experiment itself. The Health Telescope app does record such events into a part of the database that is separate from the data itself.
- Minimizing strain is important in long-term studies. Attrition rate is traditionally high in these studies, and efforts should be made to engage users, make participation simple, and clearly communicate expectations to users.

Testing

- We believe it is beneficial to set measurable, concrete goals for the system functionalities. We worked with specific, detailed use cases, that proved of great help in streamlining our repeated testing process by isolating technical issues.
- We recommend to test the software on multiple phones of different models and Android distributions during development. The stability of software often varies for different phones, in factors such as accessing specific data types, setting alarms, Bluetooth functionalities, etc.
- Bluetooth is commonly used in wearable studies. This further emphasizes the need to test the software on multiple phones, as it is not possible to test Bluetooth connection for different Android distributions through Android Studio's virtual machines.

Evaluating

- We emphasize the importance of feedback: try to involve feedback from as many people as possible in the development process. This can be colleagues, or potential participants, depending on the goal of the interaction. Pilot studies are an effective way of involving different individuals to gather feedback, and test the software on multiple devices.
- When designing a pilot study, think carefully of the things you hope to take away from it, and use this information in your design: Should the technical stability be tested? Include as many phones as possible, and set up the pilot to include these technical interactions, or stresstest the system. Should the pilot test the burden of participating? Focus on ways to capturing the user experience, by closely monitoring their actions and giving them opportunities to provide feedback.
- We advise to use systems such as TestFairy that track bugs and technical issues during testing. These systems can be used to quickly identify the specific issue when a technical problem occurs.

6.4   Conclusion

In this paper, we presented the development process of the system designed for data collection during the Health Telescope study. By detailing the steps in development, we aim to contribute to longitudinal research using smartphones and wearables. We gave a detailed look at the system architecture, and showed how it can be used to accomplish the study interventions. We displayed the role that pilot studies can play in the development of a system and showed the changes made following this pilot.

We concluded the paper by providing a list of guidelines for researchers, that we hope aid researchers interested in setting up longitudinal studies using electronic tools in developing their study designs and technical infrastructure. In doing so, we aim to show the value of sharing important lessons from developing work like ours. We encourage colleagues to share their work, to contribute to lowering the complexities in setting up longitudinal studies.

References

1. Arain, M., Campbell, M.J., Cooper, C.L., Lancaster, G.A.: What is a pilot or feasibility study? A review of current practice and editorial policy. BMC Med. Res. Methodol. **10**(1), 67 (2010)
2. Attig, C., Franke, T.: Abandonment of personal quantification: a review and empirical study investigating reasons for wearable activity tracking attrition. Comput. Hum. Behav. **102**, 223–237 (2020)
3. Benedetti, M.G., et al.: Physical activity monitoring in obese people in the real life environment. J. Neuroeng. Rehabil. **6**(1), 47 (2009)
4. Byambasukh, O., Vinke, P., Kromhout, D., Navis, G., Corpeleijn, E.: Physical activity and 4-year changes in body weight in 52,498 non-obese people: The lifelines cohort (2020)
5. Carson, T.P., Adams, H.E.: Activity valence as a function of mood change. J. Abnorm. Psychol. **89**(3), 368 (1980)
6. Case, M.A., Burwick, H.A., Volpp, K.G., Patel, M.S.: Accuracy of smartphone applications and wearable devices for tracking physical activity data. Jama **313**(6), 625–626 (2015)
7. Collins-Cope, M.: RSI-a structured approach to use cases and HCI design. Manuscrito no publicado (comunicación personal), Ratio Group Ltd. (1999)
8. Coorevits, L., Coenen, T.: The rise and fall of wearable fitness trackers. In: Academy of Management (2016)
9. Das, M., Knoef, M.: Experimental and longitudinal data for scientific and policy research: open access to data collected in the longitudinal Internet Studies for the Social sciences (LISS) panel. In: Crato, N., Paruolo, P. (eds.) Data-Driven Policy Impact Evaluation, pp. 131–146. Springer, Cham (2019). https://doi.org/10.1007/978-3-319-78461-8_9
10. El-Amrawy, F., Nounou, M.I: Are currently available wearable devices for activity tracking and heart rate monitoring accurate, precise, and medically beneficial? Healthc. Inform. Res. **21**(4), 315–320 (2015)
11. Batalas, N., aan het Rot, M., Khan, V.J., Markopoulos, P.: Using tempest: end-user programming of web-based ecological momentary assessment protocols. Proc. ACM Hum.-Comput. Interact. **2**D(EICS), 3:1–3:24 (2018). Redacted for anonymization

12. Batalas, N., Khan, V.-J., Franzen, M., Markopoulos, P., aan het Rot, M.: Formal representation of ambulatory assessment protocols in HTML5 for human readability and computer execution. Behav. Res. Methods **51**(6), 2761–2776 (2018). https://doi.org/10.3758/s13428-018-1148-y. Redacted for anonymization
13. Gimhae, G.-N.: Six human factors to acceptability of wearable computers. Int. J. Multimed. Ubiquit. Eng. **8**(3), 103–114 (2013)
14. Hallal, P.C., et al.: Global physical activity levels: surveillance progress, pitfalls, and prospects. Lancet **380**(9838), 247–257 (2012)
15. Henriksen, A., et al.: Using fitness trackers and smartwatches to measure physical activity in research: analysis of consumer wrist-worn wearables. J. Med. Internet Res. **20**(3), e110 (2018)
16. Herman, K.M., Craig, C.L., Gauvin, L., Katzmarzyk, P.T.: Tracking of obesity and physical activity from childhood to adulthood: the physical activity longitudinal study. Int. J. Pediatr. Obes. **4**(4), 281–288 (2009)
17. Hills, P., Argyle, M.: The oxford happiness questionnaire: a compact scale for the measurement of psychological well-being. Personality Individ. Differ. **33**(7), 1073–1082 (2002)
18. Janz, K.F., Dawson, J.D., Mahoney, L.T.: Tracking physical fitness and physical activity from childhood to adolescence: the Muscatine study. Med. Sci. Sports Exerc. **32**(7), 1250–1257 (2000)
19. Kurti, A.N., Dallery, J.: Internet-based contingency management increases walking in sedentary adults. J. Appl. Behav. Anal. **46**(3), 568–581 (2013)
20. L'Hommedieu, M., et al.: Lessons learned: recommendations for implementing a longitudinal study using wearable and environmental sensors in a health care organization. JMIR mHealth uHealth **7**(12), e13305 (2019)
21. McGreal, R., Joseph, S.: The depression-happiness scale. Psychol. Rep. **73**(3_suppl), 1279–1282 (1993)
22. Mercer, K., Li, M., Giangregorio, L., Burns, C., Grindrod, K.: Behavior change techniques present in wearable activity trackers: a critical analysis. JMIR mHealth uHealth **4**(2), e40 (2016)
23. Profita, H.P.: Designing wearable computing technology for acceptability and accessibility. ACM SIGACCESS Access. Comput. **114**, 44–48 (2016)
24. Quiñonez, S.G., Walthouwer, M.J.L., Schulz, D.N., de Vries, H.: mhealth or ehealth? Efficacy, use, and appreciation of a web-based computer-tailored physical activity intervention for Dutch adults: a randomized controlled trial. J. Med. Internet Res. **18**(11), e278 (2016)
25. Randriambelonoro, M., Chen, Y., Geissbuhler, A., Pu, P.: Exploring physical activity monitoring devices for diabetic and obese patients. In: Adjunct Proceedings of the 2015 ACM International Joint Conference on Pervasive and Ubiquitous Computing and Proceedings of the 2015 ACM International Symposium on Wearable Computers, pp. 1003–1008 (2015)
26. Willemse, B.J.P.C., Kaptein, M.C., Hasaart, F.: Developing effective methods for ehealth personalization: protocol for the health telescope, a prospective interventional study. JMIR Res. Protocols **9**, e16471 (2020). Author redacted for anonymization
27. Ridgers, N.D., et al.: Wearable activity tracker use among Australian adolescents: usability and acceptability study. JMIR mHealth uHealth **6**(4), e86 (2018)
28. Ryman, D.H., Biersner, R.J., La Rocco, J.M.: Reliabilities and validities of the mood questionnaire. Psychol. Rep. **35**(1), 479–484 (1974)

29. Telama, R., Yang, X., Viikari, J., Välimäki, I., Wanne, O., Raitakari, O.: Physical activity from childhood to adulthood: a 21-year tracking study. Am. J. Prev. Med. **28**(3), 267–273 (2005)
30. Van Teijlingen, E.R., Hundley, V.: The importance of pilot studies (2001)
31. Veerabhadrappa, P., Moran, M.D., Renninger, M.D., Rhudy, M.B., Dreisbach, S.B., Gift, K.M.: Tracking steps on apple watch at different walking speeds. J. Gen. Intern. Med. **33**(6), 795–796 (2018)
32. Wang, J.B., et al.: Wearable sensor/device (Fitbit One) and SMS text-messaging prompts to increase physical activity in overweight and obese adults: a randomized controlled trial. Telemed. e-Health **21**(10), 782–792 (2015)
33. Yavelberg, L., Zaharieva, D., Cinar, A., Riddell, M.C., Jamnik, V.: A pilot study validating select research-grade and consumer-based wearables throughout a range of dynamic exercise intensities in persons with and without type 1 diabetes: a novel approach. J. Diab. Sci. Technol. **12**(3), 569–576 (2018)

Design of a Mobile-Based Neurological Assessment Tool for Aging Populations

John Michael Templeton$^{(\boxtimes)}$ ⓘ, Christian Poellabauer ⓘ,
and Sandra Schneider ⓘ

University of Notre Dame, Notre Dame, IN 46556, USA
{jtemplet,cpoellab,sschnei8}@nd.edu

Abstract. Mobile devices are becoming more pervasive in the monitoring of individuals' health as device functionalities increase as does overall device prevalence in daily life. Therefore, it is necessary that these devices and their interactions are usable by individuals with diverse abilities and conditions. This paper assesses the usability of a neurocognitive assessment application by individuals with Parkinson's Disease (PD) and proposes a design that focuses on the user interface, specifically on testing instructions, layouts, and subsequent user interactions. Further, we investigate potential benefits of cognitive interference (e.g., the addition of outside stimuli that intrude on task-related activity) on a user's task performance. Understanding the population's usability requirements and their performance on configured tasks allows for the formation of usable and objective neurocognitive assessments.

Keywords: Neurocognitive tests · Parkinson's Disease · Mobile app

1 Introduction

Mobile devices are becoming more pervasive in the monitoring of individuals' health as device functionalities increase as does their overall prevalence in daily life [1]. As individuals age, the challenges associated with using these mobile health apps increase particularly due to cognitive and motor issues [2,3]. App designs for usability and monitoring need to take these factors into account considering the prevalence of cognitive decline and neurodegenerative diseases in the aging population. Traditionally, neurological conditions have been assessed in clinical settings using various accepted pen-and-paper style assessments [4]; however, technology and its capabilities allow for the collection of far more information and objective metrics than we ever could achieve using pen-and-paper style tests [5]. Cognitive screening instruments such as the Montreal Cognitive Assessment (MoCA) [6], Mini Mental State Examination (MMSE) [7], and the Menu Task Assessment (MT) [8] are usually initially given whenever a progressive or acquired neurological condition (e.g., Parkinson's Disease, dementia, stroke, etc.) is suspected. These assessment instruments consist of functional tasks such as, motor (e.g., fine and gross motor), speech, memory, and executive

© ICST Institute for Computer Sciences, Social Informatics and Telecommunications Engineering 2021
Published by Springer Nature Switzerland AG 2021. All Rights Reserved
J. Ye et al. (Eds.): MobiHealth 2020, LNICST 362, pp. 166–185, 2021.
https://doi.org/10.1007/978-3-030-70569-5_11

function all or some of which may be difficult for individuals with neurodegenerative conditions like Parkinson's Disease (PD) [9–11]. Subsequently, the transition
of cognitive assessments from paper versions to mobile devices calls for the configuration of tasks to be clear and usable by individuals with diverse abilities and
conditions as to not impair their performance or assessment results. Therefore,
a focus should be placed on mobile user interface design, task design, and overall
usability to accommodate these potential user impairments while maintaining
the requirements of the functional test [12].

The objective of this paper is to address the issues of usability and efficient assessment design to accommodate the aging population both with mild
cognitive impairment and with recognized neurodegenerative disabilities. This
paper proposes designs of the user interface, specifically testing instructions, layouts, and subsequent user interactions. In addition, functional task designs are
explored to understand the potential benefits of cognitive interference (e.g., the
addition of outside stimuli that intrude on task-related activity) on task performance. This paper focuses on individuals with Parkinson's Disease since they
demonstrate impaired functionality of both motor and cognitive tasks [13].

Individuals diagnosed with PD were compared to age matched control individuals across mobile neurocognitive assessments for both usability and task
performance. Changes in the user interface design were intended to accommodate known disease symptoms (e.g., deficits in motor function, memory, executive function, and/or speech). Usability of these neurocognitive assessments
were enhanced by modifying the overall test layout, screen interactions (e.g.,
button sizing and location), and instructions (e.g., multiple versions for complete understanding of the required task) for all types of functional tests (e.g.,
motor, memory, and executive function). In addition different methods of cognitive interference on functional areas of cognition (e.g., motor, memory, speech,
and executive function) were explored for the understanding of a user's task performance and subsequent functional task designs. Cognitive interference is the
addition of outside information that intrudes on task-related activity and serve
to reduce the quality and level of performance [14]. Cognitive interference occurs
when the processing of a specific stimulus feature impedes the simultaneous processing of a second stimulus attribute [15]. This interference can be derived from
many sources, however, maintaining testing design, layout, and desired functionality between mobile assessment versions allows for the understanding of
cognitive interference in functional task versions.

2   Related Work

2.1   Testing Layout

Functional assessments should aim to minimize any additional outside cognitive
load for the user (e.g., the used amount of working memory resources). This
allows the user to focus only on the required tasks (e.g., motor, speech, memory,
executive function, or designed dual-task assessments). This would include the

formation of simple test views (e.g., splitting information into sub-views to minimize amounts of material on the device screen) and instructional design (e.g., having only relevant information included) [2]. Further, the test layout should minimize errors caused by user screen interactions through the placement of navigation components in positions that are accessible but not error prone [16].

2.2   Screen Interactions

Touch technology on mobile devices must accommodate users with motor impairments (e.g., minimizing unwarranted button presses while a user completes a required functional task like tracing a shape on the device screen). Button location and sizing are both important factors necessary for user interface design for aging individuals and individuals with motor impairments [3,17]. Screen interactions for right-handed users, typically result in significantly more time and effort to reach the upper left and lower right corners of the device. The opposite occurs for left handed individuals (e.g., resulting in significantly more time and effort to reach the upper right and lower left corners of the device). However, many current touchscreen interfaces have essential system functionality located in these areas; especially the top and bottom corners of the device screen [16]. Further, device users tend to prefer and perceive bottom bar navigation menus better than other types (e.g., the hamburger menu), and it is seen to be more efficient [18].

2.3   Testing Instruction

As testing becomes readily available on mobile devices, it is important to maintain comprehensive instructions similar to clinical settings (e.g., having a trained clinician explain the testing protocol to the user and/or answer any clarification questions). User interpretations of instructions based on impairment, and/or language barriers may lead to possible data quality and consistency issues [4,19]. Similarly, multiple forms of instruction (e.g., short explicit texts and clear visual demonstrations of actions the user is required to perform) aid the users in understanding the required actions of the test [4,20]. The method in which these different users understand the functional assessments may change based on the assessment focus (e.g., motor function, speech, memory, executive function, or dual-task assessments) or their preferred learning style (e.g., visual or auditory).

2.4   Cognitive Interference

Since individuals with neurodegenerative conditions (e.g., Parkinson's Disease) demonstrate impaired functionality of both motor and cognitive tasks [13], the assessment of these functional areas of neurocognition should occur in multiple approaches. These can be assessed using both single and dual-task testing approaches [21,22], both of which can examine cognitive interference effects.

Table 1. Functional tasks

Functional task	Function(s)	Reference
Card matching task	Memory	[25]
Reaction time task	Motor function	[26]
Word sequence task	Speech	[27]
Trail making task	Executive function/motor function	[23]
Apraxia tasks	Motor function/speech	[28]

Single Task Interference. The purpose of single functional tasks is to focus on one primary area of neurocognition (e.g., motor function, memory, or executive function). A set of single modal tasks are seen in Table 1. Card matching, reaction time, and word sequence tests are all seen as single function tests as they monitor one main area of cognition. In the trail making task, testing configurations allow for the focus on one primary area of neurocognition (e.g., executive function), even if an individual's motor function carries out the executive function task. Structural variations (e.g., different visual cues or changing of depicted features) can lead to the implementation of cognitive interference(s) [23,24]. Understanding the extent of how these possible interference configurations affect individuals both in PD and control groups is of interest and will be explored in this work.

Dual-Task Interference. Dual-tasks involve two functional areas of neurocognition equally (e.g., walking and talking) at the same time [22]. Dual-tasks have inherent interference as the processing and/or production of each of the functional cognitive aspects (e.g., motor and speech) causes an intrusion in the other. When this method is employed for individuals with neurological conditions, it is to understand the prioritization strategies of the required activities compared to control groups [13]. Table 1 provides a depiction of dual functional tasks. Understanding different configurations of dual functional tasks for the areas of motor and speech across PD and control groups will be explored in this work.

3 Application Design

3.1 Test Layouts

As neurocognitive assessment instruments consist of multiple tasks, an assessment instrument should take into consideration the minimization of any additional outside cognitive load to the user (e.g., the used amount of working memory resources needed) during each task [2]. This can be accomplished by minimizing the number of screen interactions by the user (e.g., minimizing unwarranted button presses across assessments) [16] and maintaining all test instructions and interactions on the task application screens [4,20]. Each test layout design (Figs. 1 and 2) therefore was formatted to provide all necessary testing information without the need for navigating to other pages or requiring additional button presses by the user.

3.2   Test Instruction

Testing instructions were given to the user verbally (e.g., by a test proctor or clinician) [19] and via the tablet (e.g., short explicit texts and clear visual demonstrations of actions the user is required to perform) [4]. Figure 1 shows the instructional and interactive views of a fine motor functional tracing test. The instructional view provides the user all testing instructions and a partial demonstration (e.g., the image of an index finger with a trailing blue line). Once the user interacts with the tablet (e.g., "tap to begin"), the interactive view removes the demonstration image while the user is still shown the rest of the instructions to complete the test. Figure 2 shows samples of interactive views for gross motor function, memory, and executive function based tasks.

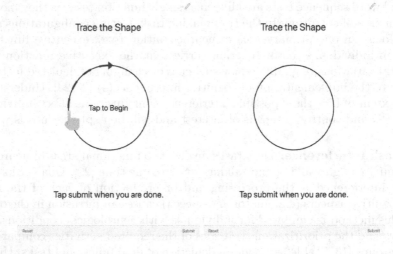

Fig. 1. Sample instructional and interactive views of a fine motor functional tracing task. (Color figure online)

3.3   Test Interactions

The partial demonstration shown in Fig. 1 depicts how the user is intended to interact with the fine motor tracing test (e.g., using their index finger to trace the shape, in a clockwise motion starting from the left). The user is to tap on the screen to enable the interactive view, and then trace the depicted shape based on the given instructions. A gross motor task would include tapping on the screen to enable the interactive view so they may manipulate the mobile device to "air"-trace a prompted shape (e.g., asking the user to hold the device directly in front of them with both hands, arms outstretched and move the device to emulate a shape). Examples of a memory test would include tapping on cards in pairs until all cards have been matched. In the trail making test the user is intended to draw a line using their index finger to connect the dots in increasing

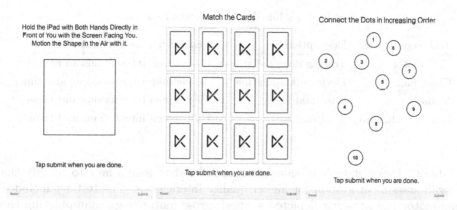

Fig. 2. Sample interactive views of gross motor, memory, and executive function tasks.

order. Finally, each of these tasks depicted visual feedback to the user from their interactions on the device screen (e.g., lines on the screen where the user has traced or the cards flipping and staying face up when matched).

3.4 Test Submission

Following the completion of any of the aforementioned tests (e.g., tracing the shape, emulating the shape, card matching, and trail making) the user is instructed to tap the submit button in the navigation bar in the bottom right corner of the screen. The submission button interaction denotes when the user feels they have finished the functional task based on the given set of instructions.

4 Methods

4.1 Usability

Participants were 40 adults between the ages of 52 and 84. These participants were divided into two groups; those with a confirmed diagnosis of Parkinson's Disease and age matched healthy controls. Participants were recruited through advertisements, physician and clinician referrals, spouses/caretakers of the diagnosed population, and prior studies in our laboratory. Inclusion criteria for the current study consisted of being age 50 years or older. Participants were excluded from the current study if they were unable to provide informed consent or if their native language was not English (as instructions and speaking tasks were all formatted in English).

All participants were required to complete the mobile versions of the tasks mentioned previously (e.g., tracing the shape, emulating the shape, card matching, and trail making) to gather objective metrics in the assessment of neurocognitive functionalities (e.g., using device sensors and screen interactions)

Table 2. Mobile device assessment features

Task type	Description	Utilized mobile device features
Fine motor	Tracing depicted shapes	User-screen interactions and timer
Gross motor	Device manipulation	Accelerometer, gyroscope, and timer
Memory	Card matching	User-screen interactions and timer
Executive function	Trail making	User-screen interactions and timer

(Table 2). Different task versions were completed to assess how to modify the overall assessment system for higher quality interactions. The test set included fine motor (e.g., tracing depicted shapes), gross motor (e.g., manipulating the device to "air"-trace a prompted shape), memory (e.g., card matching), and executive function (e.g., trail making) tasks. For usability, a focus was placed on observing user device interactions for updating the overall testing design (e.g., device task instructions and button placement).

4.2 Cognitive Interference

Since individuals with neurodegenerative conditions (e.g., Parkinson's Disease) demonstrate impaired functionality of both motor and cognitive tasks, multiple versions of each functional task were created (e.g., single and/or dual-task) to examine cognitive interference effects in mobile task design.

Single Task Interference. Single functional tasks of card matching and trail making were administered to all participants using two versions of each task.

Card Matching. Two versions of the card matching task prompt the user to match cards with different stimulus constraints. During each task the user must interact with only two cards per turn. If both cards match they remain face up and are out of play the rest of the assessment; otherwise, they are turned back over until the user matches the correct pair.

The first memory assessment (Version A) has the user match 6 pairs of cards where each pair is set to be a different shape and color combination (e.g., matching two *grey squares*, two *red triangles*, two *purple hexagons*, etc.). The second assessment (Version B) introduces visual cognitive interference. The protocol has the user match 6 pairs of cards where each pair has a different shape but only 2 colors (red and black) (e.g., matching two *red hearts*, two *red diamonds*, two *red stars*, two *black spades*, two *black clubs*, and two *black crosses*).

The overall time to complete the task (e.g., time from the user's interaction with the first card, until the last pair is matched) is collected for both versions of this test.

Trail Making. In two versions of the trail making task, the user must use their finger to draw a line connecting shapes in increasing order of numerical count.

The first trail making assessment (Version A) has the user connect the circles in increasing order from 1–10. The second assessment (Version B) introduces a visual cognitive interference. In this version the shapes are varied (e.g., circles, squares, triangles, etc.) as are their location and fill colors (e.g., white and grey). The protocol is maintained to have the user connect the shapes in increasing order from 1–10.

Metrics collected for both versions of this task include the overall time (e.g., the time from user start to user submit), the total number of points drawn, and the average distance from a true value point (e.g., the average distance between the closest point drawn by the user and the center point or 'true value' of each numbered shape).

Dual-Task Interference

Fine Motor Function with Speech. Understanding how fine motor function is affected *with* speech, it is necessary to understand fine motor function *without* speech. In a fine motor task *without* speech, the user is prompted to interact with the device screen by tracing a shape (e.g., a circle) with their finger (Version A).

In the dual-task version of the assessment of fine motor function and speech (Version B) the user is prompted to trace the same shape shown on the screen while in tandem saying the months of the year, aloud, in reverse order (e.g., December to January). The reverse ordering of months without visual cues institutes a non-automatic task that increases cognitive interference.

Metrics collected for the single and dual-task approaches of fine motor testing include the overall time (e.g., the time from user start to user submit) and the total number of points drawn.

Gross Motor Function with Speech. Similar to the dual-task assessment above, an understanding of how gross motor function is affected *with* speech, it is also necessary to understand it *without* speech. The task version *without* speech (Version A) has the user manipulating the mobile device to "air"-trace a prompted shape (e.g., a square).

In the dual-task version (Version B) of this task the user is prompted to manipulate the mobile device for the emulation of the shape in tandem with the non-automatic task of saying the months of the year, aloud, and in reverse order.

Metrics collected for the single and dual-task approaches of gross motor testing include the overall time (e.g., the time from user start to user submit) as well as the average, maximum, and minimum magnitudes of the device's acceleration.

5   Results

5.1   User Interface

The usability of the testing setup was analyzed across all participants to understand the overall quality of the design (e.g., layout, instructions, and screen interactions). This analysis was intended to allow for updating the testing process for higher usability of individuals in diagnosed populations, specifically those with Parkinson's Disease.

The overall usability was assessed by gathering the number of incorrect screen interactions between groups. An *incorrect screen interaction* was denoted as any time a user interacted with the screen incorrectly in terms of navigation (e.g., clicking submit prior to completing the test), or by interacting with the screen in a way that was not depicted by instructions or demonstrations (e.g., tapping on the screen when drawing was required). Table 3 looks at the total number of incorrect interactions by group. Individuals in the PD group interacted with the testing application incorrectly more than individuals in the age-matched control group for baseline assessments (5.02% compared to 0.35%). Further, when a representative subset of individuals in the PD group were asked to take the mobile based assessment again (e.g., with the same test instructions given both verbally and via the tablet) there were still a higher number of incorrect interactions compared to the control group (3.15% compared to 0.35%).

Table 3. Overall frequency of incorrect screen interactions

Group	Number of tests	Number of incorrect interactions	Ratio
PD baseline	598	30	5.02%
PD 2nd visit	286	9	3.15%
Control	286	1	0.35%

5.2   Test Design - Cognitive Interference

Single Task Interference

Card Matching. The analysis revealed a significant difference in both task versions for the time taken to complete the task between both groups ($p < 0.05$) with individuals diagnosed with Parkinson's Disease taking longer than the age appropriate control group (Table 4).

Table 4. Card matching metrics

Metric	Mean (SD) or p-val
Version A (without interference)	
Time (PD)	64.43 (41.93)
Time (control)	36.54 (13.73)
T-Test	$p = 0.007$
Version B (with visual interference)	
Time (PD)	62.72 (51.47)
Time (control)	38.29 (17.10)
T-Test	$p = 0.048$

Trail Making. The analysis of both trail making task versions (Table 5) revealed a significant difference ($p < 0.05$) for the metrics of time taken, and total points drawn. The metric of the average distance (e.g., the average distance between the closest point drawn by the user and the center point of a numbered shape) in the task without visual interference (Version A) yielded a significant difference between the PD and control groups ($p < 0.05$) whereas the task with visual interference (Version B) did not ($p = 0.457$).

Table 5. Trail making metrics

Metric	Mean (SD) or p-val
Version A (without interference)	
Time (PD)	17.28 (4.68)
Time (control)	12.13 (2.26)
T-Test	$p = 0.011$
Total points (PD)	387.74 (143.94)
Total points (control)	293.67 (57.85)
T-Test	$p = 0.010$
Average distance (PD)	13.56 (3.11)
Average distance (control)	10.03 (3.92)
T-Test	$p = 0.008$
Version B (with visual interference)	
Time (PD)	18.38 (8.45)
Time (control)	11.67 (2.06)
T-Test	$p = 0.001$
Total points (PD)	370.87 (103.71)
Total points (control)	252.58 (38.56)
T-Test	$p < 0.001$
Average distance (PD)	12.85 (4.26)
Average distance (control)	11.76 (3.65)
T-Test	$p = 0.457$

Dual-Task Interference

Fine Motor Function with Speech. The analysis of fine motor metrics without speech found a significant difference ($p < 0.05$) between groups for total time, and total points was found. Similarly in the dual-task version, (e.g., assessing speech and fine motor function together) a significant difference ($p < 0.05$) between groups for overall time and total points drawn by the user was found. Overall individuals diagnosed with Parkinson's Disease in both single and dual-task versions took longer and interacted with the screen more (e.g., drawing more points) than those in the control group (Table 6).

Table 6. Fine motor metrics

Metric	Mean (SD) or p-val
Version A (without interference)	
Time (PD)	9.62 (5.26)
Time (control)	6.21 (1.17)
T-Test	$p = 0.007$
Total points (PD)	216.91 (94.77)
Total points (control)	146.83 (69.07)
T-Test	$p = 0.018$
Version B (dual-task interference)	
Time (PD)	14.41 (8.58)
Time (control)	9.51 (1.97)
T-Test	$p = 0.015$
Total points (PD)	515.78 (265.30)
Total points (control)	349.17 (80.06)
T-Test	$p = 0.010$

Gross Motor Function with Speech. The single task version of the gross motor functional task yielded a significant difference ($p < 0.05$) comparing the groups for total time. All other metrics collected (e.g., the device's average, maximum, and minimum magnitudes of acceleration) were found to be non-significant ($p = 0.796$; $p = 0.220$; $p = 0.058$, respectively). The dual-task version (e.g., assessing speech and gross motor function together) revealed a significant difference ($p < 0.05$) between groups for maximum and minimum magnitude of acceleration. The metrics of overall time and average magnitude of acceleration were found to be non-significant ($p = 0.180$; $p = 0.96$, respectively). Metrics and their respective significance values for all gross motor functional testing are seen in Table 7.

6   Discussion

6.1   User Interface

The disparity in usability between PD and control groups of incorrect screen interactions depicts that updates in the user interface design need to be completed. The number of user mistakes differed notably between groups in the assessment (e.g., 5.02% compared to 0.35%). Although experience and/or training can address some of the problems had by users (e.g., the number of mistakes from a representative subset of the PD group decreased in a secondary interaction of the assessment; 3.15%), the disparity between groups calls for updates to the application to create a more usable device for all intended populations. *Incorrect screen interactions* are denoted as any time the user interacted with the screen incorrectly in terms of navigation (e.g., clicking submit prior to completing the test), or by interacting with the screen in a way that was not depicted

Table 7. Gross motor metrics

Metric	Mean (SD) or p-val
Version A (without interference)	
Time (PD)	7.88 (3.05)
Time (control)	4.97 (1.31)
T-Test	$p = 0.001$
Average magnitude (PD)	1.00 (0.01)
Average magnitude (control)	1.00 (0.01)
T-Test	$p = 0.796$
Maximum magnitude (PD)	1.27 (0.20)
Maximum magnitude (control)	1.35 (0.14)
T-Test	$p = 0.220$
Minimum magnitude (PD)	0.78 (0.14)
Minimum magnitude (control)	0.68 (0.14)
T-Test	$p = 0.058$
Version B (dual-task interference)	
Time (PD)	9.05 (2.54)
Time (control)	7.98 (1.84)
T-Test	$p = 0.180$
Average magnitude (PD)	1.00 (0.01)
Average magnitude (control)	1.00 (0.01)
T-Test	$p = 0.96$
Maximum magnitude (PD)	1.19 (0.14)
Maximum magnitude (control)	1.32 (0.17)
T-Test	$p = 0.033$
Minimum magnitude (PD)	0.832 (0.104)
Minimum magnitude (control)	0.725 (0.119)
T-Test	$p = 0.017$

by instructions or demonstrations. Those processes in the user interface design need to incur changes to reduce the number of incorrect instances of the diagnosed population. The following subsections discuss methods of updating the application to address both task instructions (e.g., re-watchable demonstrations) and navigational components (e.g., button placement) to help mitigate incorrect screen interactions.

Test Layout. Figure 3 shows a depiction of the updated fine motor functional tracing test version of the assessment for both instructional views and interactive views. Figures 4, 5, and 6 shows the updated gross motor, memory, and executive function test views. These updated test layouts allows for separated material

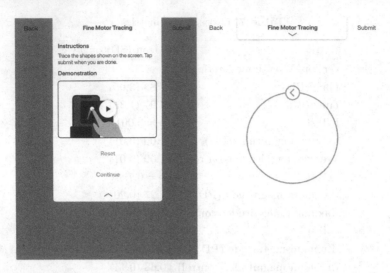

Fig. 3. Updated instructional and interactive views of a fine motor functional tracing task.

(e.g., moving the instructions to a separated screen from the interactive view) while allowing for all test instructions to be viewed by the user at any point in time through the inclusion of a drop down menu.

Test Instruction. Testing instructions for the updated versions can still be given to the user verbally (e.g., by a test proctor or clinician) and via the tablet (e.g., written in short texts in common language). The updated version also includes a video demonstration of the functional task compared to a static partial demonstration in the previous versions. Figure 7 is a depiction of this video demonstration for the fine motor tracing test where a sample shape is being traced by an animated index finger in the required direction in its entirety. These videos can be played multiple times to allow the user to understand the test completely prior to their interactions. On the interactive screen for certain tests, a smaller prompt (e.g., a small circle with an arrow pointed in the direction of intended interaction) is shown to give users a starting location and direction as described in the video demonstrations.

Test Interactions. Updates to the testing layout were also completed to enhance user test interactions. The updates of moving all buttons to the top of the screen are to help mitigate incorrect screen interactions including clicking submit prior to completing the test. Although device users prefer and perceive bottom bar navigation menus better than other types (e.g., hamburger menu), populations with motor impairments show to have unintentional interactions near the edges of the screen closest to their dominant hand (e.g., clicking submit prior to being done with the functional task). Similarly, removing the

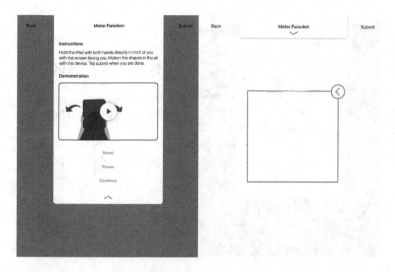

Fig. 4. Updated instructional and interactive views of a gross motor task.

instructions and bottom navigational bars allows for the user to have more room for interactions on the screen while maintaining desired functionality.

6.2   Test Design

Since individuals with Parkinson's Disease demonstrate impaired functionality of both motor and cognitive tasks, multiple versions of each functional task were created (e.g., single and/or dual-task) to examine cognitive interference effects in mobile task design. The following subsections discuss the potential benefits of these different versions for the implementation in mobile assessment instruments.

Card Matching. Memory function metrics from both versions of the card matching task showed that either task could be implemented in the formation of a new testing suite. There were no significant differences in time between the card matching tasks *with* or *without* visual interference in the case of reducing the number of unique colors from six to two for the PD group ($p = 0.902$) or control group ($p = 0.785$). Therefore either task version, A or B, could be implemented to gather necessary timing metrics for memory function of individuals with PD. An updated depiction of the card matching task is shown in Fig. 5.

Trail Making. Version B of the task showed a difference for control groups compared to its non-interference counterpart, specifically for the metric of average distance (e.g., the average distance between the closest point drawn by the user and the center point or *'true value'* of each numbered shape). The desired outcome of configured tasks is the formation of a version that separates the groups maximally (e.g., yields the highest number of significant metrics between

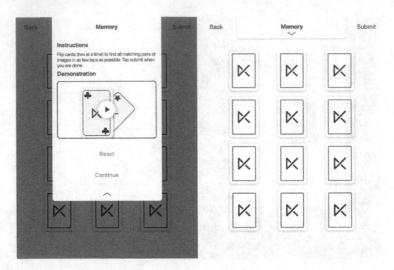

Fig. 5. Updated instructional and interactive views of a memory based task.

groups), therefore the implementation of Version A (e.g., having the user connect circles in increasing order from 1–10) should occur as Version B does not provide the maximum separation of the PD and control groups. An updated depiction of Version A is seen in Fig. 6.

Fine Motor Function with Speech. Fine motor function metrics from both singular and dual-task versions show that either version of the task could be implemented in the formation of a new testing suite, however unlike the card matching task, there are benefits to both. Version A of the fine motor task (without dual-task interference) has a significantly shorter duration than the dual-task version ($p = 0.028$ and $p < 0.001$) when comparing the PD and control groups across versions. In the formation of a dual modal task (Version B), additional information can be collected with the configuration of mobile device sensors and capabilities. As the participant is required to speak aloud during Version B of the test, the device's speech recognizers can be implemented for the accuracy count of words said. Further, audio recordings of the speech sample can be made for the subsequent analysis of frequency measures. An updated depiction of Version A is shown in Fig. 3 and Fig. 8 for Version B (dual modal).

Gross Motor Function with Speech. The collected gross motor metrics, from singular and dual-task versions, show that both are needed for the collection of significant, objective metrics. Having participants do either Version A (without dual-task interference) or Version B (with dual-task interference) alone, removes significant and objective information on the state of the person being assessed. In new testing suites, gross motor function in a dual-task versions should be added.

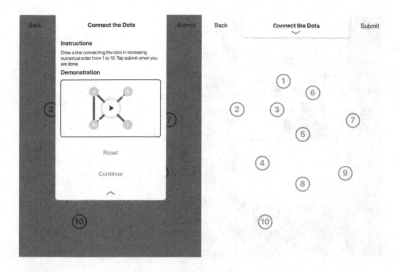

Fig. 6. Updated instructional and interactive views of an executive function based task.

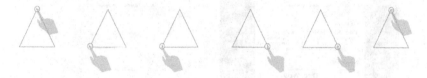

Fig. 7. Animation of fine motor tracing instructions.

An updated depiction of Version A is shown in Fig. 4 and Fig. 9 for Version B (dual modal).

Comparing Interference Types. Interference types may have different effects on overall cognitive function during assessments. Sensory interference (e.g., visual, auditory, and tactile) can be implemented as distraction mechanisms during tasks where the main goal is to see if users can minimize these distractions and complete the task at hand. Multifunctional tasks can be implemented to help understand prioritization strategies of the required tasks. Instances of tasks with fine motor components were modified to implement both sensory interference or dual-task interference. In the single modal task with visual interference, there was a decrease in the number of significant metrics collected as the difference between PD and control groups for the metric of average distance was non-significant. In a dual-task version of task interference the collected fine motor metrics remained significant and there is also the potential for a variety of other metrics to be collected. In the formation of new functional testing assessments, the implementation of the dual-task version should be added due to the collection of additional relevant metrics, unless there are impending time constraints.

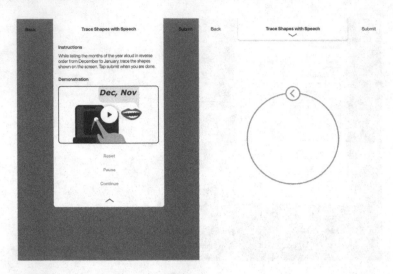

Fig. 8. Updated instructional and interactive views of a dual modal fine motor task.

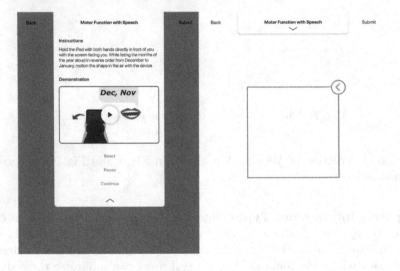

Fig. 9. Updated instructional and interactive views of a dual modal gross motor task.

Interference Modalities. Although visual interference (e.g., single task interference) and motor and speech dual-task interference were monitored in this study, there are additional ways to implement cognitive interference into testing platforms. Extensive interference processes could also be completed in the case of tri- or multi-task interference (e.g., having the user engage in three or more functional areas of interest at one time) or compounded task interference (e.g., increasing interference signals over the course of a test). Similarly, multifunctional assessments could implement one or multiple sensory interference(s) for the simulation of more real world scenarios (e.g., walking and talking with implemented sensory stimulus).

For individuals with Parkinson's Disease, visual cognitive interference in both memory and executive function did not provide additional significant metrics compared to control groups. In dual-task cognitive interference, fine motor function maintains significance for all explored metrics but ultimately allows for the collection of speech samples for further analysis and expanded metric sets. Dual-task interference for gross motor function showed varied significance metrics compared to a non-interference version. In this capacity, the use of both task versions allows for the collection of additional, relevant, and objective metrics.

7 Conclusions and Future Work

Mobile devices are becoming more prevalent in the monitoring of individuals' health in many capacities. Based on the findings in this study, a focus should be given to updating mobile assessment instruments for both usability and task performance. This should be done by changing layouts to minimize incorrect interactions (e.g., moving submission buttons, making locations for screen interaction much clearer/understood), while maintaining all necessary instructional information such that the user understands the functional task. Although healthy populations tend to be able to interact with various features across many applications, overall application development should focus on all possible users. With regards to the mobile neurocognitive assessment systems, the configuration of devices and user interactions for an aging population across diverse abilities and conditions is necessary for the monitoring of individuals task performance and can yield the highest usability and accuracy across all groups. This can be completed by updating overall user interface design, specifically testing instructions, layouts, subsequent user interactions, and task configurations. In the formation of relevant and objective task configurations, for various progressive and acquired neurological conditions, an understanding of how cognitive interference plays a roll is necessary. Different implementations should be explored to understand when cognitive interference is beneficial in different neurological task versions. This should be done across all functional neurocognitive areas of interest and against an extensive set of configurable device metrics. The understanding of new interference modalities can further aid in the formation of comprehensive assessments for all neurological conditions. Other conditions including stroke, dementia, or traumatic brain injuries may call for different user device configurations and/or different cognitive interference types across digital tests for the collection of important objective metrics. Ultimately, the formation of usable mobile neurocognitive assessment systems for digital testing can assist in the understanding of new relevant, objective, and significant metrics. Further understanding of the usability of mobile devices for individuals with neurological conditions in addition to the implementation of cognitive interference to address task performance may allow for the increase in accuracy for both diagnostic and rehabilitative monitoring purposes for all neurological conditions.

References

1. Chen, K.B., Savage, A.B., Chourasia, A.O., Wiegmann, D.A., Sesto, M.E.: Touch screen performance by individuals with and without motor control disabilities. Appl. Ergon. **44**, 297–302 (2013)
2. Vo, A.: Usability in designing a mobile application for elderly users. Technical report (2019)
3. Xiong, J., Muraki, S.: Thumb performance of elderly users on smartphone touchscreen. SpringerPlus **5** (2016). Article number: 1218. https://doi.org/10.1186/s40064-016-2877-y
4. Vianello, A., Chittaro, L., Burigat, S., Budai, R.: MotorBrain: a mobile app for the assessment of users' motor performance in neurology. Comput. Methods Programs Biomed. **143**, 35–47 (2017)
5. Byrom, B., Wenzel, K., Pierce, J., Wenzel, K., Pierce, J.: Computerised clinical assessments: derived complex clinical endpoints from patient self-report data, pp. 179–202, May 2016
6. Nasreddine, Z.S., et al.: The montreal cognitive assessment, MoCA: a brief screening tool for mild cognitive impairment. J. Am. Geriatr. Soc. **53**, 695–699 (2005)
7. Tombaugh, T.N., McIntyre, N.J.: The mini-mental state examination: a comprehensive review. J. Am. Geriatr. Soc. **40**, 922–935 (1992)
8. Al-Heizan, M.O., Giles, G.M., Wolf, T.J., Edwards, D.F.: The construct validity of a new screening measure of functional cognitive ability: the menu task. Neuropsychological Rehabil. **30**, 961–972 (2020)
9. Pettersson, A.F., Olsson, E., Wahlund, L.-O.: Motor function in subjects with mild cognitive impairment and early Alzheimer's disease. Dement. Geriatr. Cogn. Disord. **19**, 299–304 (2005)
10. Barbosa, A.F., et al.: Cognitive or cognitive-motor executive function tasks? Evaluating verbal fluency measures in people with Parkinson's disease. BioMed Res. Int. **2017** (2017). Article ID: 7893975
11. Camp, C.J., Foss, J.W., O'Hanlon, A.M., Stevens, A.B.: Memory interventions for persons with dementia. Appl. Cogn. Psychol. **10**, 193–210 (1996)
12. Ji, Y.G., Park, J.H., Lee, C., Yun, M.H.: A usability checklist for the usability evaluation of mobile phone user interface. Int. J. Hum.-Comput. Interact. **20**(3), 207–231 (2006)
13. Löfgren, N., Conradsson, D., Rennie, L., Moe-Nilssen, R., Franzén, E.: The effects of integrated single- and dual-task training on automaticity and attention allocation in Parkinson's disease: a secondary analysis from a randomized trial. Neuropsychology **33**, 147–156 (2019)
14. Sarason, I.G., Sarason, B.R., Pierce, G.R.: Cognitive interference. In: Saklofske, D.H., Zeidner, M. (eds.) International Handbook of Personality and Intelligence. PIDF, pp. 285–296. Springer, Boston (1995). https://doi.org/10.1007/978-1-4757-5571-8_14
15. Scarpina, F., Tagini, S.: The stroop color and word test. Front. Psychol. **8**, 557 (2017)
16. Wiegand, K., Patel, R.: Impact of motor impairment on full-screen touch interaction. Technical report (2015)
17. Sesto, M.E., Irwin, C.B., Chen, K.B., Chourasia, A.O., Wiegmann, D.A.: Effect of touch screen button size and spacing on touch characteristics of users with and without disabilities. Hum. Factors J. Hum. Factors Ergon. Soc. **54**, 425–436 (2012)

18. Tsiodoulos, D., Kth, D.T.: Comparison of hamburger and bottom bar menu on mobile devices for three level navigation. Technical report (2016)
19. Templeton, J.M., Poellabauer, C., Schneider, S.: Enhancement of neurocognitive assessments using smartphone capabilities: systematic review. JMIR mHealth uHealth **8**, e15517 (2020)
20. Kobayashi, M., Hiyama, A., Miura, T., Asakawa, C., Hirose, M., Ifukube, T.: Elderly user evaluation of mobile touchscreen interactions. In: Campos, P., Graham, N., Jorge, J., Nunes, N., Palanque, P., Winckler, M. (eds.) INTERACT 2011. LNCS, vol. 6946, pp. 83–99. Springer, Heidelberg (2011). https://doi.org/10.1007/978-3-642-23774-4_9
21. Di Rosa, E., Pischedda, D., Cherubini, P., Mapelli, D., Tamburin, S., Burigo, M.: Working memory in healthy aging and in Parkinson's disease: evidence of interference effects. Aging Neuropsychol. Cogn. **24**, 281–298 (2017)
22. LaPointe, L.L., Stierwalt, J.A.G., Maitland, C.G.: Talking while walking: cognitive loading and injurious falls in Parkinson's disease. Int. J. Speech-Lang. Pathol. **12**, 455–459 (2010)
23. Fellows, R.P., Dahmen, J., Cook, D., Schmitter-Edgecombe, M.: Multicomponent analysis of a digital trail making test. Clin. Neuropsychol. **31**, 154–167 (2017)
24. Salthouse, T.A., et al.: Effects of aging on efficiency of task switching in a variant of the trail making test. Neuropsychology **14**(1), 102–111 (2000)
25. Cook, D.J., Fellow, I., Schmitter-Edgecombe, M., Jönsson, L., Morant, A.V.: Technology-enabled assessment of functional health (2018)
26. Stuss, D.T., Stethem, L.L., Hugenholtz, H., Picton, T., Pivik, J., Richard, M.T.: Reaction time after head injury: fatigue, divided and focused attention, and consistency of performance. J. Neurol. Neurosurg. Psychiatry **52**, 742–748 (1989)
27. Yadav, N., et al.: Portable neurological disease assessment using temporal analysis of speech. In: BCB 2015–6th ACM Conference on Bioinformatics, Computational Biology, and Health Informatics, pp. 77–85. Association for Computing Machinery Inc., September 2015
28. Christensen, A.L.: Neuropsychological experiences in neurotraumatology. In: von Wild, K.R.H. (ed.) Re-Engineering of the Damaged Brain and Spinal Cord. NEUROCHIRURGICA, vol. 93, pp. 195–198. Springer, Vienna (2005). https://doi.org/10.1007/3-211-27577-0_34

Improving Patient Throughput by Streamlining the Surgical Care-Pathway Process

David Mc Mahon[1](✉), Joseph Walsh[2], Eilish Broderick[3], and Juncal Nogales[1]

[1] Tralee Institute of Technology Co., Kerry, Ireland
david.martin.mcmahon@research.ittralee.ie,
juncal.nogales@staff.ittralee.ie
[2] Head of School (STEM), Tralee Institute of Technology Co., Kerry, Ireland
joesph.walsh@staff.ittralee.ie
[3] Head of Department, Tralee Institute of Technology Co., Kerry, Ireland
eilish.broderick@research.ittralee.ie

Abstract. The delivery of a patient, to the operating theatre, in every hospital, consists of several heterogeneous departments working synchronously via communicating and sharing information, in relation to the current state of a patient's care, as they travel through the surgical care-path way. The surgical care-pathway typically starts at admissions and finishes as the patient is leaving recovery. The problem being, as a patient navigates the care-pathway, there are numerous risk factors in the forms of technical, environmental and human that can influence a delay in the delivery of care. This paper will discuss these risk factors and highlight different approaches taken by several authors to address such issues. Additionally, a software application will be discussed that has being developed by the author that uses portable mobile devices, to address similar issues, for a private health care provider in the south of Ireland. The results of implementing the new solution show a potential decrease in patient throughput time and an overall increase of task visibility, across the surgical care-pathway.

Keywords: Surgical care-pathway · Communication & information · Portable mobile devices

1 Introduction

Proper communication systems and methods are vital for hospitals to obtain maximum efficiency in the delivery of care [1]. When transferring a patient from one department in the hospital to another, workers depend heavily on accurate clinical information [2]. Clinical staff who make decisions about the current state of a patient's health depend on information from numerous departments inside a patients care-path-way [3]. This information needs to be non-ambiguous and accessible in order to reduce delays to a patient's care and to avoid clinical errors that place the patient's health at risk [4].

J. Nogales—Project Coordinator.

© ICST Institute for Computer Sciences, Social Informatics and Telecommunications Engineering 2021
Published by Springer Nature Switzerland AG 2021. All Rights Reserved
J. Ye et al. (Eds.): MobiHealth 2020, LNICST 362, pp. 186–207, 2021.
https://doi.org/10.1007/978-3-030-70569-5_12

In order to reduce the patient risk rate and improve the workflow and patient through-put, of the surgical care-pathway, key areas have been identified in literature that form both the problem and solution definition and can have a positive or negative influence on the patients surgical care-pathway and subsequently the hospitals throughput average. These being; communication structure [5, 6]; communication culture [7, 8]; communication quality [9, 10]; interdepartmental communication [1, 11–14]; and information sharing and collaborative systems [4, 15, 16].

In order to address the risk factors mentioned above, newer technologies such as portable communication applications have been introduced into hospitals [17–20]. These technologies offer a solution by enabling rich content of information to be shared between both individuals and departments. Additionally, these systems allow for asynchronous communication, accessibility of information at the point care and accessibility to clinical decision makers without disrupting their workflow [10]. In doing so these systems increase a patient's care by reducing delays in their care-pathway and promote inter-departmental communication, patient task visibility, task compliance and information security and distribution [21–23].

The main aims of this research paper is to; (1) identify and understand the potential negative impact of the five key risk factors mentioned above inside the patient surgical care-pathway; (2) highlight how assisitve and complementary technologies are been used to counteract these risk factors; (3) demonstrate through a case study in an elective surgery based hospital in Ireland how streamlining the surgical care-pathway using a bespoke software application can improve patient throughput.

The following sections of this paper will be formatted as follows. Section 2 will present an overview of the problems associated with communication and collaboration in the hospital environment. Section 3 will present implemented solutions taken from studies that highlight both technical and non-technical solutions to the problem space. Section 4 will present the case study and implement solution and finally Sect. 5 will highlight results of the case study with conclusions.

2   The Problem Domain

This section will now explore the problem domain of some of the key influencers to poor communication and information sharing inside the patient surgical care-path that have a negative impact on the delivery of care and patient throughput.

2.1   Interdepartmental Communication and Collaboration

Interdepartmental communication in hospitals is the process of several departments collaborating and communicating, patient care objectives, in relation to their current health status, care-pathway trajectory and assessments [16]. In doing so, clinicians can make best practice decisions, for a patient, based on their findings [1]. Issues arise, if there is no collaboration between departments which can lead to ambiguity of facts, around information shared, between departments [2]. This can delay care for a patient, or put the patient at risk, of being misdiagnosed.

Additionally, hospitals can be held liable, if it is deemed that inefficient communication methodologies are being implemented, that could potentially place a patient at risk [24]. Furthermore, inventory management is effected by poor interdepartmental communication practices. If the auditing of surgical instruments is not communicated, in a timely manner, the hospital may incur a delay, in the purchasing or ordering, of the instruments. This in turn, effects the theatre scheduling process and can cause a delay to surgery [25].

2.2 The Hierarchical Influence

Another barrier to effective communication and information sharing in the hospital environment is the hierarchical structure. This structure is unique, unlike most industries where there is one leader and all decisions and objectives filter down through, sub-teams and management groups, hospitals usually have a dual hierarchy, consisting of, the medical management group and the traditional management group [26]. These hierarchies tend to form work silos [27]. Work silos promote partitioning of services that are detrimental, to the collaborative effort, needed from all departments, to deliver the best possible care for a patient [28]. Similarly, the work culture is affected by this as staff should be represented at all levels should a strategic change happen in relation to the hospitals current business objectives [8].

2.3 Hospital Information Systems

Most hospitals use information systems to store and sort, patient information in the form of EMR (Electronic Medical Records), [15].The patient's data should be, easily accessible to the medical staff who are providing care for a patient. Information systems help to collaborate different departments who are providing care for a patient. The processing of information is vital, as it must be conducted across all departments, in order to keep all departments aligned, with the current state of the patient's care [4]. Complex systems that involve trawling through data, to obtain patient information, are counterproductive [29]. Furthermore the use of arcane legacy systems, due to the time taken to retrieve the relevant information, is not efficient [30]. This can lead, to costly software migration approaches being adopted, as the interoperability of the system, does not exist, in relation to the porting functionality, with newer systems [31]. Finally, poor logic implementation and the use of unintuitive interface design, has a negative impact on information sharing and data distribution [32].

2.4 Conventional Forms of Communication

Conventional forms of communication, involve the use of letters, wired phones, pagers, email and fax to distribute, or audit information that directly influence, a patients care. By law, hospitals must use conventional forms of communication, when signing clinical documentation in a paper format, however, the document has then to be distributed manually, to different departments, for other clinicians to read. This relaying of information is inefficient and time consuming [33]. During peak demand or capacity periods in the hospital a failure to communication the patient task status in real-time, can create a backlog of tasks to be completed, hence conventional methods of communication and human error, are one of the main causes of bottlenecks in a patients care pathway [34].

Peri-operative nurses, rely heavily on information gained, via telephone calls and written messages, to assist them in relaying important information, to the surgeon and also serve as a first phase assessment tool, for post-operative care. This is a long laborious process that can lead to ambiguity of facts, about the patients care needs and can delay surgery [35]. Communication methods such as face to face conversations, between clinical workers, are the most informative methods used, in the hospital environment. The problem with this method of communication is that department representatives, directly responsible for a specific patients care, that were not engaging in the primary conversation could now be missing vital information, about the patient. This method of conversation is not robust or transparent and can lead to ambiguity of facts and increased waiting time for patients [36].

2.5 Patient Handover and Transfers

A failure to communicate efficiently, during the clinical handover process, is recognized as the key factor that causes major incidents, in the care of patients and also contributes highly, to patient and staff dissatisfaction [10]. Additionally, a standard protocol in the transfer of care often involves, paper based check lists, consisting of patient information such as type of surgery, current allergies, medical history, frequency of medication and any immediate concerns, that the patient may have [11]. Notifications are then communicated to the workers, in the receiving department via telephone and computer email. The transfer is also logged in the unit admission transfer and discharge log sheet. This form of data capture and communication is not efficient and prone to be lost, or possibly discarded out of human error [12].

2.6 Patient Security

GDPR (General Data Protection Regulation) in hospitals, is now being implemented, as a form of patient security and patient confidentiality. Under GDPR, data is not to be made available, about patients, if it breaches, the principle of purpose limitation, guidelines. This simply means, that the amount data, should be condensed or limited, with regards to its necessity, in completing a patients-care path process [37]. For development of new applications in the health care sector under GDPR privacy by design is a new method of development whereby all data that is being collected must be anonymised.

Additionally, any algorithm's that are used in the sorting and processing of data must carry out a data protection impact statement (DPIA).This is a risk evaluation process that is mandatory to all types of data processing practices. In particular, evaluating the risk associated with the processing of sensitive patient data [38]. By adhering to the new GDPR guidelines developers need to take numerous precautions when designing applications in the healthcare sector and this can be a costly process that is difficult to police. Additionally, making existing applications GDPR compliant can cost a substantial amount of money due to the possible need to overhaul and test the entire system.

2.7   From an Irish Context

With regards to the key areas defined in Table 1 below, the National Service Plan, published in 2020, provides a strong correlation between the literature based problem domains mentioned above and the proposed priorities and actions outlined by the Office of the Chief Information Officer (OoCIO). The OoCIO are responsible for the delivery of ICT health services at a national level in Ireland. With regards to communication and collaboration, data distribution and security, the following actions have been scheduled for the implementation pillar titled Enabling Healthcare Delivery [39].

Table 1. A table representation of some of the priorities and actions under the national service plan 2020, X = not applicable to column value, 0 = applicable to column value, CC = communication & collaboration, DD = data distribution, S = security.

#	Action description	CC	DD	S
1	Design and develop the summary and shared care record	0	0	X
2	Implement digital patient records for all strands	0	0	X
3	Establish the ePharmacy and the ePrescribing programmes	X	0	X
4	Finalise the procurement of an acute floor information system	0	X	0
5	Implement the telehealth strategy	0	0	0
6	Establish an eHealth solution to support referral pathways	0	X	X
7	Deliver a single software architecture approach to promote better access and sustainability	0	0	0
8	Enhance the data dictionary to facilitate the adoption of common definitions and promote interoperability	0	0	X
8	Enhance the data dictionary to facilitate the adoption of common definitions and promote interoperability	0	0	X
9	Implement the cyber security strategy to protect sensitive patient data	X	0	X
10	Migrate older legacy systems to more sustainable software solutions	X	0	0
11	Establish a centre of excellence to support and promote the implementation of cloud based technologies	0	0	0
12	Establish the interRAI It based assessment system	0	0	0
13	Establish mobile data integration and distribution services	0	0	0

Table 1 outlines a strong correlation between the actions proposed at a national level and the findings from the literature with regards to the problem domain and how communication, collaboration information sharing and security are to be prioritized going forward into 2020.

Furthermore, it has being identified in the eHealth Strategy for Ireland 2020, that ICT sector spending needs to increase to the European rate of 2–3% from the current rate of 0.85%.This new investment will go towards the implementation and maintenance of the programs mentioned above in Table 1 and help fund key research into new approaches of improving health care via eHealth solutions [40].

2.8   From a European and American Context

Based on data obtained from the European Risk Observatory Report in relation to emerging issues and crisis in the healthcare sector, communication, collaboration and information sharing are key developments that need to be addressed. The uses of eHealth systems and mHealth frameworks are of high importance when advancing the efficiency of the collaborative effort needed to deliver positive clinical and administrative work-flows [41].With regards to cyber-security the European commission for ICT has provided funding for several pilot projects such as Serums, Secure Hospitals and Sphinx. These are all aimed at safe guarding the patients data during the storage and distribution process [42]. In the US the trend in the problem space is similar with poor communication practices and the use of arcane communication technologies leading to escalating costs in the delivery of care [43] (Fig. 1, Tables 2 and 3).

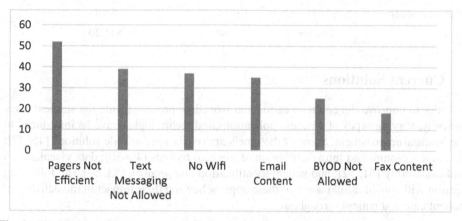

Fig. 1. The 2014 Imprivata report on the economic impact of inefficient communications in health [44]. Highlighted are the main reasons for time wasted when communicating with colleagues in US Hospitals.

Table 2. The 2014 imprivata report on the economic impact of inefficient communications in healthcare [44]. Highlighted are the cost saving estimates from adopting a mobile text messaging service to replace conventional forms of communication.

Output descriptor	Mins per patient	Mins per day	Hr per year	Annual labour cost
The collective total time spent per patient	51.2	5,223,2	31,774,5	$1,123,228
Time wasted because of communications efficiencies	33.2	3,365.1	20,592.8	$727,957
Estimated time savings using mobile text messaging	16.3	1,667.5	10,144.2	$358,596

Table 3. Continued findings from the imprivata report on the economic impact of inefficient communications in healthcare.

Workflow descriptor	Extrapolated Annual cost of Inefficient Time per hospital	Number of registered hospitals	Extrapolated annual impact for the industry (U.S. $ billions)
Patient admissions	$727,957	6.409	$4.67
Emergency response	$265,254	6.409	$1.70
Patient transfers	$753,755	6.409	$4.83
Total	$1,746,966	6.409	$11.20

3   Current Solutions

In order to improve the communication and workflow process inside the surgical care-pathway, varying types of devices applications and technologies have be introduced to the hospital environment. Some of these new approaches are mobile solutions [45–47]; the digital capture and intra distribution of medical records [48–50]; data visualization and availability [51, 52]; and patient identification and security [53, 54].The following section will now highlight some of these approaches and their impact in the delivery of patient care and patient throughput.

3.1   Mobile Based Approaches

Tran [55], identified the use of pagers, as a direct cause of bottlenecks in the patient care pathway. Not only were pagers disruptive to the workflow, they did not provide the capability, for sharing and distribution of rich content. To address this issue, Vocera communication badges were introduced. This enabled staff, to communicate on the go, without the disruptive polling of paging, and in doing so, it reduced the communication time, associated with specific tasks by 25%. O'Connor [18], also addressed the issue of team coordination and how pagers, due to their lack of functionality and their disruptive alert system, were not efficient, at coordinating team objectives. Instead a push email service was implemented, that allowing users to communicate asynchronously, without delay and provided rich content in their messaging.

Additionally, Wu [56], promoted the idea of using mobile phone applications, to address the issue of inadequate interdepartmental communication, between x-ray and oncology. The problem being that for specific x-rays, both parties needed to be present, to make clinical decisions. This would often cause bottlenecks, for patients waiting for x-ray. To address this issue, the use of mobile applications was introduced, whereby information and imagery could be shared between workers and in doing so, promote collaboration and reduce the waiting time for x-ray services.

3.2   Data Capture and Information Sharing

Abraham [14] highlighted the need to improve the hospital information systems capabilities, as the storing of patient data is essentially static and not distributed efficiently, throughout the care path-way. Additionally, these stationary systems, offer little communication capabilities, or task compliance functionality. Qiaoyu [20], re-iterated the same points and proposed the concept of, cross platform mobile technologies that are portable, and allow, for the collaboration of key decision makers to be available at all times. This reduces waiting times for patients and improves collaboration between departments and clinical workers Meijla [57].

Vezyridis [58], suggested that there is a lack of clarity in relation, to the patient data being stored. This data influences hospital workflow and if the data is inefficient or inaccurate, bottlenecks can happen in the care pathway. The use of digital whiteboards to assist nursing in their patient tasks enables nurses to view their workload in a structured manor. Additionally, the new system could be distributed throughout the care path-way, allowing a nurse to access information, view pending tasks and discuss prioritization of patients, without disrupting their workflow.

3.3 Data Visualisation

Traditionally white boards are used in hospitals, to organize staff in relation to their workload. Bossen [59], identified the use of white boards as inefficient in the scenario where, a workers tasks change, as this involves, a worker finding out what their next task is, where it is happening and with which patient. This can delay patient care and be disruptive, to the hospital workflow. To address this issue, a digital white board was implemented allowing workers to track, communicate and audit their tasks in real-time. The application could also be used to coordinate a group of workers, to specific tasks and in doing so promote, worker collaboration, compliance of tasks and improve communication. Vezyridis [58] also eluded to the same point by introducing, a digital display board to improve worker collaboration and information access.

Additionally, Kim [60], expanded the concept of digital white board to be more cognitive and interlink related information, about a patient from various departments, in the hospital. This in turn, reduced the workload and improved accessibility, to the patient's information, by efficiently tracking the patient's workflow, via event feeds and time line markers, on the display.

3.4 Patient Identification and Security

Troester [61], highlighted the need to improve interdepartmental communication and collaboration between workers. A key problem area was, the need to track medication and provide an audit trail, so the pharmacy department would know in advance, what medication was needed on a daily basis. The use of a barcode tracking and compliance application was introduced, improving the workflow and reducing waiting times for dispensing medication. In relation to QR code scanning, Wangwan [62] proposed QR codes, to track patients status in the hospital environment, improving operational efficiency. The main reason for this was, the patients chart was an inefficient medium of sharing and distributing, patient information. Furthermore, static workstations were not efficient at updating patient information, in real-time. To address the problem, RFID readers were used to provide updates via mobile device scanning.

Additionally, Anton [63], addressed the same point, by using QR codes and RFID to capture, patient data more securely via encryption and also improve the distribution of, patient data by moving away from, remote workstations and paper based patient documentation. Finally, Li-Chuan y[64] highlighted similar points in relation to QR code security and used a similar system, to track surgical equipment that needed repairing. This simplified the auditing and compliance process and helped to control inventory management in real-time.

4   Case Study – The Development of a Bespoke Software Application That Streamlines the Surgical Care-Pathway

Having explored the problem and solution domain from approaches found in the literature, this section will discuss the implementation of a new software solution to solve similar issues such as the patient throughput and delay paradigm discovered in a hospital in the south of Ireland.

4.1   Case Study Background

A hospital group in the south of Ireland wanted to improve their patient throughput by identifying and reducing the bottlenecks inside their surgical care pathway. The hospital has a capacity of 144 beds, with four theatres and typically uses an elective surgery framework. The hospital relies heavily on conventional forms of communication such as wired phones, pagers and face to face communication to receive updates about a patient's pre-post operation state, from different departments that provide a care service as the patient navigates their surgical care-pathway. The use of fixed workstations that involve complex ad-hoc querying is common through all the wards. These are typically located in corridors away from the patient's point of care.

With this information in mind, the hospital wanted to explore the concept of possibly introducing a new technology to cater for all the idiosyncrasies of each departments input into the patients surgical care pathway and in doing so, create a streamlined service that if implemented efficiently, would reduce the turnaround times for elective patients and improve the quality of care in the hospital. Additionally, the new system would serve to combine all departments under a uniformed communication system that is easy to use and relays information about a patient's state throughout the course of the patient's surgical care-pathway.

4.2   Solution Methodology Introduction

The bespoke software application was designed by implementing a hybrid of a spiral model SDLC and a water fall model. This was primarily due to the need to provide rapid prototypes to demonstrate to the stakeholders on a monthly basis. These were then critiqued and the best components were kept for the next iteration. Once enough components were finalised the waterfall model could be implemented for the final development process.

4.3 Requirements Gathering and Analysis

In order to capture and define the system user's requirements, observational research was carried out over a two-year period. This consisted of arranging to meet and interview all department staff and managers that have an influence on the patient as they navigate the surgical care-pathway. The process flow of the patients was captured by shadowing patients who were going for surgery. This shadowing proved to be a vital task, as some of the information obtained from the interview process did not correlate, with the findings from the shadowing process. By using the spiral SDLC model, these new findings could be addressed and the user requirements could be re-defined. Additionally, due to the variability of a patient's health on the day of surgery a patients workflow could alter its trajectory from the perceived norm. This had to be considered when designing the system and determining the system limitations and real-life process correlation, hence re-enforcing the importance of adopting a spiral SDLC methodology. Furthermore, meetings had to be arranged with the administrative staff with regards to the overheads required to get a software system up and running. The engagement with the hospital IT department had to start early in the project as hospital resources tend be at capacity. If a solution was to be piloted the IT department would have to dedicate resources outside of their current planned horizon and this process would need to be determined.

Finally, if the system was to use mobile technologies the Wi-Fi access points of the hospital would have to be mapped and all black-spots would have to be known. To map the hospitals coverage a mobile tracking application was used on a standard smart phone and the speed and access points along the surgical care-pathway were determined.

4.4 Application Design - Overview

Having obtained data from the iterative observational research phase, the second phase in the project was to use this data to pin-point the key areas for improvement and remove the risk of potential bottlenecks, in the surgical care-path workflow process. From the qualitative analysis of the data, it was determined, that there were five key communication points, inside the surgical care-pathway, that needed to be streamlined and at certain points the calling mechanism, needed to be automated. Additionally visibility in the surgical care-pathway needed to be improved as the patients state with regards to their admission status, current location, current and pending workflow process task status and patient transfer eligibility status was not available to all the departments connected to the patient inside their surgical care-pathway. Furthermore to identify the patients and to provide security, the system uses QR codes.

These QR codes will be added to the existing 2D barcode patient wristband and will provide unique content about the patient. Finally as access to patient data, inside the surgical care-pathway currently involves performing relatively complex ad-hoc queries, at fixed workstations, that are located away from the point of care, it is not feasible to assume, that this process is efficient, patient centric, or that the data capture, is accurate, to real-time. To address these issues, the use of mobile technologies, will allow users, to capture and distribute, patient data. This data is then securely filtered for the user, based on their role within the hospital work group (Fig. 2).

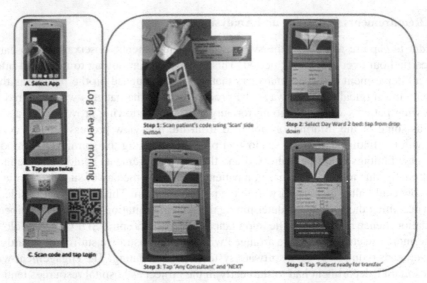

Fig. 2. The QR code scanning mobile application for the admissions process.

4.5 Application Design - Communicating Transfer Requests

The first communication process to be streamlined was a request for transfer from the theatre to the pre-op ward and porter service, for all patients, except the first patient. The second process was a patient transfer request being initiated from the anaesthetist in the ward to the theatre and the porter service. The third transfer request was from the theatre to the ward and the porter service, for the transfer of a patient to the holding bay. The fourth communication process was a request to transfer a patient from the recovery ward to their assigned returning ward. The final communication process was a request from the receiving ward to the porter service to collect the patient from the recovery ward. These transfer requests are currently all manually initiated by staff members, using conventional forms of communication such as wired phones. The proposed new system will champion the use of a push message service that alerts the application users when a transfer request has being initiated (Fig. 3). Additionally where applicable the push message service will be automated based on a task being completed. An example of this would be where a delay is initiated by the returning ward with regards to their capacity to initiate the transfer request. If the delayed time estimate is reached and the request has not being resolved the message will automatically be sent again without being initiated by the message source (Table 4).

4.6 Application Design – Task Visibility

Based on the observational research, it was concluded that task visibility, needed to be available throughout the entire surgical care-pathway, as a means to pseudo-inter-connect, all the departments that interact with the patient, during their surgery process. Additionally, the format of the visibility would have to vary, per device, device component and user. For instance, visibility in the theatre, on a large touch screen computer,

Table 4. A communication process table to be streamlined by the new system.

Request origin	Receivers	Description
Theatre	Porters, Pre-op Ward	A request to deliver the patient to the operating theatre is broadcast to the porters and the pre-op ward. Additionally all assessments have being completed
Ward/Anaesthetist	Pre-op Ward, Porters	Based on the first patient selection process the anaesthetist broadcasts a message to the ward and the porters to deliver the patient to the operating theatre
Theatre	Pre-op, Porters	A request to deliver the patient to the operating theatre is broadcast to the porters and the pre-op ward. The anaesthetic assessment has not been completed
PACU	Returning Ward	The returning ward receives a request from the PACU ward to collect a patient from their recovery bay
Returning Ward	Porters, PACU	The returning ward broadcasts a reply to the porters to collect the patient and provides compliance for the PACU ward via a verification message

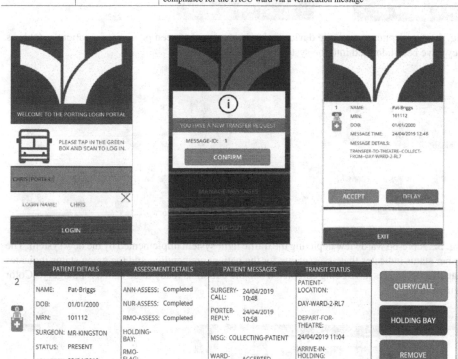

Fig. 3. An example of the porter application message acknowledge & distribution process as it relates to the theatre screen view.

of a patient who has being admitted, would be represented by, a dynamic animation in a process flow chain, that updates based on the next completed event (Fig. 4). Respectively, the same process, for the patient escort, on a mobile device, would be the dynamic addition of the patient values to a text based work-list (Figs. 5 and 6).

4.7   Application Implementation – Software and Architecture

Having finalised sections of the design and the project work break-down structure the next phase was to actually develop the application. This involved writing code for the controls

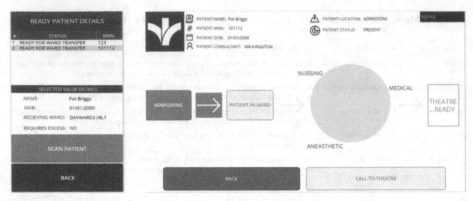

Fig. 4. A patient escort mobile device and a theatre touch-screen pc view of a patient's status as they have been admitted into the system.

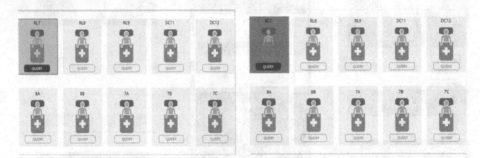

Fig. 5. A pre-op ward view depicting the traffic light system implemented by the new system. The amber status indicates that assessments for the patient are pending and the green status indicates that all assessments have being completed and the patient is ready to be called for surgery. (Color figure online)

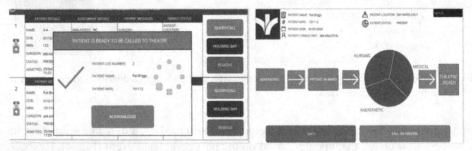

Fig. 6. A theatre view of the received popup-message that indicates that all assessments have being carried out on the patient and they are now ready to be called to surgery. (Color figure online)

for the front end components of the Microsoft Powerapps framework and connecting them to stored procedures in the back end. The stored procedures and tables associated with them were written in Microsoft SQL Server 2018. The physical devices were connected via an SQL connector API and the data XML transforms were carried out inside embedded Microsoft flow connections. To remove the load on the SQL connector the application was divided into seven different applications. This reduced the demand to poll the applications from the same source and improved efficiency. From a 'look and feel' perspective, the application design adopted a colour scheme similar to the hospital colour scheme. The application was designed to be user friendly with text prompts to inform users about the next process. The scanning process has a colour system whereby a patient would be scanned with a green theme in the application screen and the patient location would be scanned using an amber theme. This theme was further developed in the pre-op-ward screen and the PACU unit screen, where a traffic light system was used to signal, if the patient had, processes to be completed (Amber), was delayed (Red), was ready for the next phase of process (Green).These processes varied as the patient navigated the surgical care-pathway, however, the colour theme remained uniform. With regards to security, most of the stored procedures had input validation to prevent SQL injection, and there was additional client-side validation, on the QR code scanning component as well. Finally, every selection component is either a drop-down menu of controlled content or a checkbox. This further re-enforced the security of the application by not allowing the user to type bad input data into the system (Fig. 7).

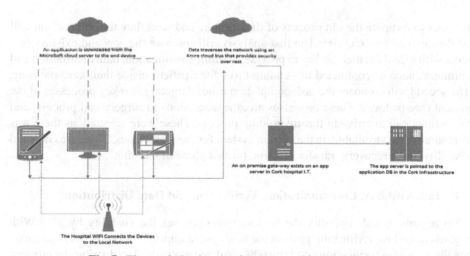

Fig. 7. The newly implemented systems architectural design.

4.8 Application Implementation - Hardware

The new system consists of two large medical grade touch screen computers that are used in a day ward and an operating theatre. Additionally based on the observational research eight medical grade handheld devices will be used by various personnel throughout the surgical care path-way. Furthermore, five tablets are dispersed throughout a recovery ward to provide alerts and compliance for messages from the PACU to collect patients.

These additional tablets were based on new features which form the basis of the second case study which is outside of the scope of this paper.

4.9 Application Testing

Once the local and remote testing phases were completed the system was now ready to be piloted in a hospital environment. The first phase of the pilot ran over four months, from September 2019, until December 2019. The pilot covered the care-pathway from admissions to recovery, for all paediatric patients, who were being operated on, by a particular consultant, in a set theatre. It was observed, that the paediatric patients, can have varying times of admission and the average time of surgery, due to the complexity, of the surgery type, is hard to define. This was a robust test for the new system, as most of the functionality, would be used, throughout the course of the pilot. Additionally, only patients that were admitted on the day of surgery were tested by the pilot. This was primarily due to the need to form comparative analysis, of admission times, versus patient surgery arrival times. The system was piloted three days a week, typically starting at 7:30 am and finishing at 8:00 pm.

5 Results

In order to compare the old process of data capture and workflow the comparison will be divided into two sections. The first analysis will compare the new and existing systems with regards to their ability to provide, visibility, verification, data distribution and communication of completed or pending tasks for a patient inside their care-pathway. The second will compare the task completion times, targeting two key processes of the patient care-pathway. These processes are, the admissions to surgery call process, and the surgery call to arrive in theatre holding process. These were selected, as there was comparative data available, in the current system for these processes. There was no valid visibility of the recovery transfer process, for this phase of the pilot.

5.1 Task Visibility, Communication, Verification and Data Distribution

With regards to task visibility the new system improves the visibility by 80%.With regards to the task verification process the new system improves this process by increasing the amount of verification points by 60%.With regards to the data distribution process, the new system increased the distribution of data by 60% throughout the patient surgical care-pathway. Finally the new communication process automates the entire patient calling process. This reduces the need to constantly poll wards for acknowledgement and verification and in doing so increases incidence of proactive communication by 80%. Table 5 is an example of how the new system when implemented in the admissions process generated an increase of over 50% more incidents of process capture, task visibility and data distribution across three separate scenarios'.

Table 5. A data capture comparison table of the old and new system for the pre-op patient transfer call process with pending anesthetic assessment 0 = yes X = no

Sceanario	Stake holders	Process capture	Old sys	Pilot sys
A theatre worker selects a patient to transfer to the holding bay for surgery	Current ward Theatre Porters	1. Call verification	0	0
		2. Call time	0	0
		3. Ward verification	X	0
		4. Porter verification	X	0
		5. Patient departure time	X	0
		6. Patient arrival time	0	0
A theatre worker selects a patient to transfer to the holding bay for surgery pending an anaesthetic assessment	Current ward Theatre Porters	1. Call verification	0	0
		2. Call time	0	0
		3. Ward verification	X	0
		4. Porter verification	X	0
		5. Patient departure time	X	0
		6. Patient arrival time	0	0
		7. Patient pending assessment status	X	0
A porter receives a notification and collects the patient from the ward	Current ward Operating Porters PACU	Call verification	X	0
		Call time	X	0
		Patient location	X	0
		Patient name	X	0
		Delay patient transfer	X	0
		Patient arrival time	0	0
		Patient pending assessment status	X	X

5.2 A Time Comparison of the New and Old System from Admission to Surgery Transfer Request

The results of this process comparison suggest several assumptions about the new system. The first being, the new pilot system was more efficient in the numerical sense, however, it is still limited to the process flow of the current hospital workflow (Table 6). With more training and possible process change, the system should deliver higher turnaround times. Secondly, even though there was an increase of 80% in the visibility and verification of tasks, there remained a high correlation between the old system and the new system (Fig. 8). This would again re-iterate the influence of process change and additionally suggest the accuracy of the data being captured by the current system is prone to error. Finally, overall the new pilot system navigated a patient 9.3 min faster than the current system from admissions to the surgery transfer request phase of the surgical care-pathway. The impact that time alone, if repeated for all surgical cases, would mean significant increase in patient throughput, which in turn generates more revenue for the hospital and improve the patient care experience.

Table 6. A time capture comparison between the new and old system based on the time taken to admit the patient and the theatre calling the patient to surgery. The data here is based on patients who were admitted between 7:00 am and 7:45 am. All of the patients are from a specific surgeon who had booked a block of time in a specific operating theatre. All surgical procedures are of a similar type. The larger times found in patients 7–10 are based on patients who were admitted early even though they were scheduled to operate on in the afternoon.

Patient#	Manual time	Pilot time
1	68 min	44 min
2	73 min	90 min
3	118 min	61 min
4	111 min	118 min
5	107 min	84 min
6	74 min	48 min
7	78 min	97 min
8	174 min	180 min
9	334 min	334 min
10	139 min	127 min

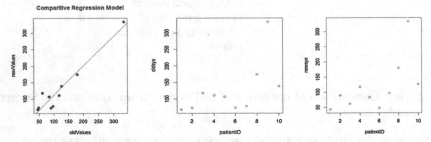

Fig. 8. A regression model built in R studio depicting a strong correlation between the old and new system times for the admissions to surgery request process.

5.3 A Time Comparison Between the New and Old System from Surgery Transfer Request to Theatre Arrival

Based on the results, it can be concluded than the communication system is far more efficient than the current system in the navigation of a patient from the pre-op ward to the surgery holding bay (Table 7). With an improvement of 80% more visibility and task verification this new communication system, once fully implemented, should create even more efficient task turnaround times. Due to the highly complex multitasking nature of the work inside the surgical care-pathway it extremely difficult to connect key decision makers and influencers at the same time. The new system streamlines the communication process by connecting the right people to the right process at the same time. The system additionally provides security via patient identification in the transfer process and also allows for the user to issue a delay in the transfer process. This delay is then broadcast to the appropriate departments and allows the user to handle this delay. In doing so, the repetitive and costly process of polling departments for service is eliminated. Finally, the impact of reducing the patients transfer time by 22 min is highly cost effective, taking into consideration the cost of overheads for a delay to surgery, and this also serves to improve the patients overall care experience inside their surgical care-pathway (Fig. 9).

Table 7. A time capture comparison between the new and old system based on the time taken to call the patient and deliver them the patient to surgery.

Patient #	Manual time	Pilot time
1	25 min	6 min
2	40 min	7 min
3	12 min	6 min
4	15 min	9 min
5	14 min	6 min
6	18 min	9 min
7	19 min	11 min
8	59 min	7 min
9	18 min	4 min
10	69 min	4 min

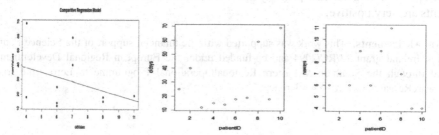

Fig. 9. A regression model built in R studio depicting a weak correlation between the old and new system times for the admissions to surgery request process.

6 Conclusion

This paper has examined how the streamlining of the surgical care-pathway can improve patient throughput by; enhancing task visibility and verification; promote interdepartmental communication and successional task compliance; securely identify and locate a patient for assessment processing and transfer; communicate with and integrate services autonomously based on adopting a task workflow completion messaging mechanism. This approach was devised from firstly exploring the varying problem domain that was identified in several studies and current government initiatives from an Irish, European and American context. Then, through several months of observational research and data analysis in a hospital in the south of Ireland, similar trends were discovered that correlated to problem domain. From here, a software solution was developed, tested and deployed and returned positive results in relation to improvements on the time taken to navigate the pre-op sections of the surgical care-pathway.

Finally, efficient patient calling in the surgical care-pathway can only be achieved by efficient interdepartmental communication at the point of patient transfers. The effect that technology has in relation to improving communication is difficult to measure. Once a technology has promoted and addressed the lack of communication and this issue has being addressed via process change, the technology may become obsolete again. Most of the technologies in the literature are aimed at improving the current state of communication. Additionally, as the surgical care-pathway is interconnected to a least 4 departments, the technical solution are not merely a messaging service to replace wired phones. This was evident in the pilot whereby every process that lead to making a wired phone request for transfer had to be, documented, digitized and re-engineered to match the existing workflow. Whether the pilot will prove to be efficient across the post-operative surgical care-pathway process remains to be seen, however the current results are very positive.

Acknowledgements. This work was supported with the financial support of the Science Foundation Ireland grant 13/RC/2094 and co-funded under the European Regional Development-Fund through the Southern & Eastern RegionalOperational Programme to Lero - the Irish SoftwareResearch Centre (www.lero.ie).

References

1. Junge, T.L.: Surgical Technology for the Surgical Technologist, p. 18. Taylor & Francis (2004)
2. Li, P.: A prospective observational study of physician handoff for intensive-care-unit-to-ward patient transfers. Am. J. Med. **124**(9), 860–867 (2011)
3. Fairbanks, R.J.T., Bisantz, A.M.: Interpersonal communication and public display tools in the emergency department. In: Proceedings of the 2005 Systems and Information Engineering Design Symposium, p. 1–4 (2005)
4. Haux, R.: Strategic Information Management in Hospitals: An Introduction to Hospital Information Systems, p. 14. Springer, Heidelberg (2013)
5. Sharma, D.K.: Hospital Administration and Human Resource Management. PHI Learning (2017)

6. Weimann, E.: High Performance in Hospital Management: A Guideline for Developing and Developed Countries, pp. 93–94. Springer, Heidelberg (2017). https://doi.org/10.1007/978-3-662-49660-2

7. Rosiek, A.: Organizational Culture and Ethics in Modern Medicine. IGI Global (2015)

8. Langabeer, J.R.: Competitive Business Strategy for Teaching Hospital, pp. 211–212. Creenwood Publishing Group (2000)

9. Sears, K.: Influencing the Quality, Risk and Safety Movement in Healthcare: In Conversation with International Leaders, pp. 171–172. Ashgate, Farnham (2015)

10. Suzanne, E.: Effective Communication in Clinical Handover: From Research to Practice, pp. 17–18. Walter de Gruyter GmbH & Co KG (2016)

11. Zaoutis, L.B.: Comprehensive Pediatric Hospital Medicine, p. 62. Elsevier Health Sciences, Amsterdam (2007)

12. Gillingham, E.A.: LaFleur Brooks' Health Unit Coordinating, pp. 355–356. Elsevier Health Sciences, Amsterdam (2013)

13. Edward, M.D.: Financial Management Strategies for Hospitals and Healthcare Organizations: Tools Techniques Checklists and Case Studies, pp. 59–60. CRC Press, Boca Raton (2013)

14. Abraham, J.: Challenges to inter-departmental coordination of patient transfers: a workflow perspective. Int. J. Med. Inform. **79**, 112–122 (2010)

15. Dudeck, K.: New Technologies in Hospital Information Systems. IOS Press (1997)

16. Association of Surgical Technologists: Surgical Technology for the Surgical Technologist, p. 100. Cengage Learning (2016)

17. Arisaka, N.: Trial of Real-Time Locating and Messaging, pp. 689–699. IOS Press (2016)

18. O'Connor, C.: The use of wireless e-mail to improve healthcare team communication. J. Am. Med. Inform. Assoc. **16**(5), 705–711 (2009)

19. Hanada, E.: Managing the availability of hospital wireless communication systems. In: URSI Asia-Pacific Radio Science Conference (URSI AP-RASC), pp. 737–739 (2016). From the viewpoint of the electromagnetic environment

20. Sun, Q.: Application of wireless local area network in hospital information system. In: 2017 IEEE 2nd Advanced Information Technology, Electronic and Automation Control Conference (IAEAC), pp. 263–266 (2017)

21. Johnston, M.: Requirements of a new communication technology for handover and the escalation of patient care: a multi-stakeholder analysis. J. Eval. Clin. Pract. **20**(4), 486–497 (2014)

22. Cavada, D.: A multi-functional mobile information system for hospital assistance, pp. 1–6. IEEE (2013)

23. Vinu, M.: The use of a digital structured format for nursing shift handover to improve communication. In: 2016 IEEE 29th International Symposium on Computer-Based Medical Systems (CBMS), pp. 71–74 (2016)

24. Giesen, D.: International Medical Malpractice Law: A Comparative Law Study of Civil Liability Arising from Medical Care, p. 65. BRILL Publishings (1988)

25. Marcinko, D.E.: Financial Management Strategies for Hospitals and Healthcare Organizations, Tools, Techniques, pp. 59–60. Checklists and Case Studies. CRC Press, Boca Raton (2013)

26. Greenwald, H.P.: Health Care in the United States, Organization, Management and Policy, p. 121. Wiley, San Francisco (2010)

27. Hall, R.: Patient Flow: Reducing Delay in Healthcare Delivery, pp. 102–103. Springer, Heidelberg (2006). https://doi.org/10.1007/978-0-387-33636-7

28. Rosenstein, M.: Professional communication and team collaboration. In: Patient Safety and Quality: An Evidence-Based Handbook for Nurses, Rockville, vol. 2, pp. 271–274 (2015)

29. Wen, D.: The challenges of emerging HISs in bridging the communication gaps among physicians and nurses in China: an interview study. BMC Med. Inform. Decis. Making **17**, 1–11 (2017)
30. Ward, D.M.: Issues in Cost Accounting for Health Care Organizations, p. 335. Jones & Bartlett Learning (1999)
31. Tsujii, H., Kamada, T., Shirai, T., Noda, K., Tsuji, H., Karasawa, K. (eds.): Carbon-Ion Radiotherapy. Springer, Tokyo (2014). https://doi.org/10.1007/978-4-431-54457-9
32. Graban, M.: Lean Hospitals: Improving Quality, Patient Safety, and Employee Engagement, 3rd edn., p. 97. CRC Press, Boca Raton (2016)
33. Fordney, M.T.: Administrative Medical Assisting, p. 211. Cengage Learning (2007)
34. Charles, P.: Leveraging Lean in Ancillary Hospital Services: Creating a Cost Effective, Standardized, High Quality, Patient-Focused Operation, p. 142. CRC Press, Boca Raton (2014)
35. Rothrock, J.C.: Alexander's Care of the Patient in Surgery, p. 7. Elsevier, Amsterdam (2010)
36. Ramlaul, A.: Patient Centered Care in Medical Imaging and Radiotherapy, p. 25. Elsevier Health Sciences, Amsterdam (2013)
37. Dixit, S.: Human Bond Communication: The Holy Grail of Holistic Communication and Immersive Experience, p. 192. Wiley, Hoboken (2017)
38. Yuan, B.: The policy effect of the general data protection. Int. J. Environ. Res. Public Health 1–15 (2019)
39. HSE: eHealth Strategy for Ireland. Department of Health an EU Commission On Helath (2020)
40. HSE. National Service Plan 2018. HSE (2018)
41. de Jong, T.: European Risk Observatory. Publications Office of the European Union, Luxemburg (2014)
42. Directorate-General for Communications Networks, Content and Technology: Research and Innovation in the Field of ICT for Health. Digital Society, Trust and Cybersecurity (2019)
43. Khosrow-Pour, M.: Advanced Methodologies and Technologies in Medicine and Healthcare, p. 289. IGI Global (2018)
44. Ponemon Institute: The Imprivata Report on the Economic Impact of. Ponemon Institute (2014)
45. Karahoca, A.: Advances and Applications in Mobile Computing, p. 162. BoD – Books on Demand (2012)
46. Househ, M.: Social Media and Mobile Technologies for Healthcare, pp. 48–55. IGI Global (2014)
47. Kornak, A.: Enterprise Guide to Gaining Business Value from Mobile Technologies, pp. 185–186. Wiley, Hoboken (2004)
48. Sinha, P.K.: Electronic Health Record Standards, Coding Systems, Frameworks, and Infrastructures. Wiley, Hoboken (2012)
49. Cruz-Cunha, M.M.: Handbook of Research on Developments in E-Health and Telemedicine: Technological and Social Perspectives: Technological and Social Perspectives, p. 414. IGI Global (2009)
50. Harrington, L.: Usability Evaluation Handbook for Electronic Health Records, p. 46. HIMSS (2014)
51. Patel, V.L., Kannampallil, T.G., Kaufman, D.R. (eds.): Cognitive Informatics for Biomedicine. HI, p. 225. Springer, Cham (2015). https://doi.org/10.1007/978-3-319-17272-9
52. Ugon, A.: Building Continents of Knowledge in Oceans of Data: The Future of Co-Created eHealth, pp. 283–284. IOS Press (2018)
53. Patton, R.M., Zalon, M.L., Ludwick, R. (eds.): Nurses Making Policy: From Bedside to Boardroom, p. 348. Springer, New York (2014). https://doi.org/10.1891/9780826198921

54. Schreier, G.: Health Informatics Meets eHealth. In: Proceedings of the 12th eHealth Conference, p. 276. IOS Press (2018)
55. Tran, K.: Effects of clinical communication interventions in hospitals: a systematic review of information and communication technology adoptions for improved communication between clinicians. Int. J. Med. Inform. **81**(11), 723–730 (2012)
56. Wu, V.: Development of a prototype of the tele-localisation system in radiotherapy using personal digital assistant via wireless communication. J. Med. Imaging Radiat. Oncol. **57**(1), 113–118 (2013)
57. Mejĺa, D.A.: Understanding and supporting lightweight communication in hospital work. IEEE Trans. Inf. Technol. Biomed. **14**(1), 140–146 (2009)
58. Vezyridis, P.: Going paperless at the emergency department: a socio-technical study of an information system for patient tracking. Int. J. Med. Inform. **80**(7), 455–459 (2011)
59. Bossen, C.: Implications of shared interactive displays for work at a surgery ward: coordination, articulation work and context-awareness, pp. 464–469. IEEE (2008)
60. Kim, T.: Assessing the usability of a prototype EMP centered EHR display. In: 2018 IEEE Conference on Healthcare Informatics, pp. 1–22. IEEE (2018)
61. Troester, S.: Drive nursing activities to the bedside with a closed-loop system. Nurs. Manag. **37**(12), 18–20 (2006)
62. Sangwan, R.: Using RFID tags for tracking patients, charts and medical equipment within an integrated health delivery network, pp. 1–13. IEEE (2005)
63. Anton, F.D.: QR code indentify replace paper based system information sharing using a technical platform, pp. 1–14. IEEE (2018)
64. Chu, L.-C.: Applying QR code technology to facilitate hospital medical equipment repair management. In: 2012 International Conference on Control Engineering and Communication Technology, pp. 856–858. IEEE (2012)

Connect - Blockchain and Self-Sovereign Identity Empowered Contact Tracing Platform

Eranga Bandara[1]([⊠]), Xueping Liang[2], Peter Foytik[1], Sachin Shetty[1],
Crissie Hall[4], Daniel Bowden[4], Nalin Ranasinghe[3], Kasun De Zoysa[3],
and Wee Keong Ng[5]

[1] Old Dominion University, Norfolk, VA, USA
{cmedawer,pfoytik,sshetty}@odu.edu
[2] University of North Carolina at Greensboro, Greensboro, NC, USA
x_liang@uncg.edu
[3] University of Colombo School of Computing, Colombo, Sri Lanka
{dnr,kasun}@ucsc.cmb.ac.lk
[4] Sentara Healthcare, Norfolk, VA, USA
{cehallre,dsbowden}@sentara.com
[5] School of Computer Science and Engineering, Nanyang Technological University,
Singapore, Singapore
awkng@ntu.edu.sg

Abstract. The COVID-19 pandemic in 2020 has resulted in increased fatality rates across the world and has stretched the resources in healthcare facilities. There have been several proposed efforts to contain the spread of the virus among humans. Some of these efforts involve appropriate social distancing in public places, monitoring and tracking temperature at the point of access, etc. In order for us to get back to the "new normal", there is a need for automated and efficient human contact tracing that would be non-intrusive and effective in containing the spread of the virus. In this paper, we have developed "Connect", a Blockchain and Self-Sovereign Identity (SSI) based digital contact tracing platform. "Connect" will provide an automated mechanism to notify people in their immediate proximity of an occurrence of a positive case and would reduce the rate at which the infection could spread. The platform's self-sovereign identity capability will ensure no attribution to a user and the user will be empowered to share information. The ability to notify in a privacy-preserving fashion would provide businesses to put in place dynamic and localized data-driven mitigation response. "Connect's" SSI based identity wallet platform encodes user's digital identities and activity trace data on a permissioned blockchain platform and verified using SSI proofs. The user activities will provide information, such as places travelled, travel and dispatch updates from the airport etc. The activity trace records can be leveraged to identify suspected patients and notify the local community in real-time. Simulation results demonstrate transaction scalability and demonstrate the effectiveness of "Connect" in realizing data immutability and traceability.

© ICST Institute for Computer Sciences, Social Informatics and Telecommunications Engineering 2021
Published by Springer Nature Switzerland AG 2021. All Rights Reserved
J. Ye et al. (Eds.): MobiHealth 2020, LNICST 362, pp. 208–223, 2021.
https://doi.org/10.1007/978-3-030-70569-5_13

Keywords: Blockchain · COVID-19 · Contract tracing · E-Health · Big data

1   Introduction

The COVID-19 pandemic has challenged countries to invest in resources to control the spread of the virus. The number of positive COVID-19 cases have been rising all over the world, with the majority of the confirmed cases found in the U.S. The reasons for the rapid spread through humans have been attributed to symptomatic, pre-symptomatic and asymptomatic cases [30]. The current approaches to limit the spread of the virus includes various methods to enforce safe social distancing and limiting air travel. Though these approaches have value, there is a need for a platform that can alert the presence of a positive case to a regional community in a timely and privacy-preserving fashion.

Organizations are working on "safe back to work" policies to realize a "new normal working environment", that would provide a data-driven mitigation response to limit the spread of the virus. These "back to work" policies are not just limited to COVID-19 and will also be effective against any infectious disease. It has been acknowledged that an effective means to limit the spread of the virus is to continuously track user activities at various points of visit and access [15] and notify potential cases or exposure to local and regional communities. The resultant data-driven insights would help organizations to operate safely and people to access public spaces.

However, on the flip side, current approaches that provide capabilities to address the aforementioned need are plagued with data centralization, privacy concerns and location tracking concerns. The centralization of user data in a cloud environment can be vulnerable to adversarial attacks. The privacy concern for both potential patient and the people they could come in contact should be preserved [2].

In this paper, we propose "Connect", a "back to work safely" system based on a blockchain and self-sovereign identity (SSI) empowered digital contract tracing platform. The platform keeps employees' digital identities and events related to testing/symptoms on a blockchain platform using SSI [27] proofs. The employer can use a mobile app to self-report the requested information that uses SSI to record results anonymously and without location tracking. The employer can use the back end analytics to monitor workplace conditions and use a data-driven approach to inform workplace safety policies and guidelines. The main contributions of "Connect" are as follows.

1. Blockchain and SSI empowered digital contact tracing platform to realize decentralized and privacy-preserving digital contact tracing
2. SSI based identity wallet to capture/verify the user identity proofs and activity trace record proofs.
3. Store user identity data and activity trace record data on blockchain platforms by using self-sovereign identity proofs.

4. Self-sovereign identity proof-based identity and activity trace storage address the common issues in cloud-based data storages (e.g. lack of data privacy, lack of data immutability, lack of traceability, lack of data provenance [25,35]).

The rest of the paper is organized as follows. Section 2 discusses the architecture of the Connect platform. Section 3 implementation details of the Connect platform. Section 4 performance evaluation, Sect. 5 surveys related work. Section 6 concludes the Connect platform with suggestions for future work.

2 Connect Platform

2.1 Overview

Connect is a blockchain, self-sovereign identity-based user identity, and activity tracking platform. It can be used to track the activity of COVID-19 suspected patients during a quarantine process. The Connect platform is built using a layered architecture shown in Fig. 1 containing four main layers.

1. Distributed ledger - Where all user cryptographic artifacts for identity (DIDs) and proofs of activity are stored.
2. DID communication layer - Where peer to peer data exchange between user identity wallets happens within the DID communication layer.
3. Credential layer - Where different entities in the platform (users, admins) create and exchange credentials for verification via credential layer.
4. Activity trace layer - Where user activity trace recording and verification happens.

Distributed ledger is the blockchain-based peer to peer storage system used in the Connect platform. The blockchain can be deployed among multiple organizations such as government organizations, hospitals, airport/port customer offices, banks, identity authorities etc. Each organization in the network can run its own blockchain node connected as a ring cluster, Fig. 8. It stores all user digital identity proofs (which are identified as DID or decentralized identity proof [6]) and user activity trace record proofs on Connect platform.

The DID communication layer is used to exchange the actual credential information (such as user image, id numbers, etc.) between the credential approvers/versifiers (admins) mobile wallet and the credential owners (users) mobile wallets. Peer to peer data exchange between user identity wallets happens in this layer. When a user's identity needs to be verified/approved, the admin requests proof of identity from the holder, the holder consents and shares data along with cryptographic proof stored on the blockchain. The Connect mobile app fetches the identity information stored in local storage to send to the admins Trace mobile wallet. The admin can do further verification/approvals based on this information.

There are two main types of entities (users) in the connect platform, credential owners, credential verifiers (admins). Connect provides a self-sovereign

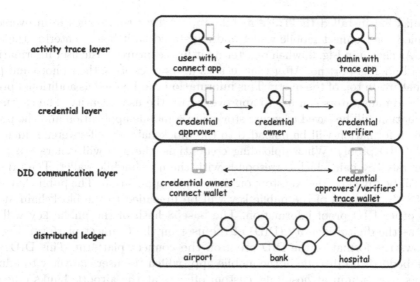

Fig. 1. Connect platform layered architecture. Distributed ledger used to store DIDs. Peer to peer data exchange between user identity wallets happens in the DID communication layer. Credential create, verification happens in Credential layer. User activity trace recording and verification happens in the activity trace layer.

identity based mobile wallet application for each type of user. Credential owners use "Connect mobile wallet" and admins use "Trace mobile wallet". Credential owners register their DID proofs on blockchain and enroll in the Connect platform with the Connect mobile application. Admins verify credentials (DID proofs) via Trace mobile wallet. The credential exchange process happens in the Credential layer, where credential owners and admins exchange the credentials for verification.

All user activity trace data in the Connect platform are stored in the blockchain ledger based on an SSI approach. When a user goes to a specific place (e.g. airport, bank, hospital, office) the admin officers there can verify the identity of the user and create an activity trace record for the user on the blockchain. This identity verification and activity trace data creation process is done via Trace mobile wallet application given to the admin officers. Admins also can fetch user activity trace records which are stored in the blockchain when consent is given, verify them, and view through the Trace mobile application. Trace mobile app comes with a QR code scan-based identity and activity trace data verification process. All activity trace data is handled with functions (activity trace data creation, activity trace data verification) implemented in the Activity trace layer.

2.2 Functionality

Consider a scenario where a blockchain network is deployed at the Airport, Hospital network, Government Bank and Identity office. The admin officers at each organization installed the Trace mobile app. A user who comes from overseas installed the Connect mobile wallet and registered on it before entering the airport. As shown in Fig. 3, when registering it first captures basic user information with Id no/Passport no. After that, it asks users to capture their photo and put a signature on top of the photo. This information can be used as additional proof which administrators can use to approve/verify the user identity. The captured information will be saved in secure storage in a mobile application and the proof of this information will be uploaded to the blockchain as self-sovereign identity proof (DID proof). When uploading credentials, the app will generate a public/private key pair which corresponds with the user/mobile wallet. The private key will be saved on the Keystore on the mobile application. The public key and base58 [16,28] hash of the public key will be uploaded to the blockchain along with other DID proof information. The base58 hash of the public key will be used as the digital identity (DID) of the user on the Connect platform. Figure 2 shows the format of the DID proof on the connect platform. This DID will be embedded to QR code in the mobile app, which the user can show to admin officers (e.g. admin at hospitals, custom officers at the airport, banks officers) for verification, Fig. 3.

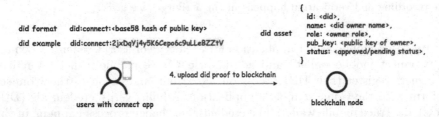

Fig. 2. DID format which generated in Connect app and DID asset format which stored in blockchain.

Assume a user comes from an overseas country and installed the Connect wallet on his/her mobile phone. When the user comes to the airport he/she needs to show the QR code identity which is embedded in the Connect mobile wallet to the admin officer (e.g. customer officer) at the airport in order to have their digital identity issued, Fig. 3. The officer will scan the QR code via Trace application and fetch the user identity proofs which are saved in the blockchain. After that, it requests for consent to specific data and connects to users through the "Connect mobile wallet" application. This process is achieved via push notification (DID communication layer) in order to fetch the actual user identity information (e.g. Id numbers, photo, signature) to the Trace mobile app, Fig. 4. Then the admin could check the information against the passport/id card of the user. If the data is correct according to the passport/id card, the admin approves the identity of the user. When approving, it updates the status of users' digital identity in the blockchain. This is the first-time vetting process which needs to

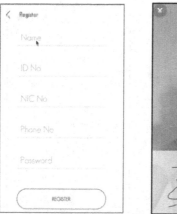
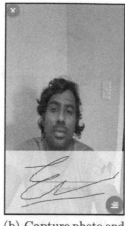

(a) Add identity information

(b) Capture photo and signature

(c) Connect identity in QR code

Fig. 3. Connect mobile wallet application. It will embed users' digital identity on QR code.

be done in order to approve the user identity saved in the blockchain is authentic and verified by a trusted source. Once identity is approved by an authorized administration user can use his/her identity wallet in any other place to prove his/her identity (ex in a bank, hospital etc.). When approving the identity, it will use the Identity smart contact. After identity approved blockchain will create an activity trace record (along with user digital identity/DID, date/time and location) by using Trace smart contract. This activity trace record specifies the user is dispatched from the airport. Once the activity trace record is created in the blockchain node at the airport, it will be available to other blockchain nodes at hospitals and banks.

For example, assume the user goes to a bank a few days after he/she enters the country. User needs to show his/her identity wallet QR code in order to prove identity at the bank. Then the admin at the bank scans the QR code, fetches the identity proof of the blockchain and verifies the user. At the end of this process, blockchain will save another activity trace record which mentions that the user came to the bank with date/time and location, Fig. 5. In this way, the connect platform traces all the user activities as self-sovereign identity proofs (or proof of location). Now assume the user goes to the hospital for some various treatment. The user shows the identity wallet with QR code, then an officer at the hospital scans it and fetches the user identity proof with all user activity record proofs from the blockchain. The activity trace contains an activity that mentions the user came from a foreign country and dispatched from the airport on a specific date, Fig. 4. With this information, it can be easily identified if a person could be suspected of Covid-19. Further precautions can be taken before spreading the virus to more people.

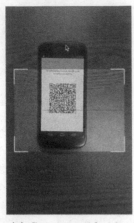 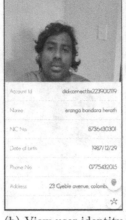 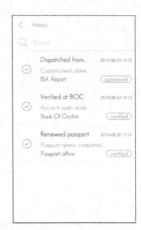

(a) Scan user identity   (b) View user identity   (c) View activity trace

Fig. 4. Trace mobile application. It can view users' identity information and activity trace.

By recording an activity trace of users, Connect platform can support in identifying spread from three main transmission methods of Covid-19 virus, Symptomatic transmission (direct transmission from an asymptomatic individual), Pre-symptomatic transmission (direct transmission from an individual that occurs before the source individual experiences noticeable symptoms), Asymptomatic transmission (direct transmission from individuals who never experience noticeable symptoms).

2.3 Contact Tracing

The users in the Connect platform can be notified via the peer to peer notification system. These notifications can be used to notify the users who are at risk of getting infected with Covid-19 virus. For example, assume a user who has registered in the Connect platform is diagnosed as a Covid-19 infected person. The medical officer at the hospital can report the patient to the Connect platform via Trace mobile application. Additionally, the Connect mobile wallet provides a feature to self-report the diagnosis of the users. This diagnosis information will be uploaded and stored in the blockchain. Once Covid-19 case is reported, the Connect platform can identify all places where the patient has visited (during the last 14 d) by using the activity trace data in the blockchain. The activity trace data contains information about user identity (DID), times and location (latitude, longitude) the diagnosed person has visited. Based on these activity trace information, it can identify the other users who have been in these places at the same time with Covid-19 infected person without revealing personal information. Then Connect platform can send the notifications to these users mentioning there is a risk of contact with Covid-19 since they have been in a place where Covid-19 infected person visited,

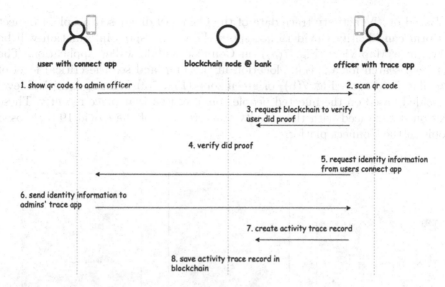

Fig. 5. Admin officer scans QR code identity of the user and creates activity trace record in the blockchain. The trace record contains the information about user identity (DID), time and location (latitude, longitude)

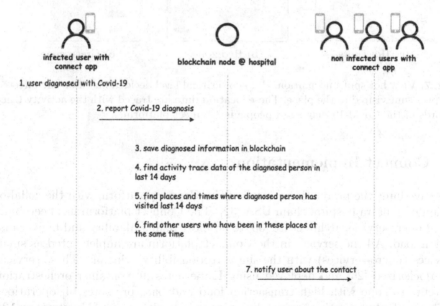

Fig. 6. Covid-19 contact tracing. Once a user is identified as Covid-19 infected person, Connect platform finds the other users who have contacted that person and notify them.

Fig. 6. With the notification function, the user can be aware of the risks in time and take some actions accordingly.

Based on the activity trace data of the Covid-19 diagnosed people, Connect platform can identify Covid-19 hot spots. These hot spots information will be shown in a Map view (Fig. 7(a)) on Connect mobile wallet application. The users can search for a specific location in the map and see the critical level of that place, red zone (Fig. 7(b)) or green zone (Fig. 7(c)). Hot spot critical level is decided based on the infected people count visited that place recently. These location data traced with the activity trace records of the Covid-19 diagnosed people in the Connect platform.

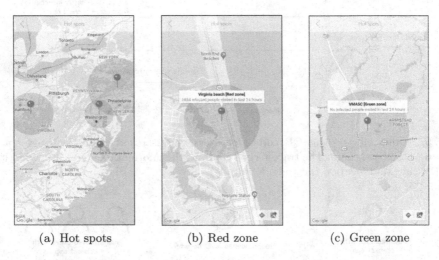

(a) Hot spots   (b) Red zone   (c) Green zone

Fig. 7. View hot spot information. Hot spot critical level decided based on the infected people count visited to the place. These location data are traced with the activity trace records of the Covid-19 diagnosed people in Connect platform.

3   Connect Implementation

We have built the production version of the Connect platform with the collaboration of Sentara hospital chain USA [32]. The Connect platform has been built using microservices architecture [33] to support high scalability and high transaction load. All the services in the Connect platform are implemented as small services (micro-services) with the single responsibility principle. These services are dockerized [26] and deployed using Kubernetes [9] container orchestration system. To cope with high transaction load and back-pressure [14] operations we have adopted reactive streams based approach with using Akka streams [12]. All the microservice communications are handled via Apache Kafka [20,23] message broker. We run 3 Kafka broker nodes with 3 Zookeeper nodes in Connect. The platform is running as a permissioned blockchain system in a private cloud. Figure 8 shows the architecture of the Connect platform.

Rahasak blockchain has been used to implement the functionalities of the Connect platform. Rahasak blockchain [7] comes with concurrency enabled Aplos smart contacts [8] which are written with Scala [1,29] and Akka actor-based [4] concurrency handling [18,19]. All the functionalities of blockchain implemented with Aplos smart contracts. There are four main smart contracts a) identity contract, b) asset contract c) notification contract d) verification contract. "Connect" and 'Trace" mobile wallets are the client applications on the Connect platform. The functions which are implemented in the blockchain smart contracts will be invoked by Mobile clients. The requests generated from Mobile apps will be directed to blockchain smart contracts via Connect gateway service which is HTTPS REST API [3] built with Golang [31]. There is a peer to peer communication channel between "Connect" and "Trace" mobile wallets (to exchange the credential data). Firebase push notification service [22] has been used to implement the peer to peer communication between mobile wallets. Client authentication/authorization will be handled by JWT-based [21] auth service in the Connect platform. Client credential information will be stored in auth-storage (database) in the auth service.

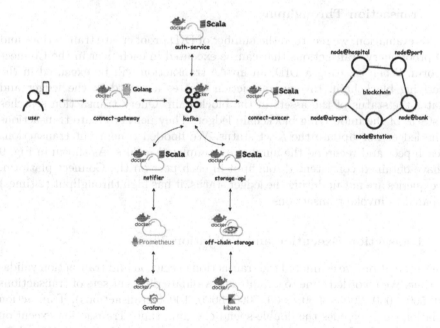

Fig. 8. Connect platform's microservices based architecture. All the services are dockerized and available to deploy with kubernetes.

4   Performance Evaluation

Performance evaluation of Connect was completed and is discussed. To obtain the results, we deployed the Connect platform with multi peer Rahasak blockchain cluster in AWS 2xlarge instances (16 GB RAM and 8 CPUs). Rahasak blockchain runs with 4 Kafka nodes, 3 Zookeeper nodes and Apache Cassandra [24] as the state database. The smart contracts on the Rahasak blockchain implemented with Scala functional programming and Akka actor based Aplos [8] smart contract platform. The evaluation results are obtained for the following, with a varying number of blockchain peers (1 to 5 peers) used in different evaluations.

1. Transaction throughput
2. Transaction execution and validate time
3. Transaction scalability
4. Transaction execution rate
5. Block generate time

4.1   Transaction Throughput

For this evaluation, we recorded the number of DID proof create transactions and DID proof query transactions that can be executed in each peer in the Connect platform. When creating a DID, an invoke transaction will be executed in the underlying blockchain. Invoke transaction creates a record in the ledger and updates the status of the assets in the blockchain. Query transaction searches the status of the underlying blockchain ledger. They neither create transactions in the ledger nor update the asset status. We flooded concurrent transactions for each peer and recorded the number of completed results. As shown in Fig. 9 we have obtained consistent throughput in each peer on the Connect platform. Since queries are not updating the ledger status, it has high throughput (2 times) compared to invoke transactions.

4.2   Transaction Execution and Validation Time

In this evaluation, we evaluated the transaction execution and transaction validation time. We recorded time to execute and validate different sets of transactions (100, 500, 1000, 2000, 3000, 5000, 7000, 8000, 10000 transactions). Transaction validation time includes the double-spend checking time. Transaction execution time includes the double-spend checking time, ledger update time, data replication time. Figure 10 shows how transaction execution time and validation time varies in different transaction sets.

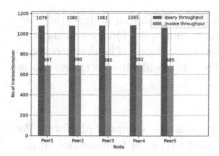

Fig. 9. Invoke transaction throughput and query transaction throughput of Connect blockchain.

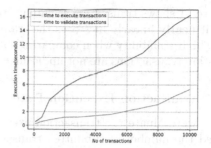

Fig. 10. Time to execute transactions and validate transactions in the Connect platform.

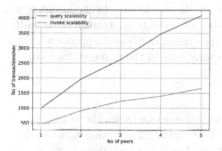

Fig. 11. Transaction scalability of Connect blockchain.

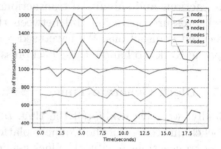

Fig. 12. Transaction execution rate with no of peers in the Connect blockchain.

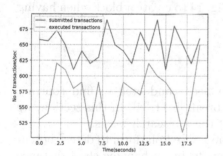

Fig. 13. Transaction execution rate and transaction submission rate in a single blockchain peer.

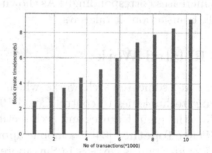

Fig. 14. Block creation time against the no of transactions in the block.

4.3 Transaction Scalability

For this evaluation, we recorded the number of transactions that can be executed (per second) over the number of peers in the network. We flooded concurrent transactions in each peer and recorded the number of executed transactions.

Figure 11 shows transaction scalability results. When adding a node to the cluster, it nearly linearly increases the transaction throughput. Query transactions have high scalability when comparing to invoke transactions. The main reason is question transactions are not updating the ledger status like invoke transactions.

4.4 Transaction Execution Rate

Next, we evaluate the transaction execution rate in the Connect platform. We tested the number of submitted transactions and executed transactions in different blockchain peers recording the time. Figure 12 shows how transaction execution rate varies when having a different number of blockchain peers in the Connect platform. When the number of peers increases, the rate of executed transactions is increased relatively. Figure 13 shows the number of executed transactions and submitted transactions in a single blockchain peer. There is a back pressure operation [14] between the rates of submitted transactions and executed transactions. We have used a reactive streaming-based approach with Apache Kafka to handle these backpressure operations in the Connect platform.

4.5 Block Generate Time

Finally, we have evaluated the time taken to create blocks in the underlying blockchain storage of the Connect platform. The statistics recorded against the no of transactions in a block. Block generate time depends on a). data replication time b). Merkel proof/block hash generate time c). transaction validation time. When the transaction count increases in the block, these factors will be increased. Due to this reason, when the transaction count increases, block generation time also increases correspondingly. As shown in Fig. 14 to create a block when having a 10k transaction, it takes 8 s.

5 Related Work

There are some research works which have been conducted to find contract tracing technologies to control Covid-19 outbreak [5,11,34]. In this section, we outline the main features and architecture of these research works.

TraceTogether [34] is a mobile application-based platform to detect potential Covid-19 virus carriers in Singapore. It works by exchanging short distance Bluetooth signals with other users of the app, giving officials a database to track potential Covid-19 carriers. If a user is diagnosed with Covid-19, the respiratory illness caused by the coronavirus, they could allow Singapore's health ministry to access their app data to identify people who had close contact with the infected individual. Then the app alerts those who come in contact with someone who has tested positive or is at high risk for carrying the coronavirus.

Google/Apple Contact Trace [17] Google and Apple recently announced a joint initiative to build a contact tracing application to help contain the Covid-19 spread. They will be launching a comprehensive solution that includes application programming interfaces (APIs) and operating system-level technology to assist in enabling contact tracing. Their system uses Bluetooth, a standard way for most mobile devices to communicate with each other. Apple and Google stressed that their system preserves users' privacy. Consent is required and location data is not collected. The technology also won't notify users who they came into contact with, or where that happened.

WeTrace [13] is a fully privacy-preserving approach and application, which built on top of BTE (Bluetooth Low Energy). This solution meets major GDPR (General Data Protection Regulation) requirements, which are in force in certain European countries. WeTrace here fulfils exactly this key requirement on privacy-preserving for arbitrary mobile devices, being able to communicate via BTE and being used by their owners in a once-used, once-associated manner. The application of low-range BTE communications determines a highly suitable coincidence between the COVID-19 "social distancing" requirements and the communications technology.

COVID Credentials Initiative (CCI) [10] is a collaboration of more than 60 organizations working to deploy self-sovereign identity (SSI) based verifiable credential solutions to help stop the spread of COVID-19. The goal of CCI is to build an "immunity passport", which is a digital certificate that lets individuals prove (and request proof from others) that they have recovered after testing negative, have tested positive for antibodies, or have received a vaccination once one is available. These digital certificates would be issued by health care institutions but controlled by the user and shared in a peer-to-peer manner. The CCI group includes individuals who are part of Evernym, ID2020, uPort, Dutch research organization TNO, Microsoft, ConsenSys Health and consultants Luxoft.

The comparison summary of these platforms and the Connect platform is presented in Table 1. It compares Architecture (Centralized/Decentralized), Running blockchain, Supported credential types (e.g. biometric), SSI support, Activity trace support, Privacy level details.

Table 1. Self-sovereign identity and activity trace tracking platform comparison

Platform	Architecture	Running blockchain	Credential type	SSI support	Activity trace support	Privacy level
Connect	Decentralized	Rahasak	Any	Yes	Yes	High
TraceTogether	Centralized	N/A	Any	No	Yes	Low
Google and Apple Contact Trace	Centralized	N/A	N/A	No	Yes	Mid
WeTrace	Centralized	N/A	N/A	No	Yes	High
CCI	Decentralized	Sovrin	Medical	Yes	No	High

6   Conclusions and Future Work

In this paper, we have presented "Connect", a Blockchain and SSI empowered digital contract tracing platform that can leverage the information on positive cases and let people in the immediate proximity be notified, which would thereby reduce the rate at which the infection could spread. This would particularly be effective if sufficient people use the platform and benefit from the targeted recommendations. The recommendations would be made in a privacy-preserving fashion and contain the spread of the virus without the need for an extended period of lockdown. We have developed a prototype for the proposed platform and conducted simulations to evaluate scalability and transaction throughput.

Acknowledgements. This work was funded by the Department of Energy (DOE) Office of Fossil Energy (FE) (Federal Grant #DE-FE0031744).

References

1. The scala programming language. https://www.scala-lang.org/
2. Abeler, J., Bäcker, M., Buermeyer, U., Zillessen, H.: Covid-19 contact tracing and data protection can go together. JMIR mHealth and uHealth **8**(4), e19359 (2020)
3. Adamczyk, P., Smith, P.H., Johnson, R.E., Hafiz, M.: Rest and web services: in theory and in practice. In: REST: From Research to Practice, pp. 35–37. Springer, New York (2011)
4. Akka: Akka documentation. https://doc.akka.io/docs/akka/2.5/actors.html
5. Allam, Z., Jones, D.S.: On the coronavirus (covid-19) outbreak and the smart city network: universal data sharing standards coupled with artificial intelligence (AI) to benefit urban health monitoring and management. In: Healthcare, vol. 8, p. 46. Multidisciplinary Digital Publishing Institute (2020)
6. Baars, D.: Towards self-sovereign identity using blockchain technology. Master's thesis, University of Twente (2016)
7. Bandara, E., et al.: Mystiko—blockchain meets big data. In: 2018 IEEE International Conference on Big Data (Big Data), pp. 3024–3032. IEEE (2018)
8. Bandara, E., Ng, W.K., Ranasinghe, N., De Zoysa, K.: Aplos: smart contracts made smart. In: Zheng, Z., Dai, H.-N., Tang, M., Chen, X. (eds.) BlockSys 2019. CCIS, vol. 1156, pp. 431–445. Springer, Singapore (2020). https://doi.org/10.1007/978-981-15-2777-7_35
9. Burns, B., Grant, B., Oppenheimer, D., Brewer, E., Wilkes, J.: Borg, omega, and kubernetes. Queue **14**(1), 70–93 (2016)
10. CCI: Cci. https://www.covidcreds.com/
11. Cho, H., Ippolito, D., Yu, Y.W.: Contact tracing mobile apps for covid-19: privacy considerations and related trade-offs. arXiv preprint arXiv:2003.11511 (2020)
12. Davis, A.L.: Akka streams. In: Reactive Streams in Java, pp. 57–70. Apress, Berkeley, CA (2019). https://doi.org/10.1007/978-1-4842-4176-9_6
13. De Carli, A., et al.: Wetrace–a privacy-preserving mobile covid-19 tracing approach and application. arXiv preprint arXiv:2004.08812 (2020)
14. Destounis, A., Paschos, G.S., Koutsopoulos, I.: Streaming big data meets backpressure in distributed network computation. In: IEEE INFOCOM 2016-The 35th Annual IEEE International Conference on Computer Communications, pp. 1–9. IEEE (2016)
15. Ferretti, L., et al.: Quantifying SARS-CoV-2 transmission suggests epidemic control with digital contact tracing. Science **368**, 6491 (2020)
16. Fisher, J., Sanchez, M.H.: Authentication and verification of digital data utilizing blockchain technology, US Patent App. 15/083,238, 29 September 2016
17. Google, Apple: Privacy-Preserving Contact Tracing. https://www.apple.com/covid19/contacttracing (2020)

18. Hewitt, C.: Actor model of computation: scalable robust information systems. arXiv preprint arXiv:1008.1459 (2010)
19. Hoare, C.A.R.: Communicating sequential processes. Commun. ACM **21**(8), 666–677 (1978)
20. Hunt, P., Konar, M., Junqueira, F.P., Reed, B.: Zookeeper: wait-free coordination for internet-scale systems. In: USENIX Annual Technical Conference, vol. 8. Boston, MA, USA (2010)
21. Jones, M.B.: The emerging JSON-based identity protocol suite. In: W3C Workshop on Identity in the Browser, pp. 1–3 (2011)
22. Khawas, C., Shah, P.: Application of firebase in android app development-a study. Int. J. Comput. App. **179**(46), 49–53 (2018)
23. Kreps, J., Narkhede, N., Rao, J., et al.: Kafka: a distributed messaging system for log processing. In: Proceedings of the NetDB, pp. 1–7 (2011)
24. Lakshman, A., Malik, P.: Cassandra: a decentralized structured storage system. ACM SIGOPS Oper. Syst. Rev. **44**(2), 35–40 (2010)
25. Liang, X., Shetty, S., Zhao, J., Bowden, D., Li, D., Liu, J.: Towards decentralized accountability and self-sovereignty in healthcare systems. In: Qing, S., Mitchell, C., Chen, L., Liu, D. (eds.) ICICS 2017. LNCS, vol. 10631, pp. 387–398. Springer, Cham (2018). https://doi.org/10.1007/978-3-319-89500-0_34
26. Merkel, D.: Docker: lightweight linux containers for consistent development and deployment. Linux J. **2014**(239), 2 (2014)
27. Mühle, A., Grüner, A., Gayvoronskaya, T., Meinel, C.: A survey on essential components of a self-sovereign identity. Comput. Sci. Rev. **30**, 80–86 (2018)
28. Nakamoto, S.: Bitcoin: a peer-to-peer electronic cash system (2008)
29. Odersky, M., et al.: An overview of the scala programming language. Technical report (2004)
30. Organization, W.H.: Coronavirus disease 2019 (covid-19) situation report. https://www.who.int/docs/default-source/coronaviruse/situation-reports/20200402-sitrep-73-covid-19.pdf?sfvrsn=5ae25bc7_2
31. Schmager, F., Cameron, N., Noble, J.: Gohotdraw: evaluating the Go programming language with design patterns. In: Evaluation and Usability of Programming Languages and Tools, p. 10. ACM (2010)
32. sentara: sentara. https://www.sentara.com/hampton-roads-virginia
33. Thönes, J.: Microservices. IEEE Softw. **32**(1), 116–116 (2015)
34. TraceTogether: Tracetogether. https://www.tracetogether.gov.sg/
35. Yu, Y., et al.: Identity-based remote data integrity checking with perfect data privacy preserving for cloud storage. IEEE Trans. Inf. Forensics Secur. **12**(4), 767–778 (2016)

EAI International Workshop on Medical Artificial Intelligence 2020

Expanding eVision's Granularity
of Influenza Forecasting

Navid Shaghaghi[✉][iD], Andres Calle, George Kouretas, Supriya Karishetti,
and Tanmay Wagh

BioInnovation and Design Laboratory, Santa Clara University, Santa Clara,
CA 95053, USA
{nshaghaghi,acalle,gkouretas,skarishetti,twagh}@scu.edu

Abstract. According to the United States' Center for Disease Control
and Prevention (CDC) between 39 and 56 million people in the US suffered from Influenza Like Illnesses (ILI) in the 2019-20 flue season. From
which, 410 to 740 thousand were hospitalized and 24 to 62 thousand
succumbed to the disease. Therefore, the existence of an early warning
mechanism that can alert pharmaceuticals, healthcare providers, and
governments to the trends of the influenza season well in advance, would
serve as a significant step in helping combat this communicable disease
and reduce mortality from it.

As reported in the [ACM Special Interest Group in Computers
and Society (SIGCAS) 2020 Computers and Sustainable Societies
(COMPASS)], [IEEE Technology and Engineering Management Society (TEMS) 2020 International Conference on Artificial Intelligence for
Good (AI4G)], and [IEEE Global Humanitarian Technology Conference
(GHTC) 2020] Long Short-Term Memory (LSTM) neural networks are
utilized by Santa Clara University's EPIC (Ethical, Pragmatic, and Intelligent Computing) and BioInnovation & Design laboratories for continued research and development of an eVision (Epidemic Vision) machine
learning tool to predict the trend of influenza cases throughout the flu
season.

There we reported eVision's success in making 3, 7, and 14 weeks
in advance predictions for the 2018–2019 United States flu season with
88.11%, 88%, and 74.18% accuracy respectively and delineated future
steps of expanding eVision's granularity by 1) adding state level predictions in order to enhance national predictions and 2) utilizing metropolitan area keyword trends to improve both state level and national predictions. This resulted in the improvement of the model's accuracy to
90.38%, 91.43%, and 81.74% for 3, 7, and 14 weeks in advance predictions respectively. This paper is to report on the methodology of obtaining these improved results.

Keywords: Flu trend prediction · Google Trends · Health care
technology · Influenza incident rate forecasting · Long Short-Term
Memory (LSTM) neural networks · Medical machine learning

© ICST Institute for Computer Sciences, Social Informatics and Telecommunications Engineering 2021
Published by Springer Nature Switzerland AG 2021. All Rights Reserved
J. Ye et al. (Eds.): MobiHealth 2020, LNICST 362, pp. 227–243, 2021.
https://doi.org/10.1007/978-3-030-70569-5_14

1   Introduction

Influenza (a.k.a. the flu) is a pervasive respiratory infection caused by Influenza viruses with an estimated 3 to 5 million severe cases annually, which lead to between 290 to 650 thousand respiratory deaths world wide [12]. For the 2019–2020 US flu season, which started October 1, 2019, and ended April 4, 2020, the United States' Center for Disease Control and Prevention (CDC) estimates between 39 and 56 million cases of flu illness, which led to between 410 and 740 thousand hospitalizations and between 24 and 62 thousand deaths [2].

During the 2018–2019 flu season, influenza vaccines prevented between 3.4 and 7.1 million flu cases and, thus, prevented 30 to 156 thousand hospitalizations as well as 1 to 13 thousand deaths [3]. At the time of this writing, the 2019–2020 flu season's flu vaccine effectiveness statistics were not yet finalized and released by the the CDC.

Since Influenza vaccination is the primary strategy to prevent influenza [16], an accurate prediction model is essential for pharmaceutical companies and healthcare providers to be able to properly prepare for an upcoming flu season. For instance, vaccine manufacturers in the US rely heavily on seasonal influenza data provided by the CDC [1] which, due to the two-week reporting lag of the CDC, leaves the vaccine manufacturers insufficient time to produce enough flu vaccines for the appropriate flu strains that can be distributed through the health care network in time.

However, the CDC only collects US data and thus for the rest of the countries the World Health Organization (WHO)'s global estimates must be used as a basis for a prediction model. Though, improvements are required to gain more accurate results, as the WHO only extrapolates based off of the limited data it receives from the countries [12].

2   Related Work

Between 2008 and 2015, the Google Flu Trends project provided an influenza activities forecaster with a linear model [9]. The idea being that since many potential patients or relatives and friends of potential patients will use Google Searches as a first attempt at diagnosis, by monitoring a region's population's Google search queries into influenza related terminology and symptoms, the presence of ILI in the population of that region may be predicted. However, no actual flue statistics from the CDC or WHO were used to validate or enhance the predictions.

Ginsberg et al. estimated weekly influenza activities by finding and monitoring Google search queries that are highly correlated with CDC data, achieving an accurate estimate with a one-day reporting lag [8]. However, their aim was only to overcome the two week reporting lag of the CDC. No attempt was made to help predict future numbers of ILI cases.

Dugas et al. applied a generalized linear model to Google Trends data [6] on a city level. Similarly to Ginsberg et al. predictions of future influenza trends was not within the scope of the research.

Paul et. al. used both Google Trends and Twitter data to forecast influenza outbreak, but because people usually only tweet about influenza after the outbreak has happened, their research can only be used for post-verification [17].

Xie used a vector auto-regression model which factors state population density, weekly temperature, and precipitation as predictors to forecast ILI incidence rate based on the Google Flu Trends and the CDC ILI incidence [23]. However, the goal of her project was not as narrowly focused as eVision. It does not aim to provide companies and health providers with an easily understood forecast of an upcoming influenza season, and as such it cannot provide a long term forecast.

3 Vector Autoregression (VAR) Model

Regression modeling is a technique which provides a relationship between dependent and independent variables. One such model is the Vector Auto Regression (VAR) model, which generalizes the uni-variate auto regression model by allowing it to include more than one predictor variable. The VAR model is thus an extension of the Autoregression model that is used to predict multiple time series variables using a single core model. Therefore, VAR helps in performing multivariate time series forecasting between multiple predictors and a response variable. This model works on the concept of lags, which means that each variable is a linear combination of past lags of itself and past lags of the other variables [18].

For example to measure three different time series variables, denoted by $x_{t,1}, x_{t,2}, x_{t,3}$, the Vector Autoregression model of order 1, denoted as VAR(1), is as follows:

$$x_{t,1} = \alpha_1 + \phi_{11}x_{t-1,1} + \phi_{12}x_{t-1,2} + \phi_{13}x_{t-1,3} + w_{t,1}$$
$$x_{t,2} = \alpha_2 + \phi_{21}x_{t-1,1} + \phi_{22}x_{t-1,2} + \phi_{23}x_{t-1,3} + w_{t,2}$$
$$x_{t,3} = \alpha_3 + \phi_{31}x_{t-1,1} + \phi_{32}x_{t-1,2} + \phi_{33}x_{t-1,3} + w_{t,3}$$

3.1 Utilization of the VAR Model for Flu Prediction

The VAR model was built in MATLAB. It was entirely constructed with the functions provided by MATLAB's Econometric Toolbox. Initial pre-processing of the data was carried out and then the VAR(4) model was created. The model was constructed using a function called varm() provided in the aforementioned toolbox, which returns a varm object, which in turn characterizes the model [14].

The VAR model was constructed to take in the same data as the eVision model to predict across the same distances. However, as the results (depicted in Sect. 6.1) show, this model does not perform as accurately as eVision's LSTM model described below (with results in Sect. 6.2).

4   Modifications to eVision

Prior work on eVision has established the base LSTM model which takes in the number of ILI reported cases along with Google Trends data to make long-term forecasts on the number of cases [20–22]. While work had previously been done on making national level predictions using state-level data, the optimal selection of states was not yet found and the effects of lower level division data were not explored.

4.1   Selecting States

Adding states was the first step in augmenting national level forecasts with more granular data.

The CDC, in addition to national level influenza statistics, provides statewide statistics for influenza. Similarly, Google Trends provides popularity of keywords by state. Thus eVision is capable of incorporating these state level indicators as features to augment its predictions.

4.2   Adding Metropolitan Data

Adding metropolitan data was done as an attempt to see if the granulation of Google Trends data would correlate to a higher level of prediction accuracy.

The municipalities on Google Trends are broken up into what were known as Designated Market Areas (DMA). DMA are 210 regions in the Unites States which receive the same radio and television options created by the Neilsen Media Research firm [11]. Having the option of a metropolitan level, it allows further testing to see if the granulated Google Trends data leads to more accurate predictions. Each of these DMA has a distinct three digit code, which Google Trends used to differentiate the different metropolitan areas from one another.

5   Data Acquisition

5.1   Google Trends

Google Trends data was used as the basis for the LSTM and VAR models. It provided a great level of flexibility because of the volume and scope of Google searches that people frequently make. Google Trends data is presented in time intervals that can range from the last 24 h to the last 10 years. The data in Google Trends is normalized from data points that correspond to searches at a given time and place. The data is normalized on a scale of 0–100 with respect to the time interval allocated, with time periods of higher search frequency corresponding to a higher number [10].

Google Trends provides data on three levels: region-wide, state-wide, and metropolitan. The region-wide levels consist of countries across the world and the state-wide areas consist of the 50 states plus the municipality of the District of Columbia.

5.2   Google Search Keywords

eVision uses four key terms: cough, flu, sore throat, and tamiflu. The search frequency for these influenza related terms strongly correlate to the frequency of influenza cases, making them an excellent source of information for training the model.

5.3   Data Acquisition Accommodations Due to COVID-19

The current COVID-19 pandemic has severely skewed data for many of our relevant search terms. As mentioned earlier, Google Trends comparatively ranks search frequency on a normalized scale from 0–100. When a significant and irregular event occurs, such as a pandemic, there is usually a corresponding alteration in search frequency for relevant terminology. This has caused an intense spike in the number of searches for virus related keywords (cough, flu, etc.), which due to Google's data post processing, eliminates the variance in weekly data.

A prime example of this is the search term "fever", which is a common symptom for both COVID-19 and influenza. Figure 1 illustrates this discrepancy by showing search frequency for a given time before and after COVID-19. When using a custom time range that does not encroach upon the hysteria of COVID-19 related Google searches, its magnitude becomes comparatively much smaller than the time range which includes COVID-19 related searches.

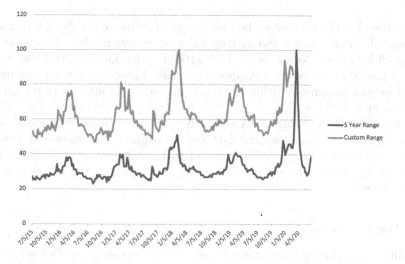

Fig. 1. Past 5 Years (blue) vs. Custom Date Range (orange) Search Frequency for Search Term "fever" (Color figure online)

The date range used for testing was a five year interval between February 16, 2015 to February 16, 2020, who's difference with modern data can be seen in Fig. 1.

5.4 Python Scraper

To obtain data from Google Trends, the publicly available Google Trends API was utilized. Using this API, a scraper was created that was able to extract selected data from Google Trends.

An older scraper created for the previous version of eVision [21], did not meet all requirements for the new additions to eVision. The main features implemented for the scraper were to allow for settings that can be toggled in order to extract results by the regional levels that Google supported: state, metropolitan, and country. It allows for the mass extraction of search data from any region in a matter of seconds.

Geographical codes were needed in order to successfully distinguish between the different regions being scraped. Since there are different scopes of regions that can be searched, Google Trends differentiates the geographical scopes in distinct ways. The way that the API accepts inputs for search terms such as geographical region, date range, etc., is by the URL of a search term on the Google Trends site as depicted in Fig. 2.

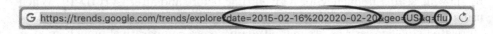

Fig. 2. Standard URL for Google Trends search

In order for the scraper to be able to yield data from different regions, a database of country, state, and metropolitan codes was needed. This is because Google differentiates locations by ISO 3166-2 codes for countries and states, while using DMA codes for metropolitan areas. These codes would be needed as an essential parameter within the scraper that would allow it to scrape data from any area in the world.

A list of all the existing DMA codes in the United States was found online [15], along with a comprehensive database of country and state codes from a public GitHub repository [7]. This proved to be sufficient to allow the scraper to swiftly and efficiently extract data from any region in the US recorded by Google Trends.

5.5 Data Selection

In addition to including a national forecast without any states and a forecast with all states to serve as comparative baselines, two main approaches for selecting states with which to make the prediction were undertaken: selecting states with the highest population and selecting those which are the largest transit hubs with the highest level of traffic.

For selecting the states that have the highest level of international transportation, it was decided that the largest ports of entry and the states with the busiest airports would be used. To find the busiest airports, the total number of passengers each airport reported to have serviced in the year 2019 was studied, and the six airports that serviced over 60 million passengers that year were selected. These airports were located in the states of Georgia, California, Illinois, Texas, Colorado, and New York.

Airports were selected as they represent the most rapid and commonly used method of transportation into the United States, especially from countries that do not directly border it. As such, it represents a major vector of disease transmission from abroad, and it could be argued that these busiest transit states would exhibit a growth in infections before the national average begins to in any significant way. Thus, under this hypothesis, data of infections in these states would be useful for predicting the total amount of infections in the future.

Data on the busiest ports of entry into the United States from Mexico and Canada was gathered from the Department of Transportation's Bureau of Transportation Statistics. Data from 2019 shows that San Ysidro, California and El Paso, Texas were by far the largest ports of entry with Buffalo, New York coming in as a distant third. The logic behind these three states serving as useful precursors to a national epidemic is the same as with airports.

The six highest population states were chosen to contrast with the airport selection, with an anomaly in the Floridian data resulting in two versions being created with and without the state. The anomaly in question is that in the CDC FluView state by state records of influenza like illnesses, data from Florida is not included resulting in it appearing as if it has always had no cases. While this does not prevent data gathered on the google keyword trends in Florida, it was determined that this could be harmful to the model and a version of the data without Florida was generated to determine if this was the case.

As previous research has determined that national level predictions can be enhanced with state level data, it raised the question of whether or not metropolitan level data could enhance these predictions further.

In order to explore this possibility, four data sets were made consisting of the top five, ten, fifteen, and twenty most populated metropolitan areas in the United States and their Google keyword search results. National level predictions were made using only national data and the metropolitan data sets. Predictions were run with and without state data as well to observe the effect of including all three levels.

For the purposes of investigating the ability for metropolitan level data to boost state level predictions, a simple set of predictions were made for California, Texas, and New York, using the state data sets alone for each of them, followed by collecting metropolitan data sets for every metropolitan area that Google Trends collected data for in each state.

6   Results

The calculation error is measured using the same metrics established in the previous paper on eVision [21]. Originally Mean Absolute Percentage Error (MAPE) [4] was used to determine error, but after review it was determined that Symmetric Mean Absolute Percentage Error (SMAPE) [13] would be a more effective metric to make use of. The methodology behind the construction of the confidence intervals in use for the LSTM results were also not changed from the aforementioned paper.

6.1   VAR Results

Various forecasts were conducted with the VAR model in order to compare its results with the ones of the LSTM model. Table 1 contains the series of national VAR forecasts, including SMAPE scores for 3, 7, and 14 weeks ahead predictions.

Table 1. VAR national forecast results

Forecast	States	3 week SMAPE	7 week SMAPE	14 week SMAPE
National all	All states	28.31	36.98	41.21
National ports of entry	CA, TX, NY	30.12	43.98	51.15
National population	CA, TX, FL, NY, PA, IL	32.96	48.10	67.80
National only	N/A	32.10	40.79	72.22

The best results were obtained for the national level prediction when all the states were included. Across every forecast, the level of error increased the further out the prediction was made. The best national results given by VAR was an error rate of 28.31%, 36.98%, and 41.21%, for 3, 7, and 14 weeks respectively. In the case of a curated selection of states, the Top 3 largest Ports of Entry proved to be a better selection of states than using the 6 largest population states. The results for 3 weeks ahead prediction between both selections was 2.84%, and the difference only rose to 4.12% for 7 weeks, but for the 14 week forecast the difference became a significant 16.65%.

Finally, the model provided with national data only had the most varied performance. With SMAPE errors of 32.1%, 40.79%, and 72.22% for 3, 7, and 14 weeks, its placement varies from third to second to last place respectively. The resulting graphs produced by these predictions can be seen in Fig. 3 For all the results obtained, it can be seen that the forecast for initial weeks matched the number of cases but completely missed the peak period, leading to high SMAPE as compared to the LSTM model.

The results in Fig. 3 were promising for 3 weeks ahead predictions but failed as the length of the prediction was increased. Considering different combinations of states for forecasting on the National level, the results were almost the same. For all the results, the model is unable to predict the peaks at the expected time interval.

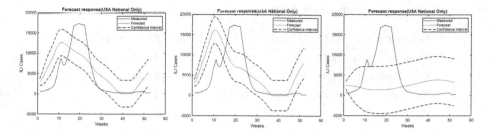

Fig. 3. National only (3, 7, 14 weeks)

State Level Forecast. Forecasts were also created to for state level predictions using no further outside data to augment them. The states selected for examination were California, Texas, and New York as they are held in common between the population selection and the ports of entry selection.

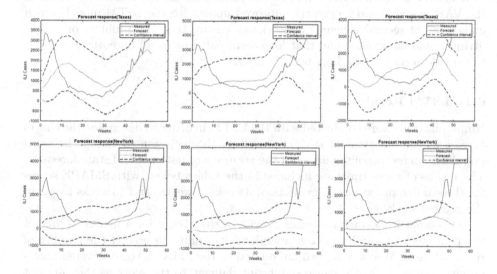

Fig. 4. Top: Texas only (3, 7, 14 weeks) Bottom: New York only (3, 7, 14 weeks)

The following Table 2 contains the SMAPE scores for the state forecasts at 3, 7, and 14 weeks ahead predictions.

Figure 4 demonstrates the results for the Texas and New York predictions. It should be noted that although the Texas forecasts have significantly higher SMAPE scores than the New York forecasts, the utility of the predictions generated are both abysmal as can be seen in the figure. Although both California and Texas manage to obtain error rates of 30% in their 3 week forecasts, and 7 week forecast, in the case of California these forecasts fail to consistently provide accurate information on the start, peak, and magnitude of an influenza outbreak.

Table 2. VAR state forecast results

Forecast VAR	SMAPE 3 week	SMAPE 7 week	SMAPE 14 week
California only	23.52	27.00	41.62
New York only	56.16	57.17	61.76
Texas only	27.43	31.69	47.64

Overall Model Analysis. The regression model used here generates hypothesis functions which produce a nonlinear curve. From the results obtained, it can be seen that the model was unable to predict the peak week of an outbreak, missing its mark by 10 weeks when it predicts an outbreak at all.

Therefore, it can be inferred from these results that this model under-fits on the data, and as such fails to extrapolate useful patterns with which it can create accurate predictions. It even fails to capture patters as basic as continuing a steady rise in cases until a shift downwards is noticed. All results generated in the VAR model would be greatly improved upon with the LSTM model, which makes use of recursive neural networks to ensure that the problem of under-fitting would be avoided and that long term patterns could be noticed in order to provide accurate, and long term forecasts.

6.2   LSTM Results

Numerous trails were conducted with the LSTM in order to determine the effects of various combinations of states, as well as the inclusion of Google keyword popularity in metropolitan areas on the accuracy of national and state forecasts. The results of these trails are included in the tables below, with SMAPE scores for three different extents of prediction, 3 weeks, 7 weeks, and 14 weeks ahead of the present week.

Two other important measures consist of the ability for a model to predict the peak week of a influenza outbreak, and its ability to predict the number of reported cases. While these two are related to the SMAPE score, severe failures on either measure would cause significant damage to the score as they are not directly related and it is possible for one model to have a higher SMAPE score than another yet fall behind on other metrics.

Most Effective State Selection for National Forecast. While there is no one selection of states that performed the best across all levels of forecasts, in fact each level performs best with a different selection, there are some important patterns that can be gleaned from the data.

The first point that stands out is the clustering that occurs in the accuracy between the levels of forecast. Across every national forecast, the difference between the SMAPE score for the 3 week and 7 week forecasts are less than the difference between either level of forecast and the 14 week forecasts.

Table 3. State selection for national forecast

Forecast	States	3 weeks SMAPE	7 weeks SMAPE	14 weeks SMAPE
National airports	GA, CA, IL, TX, CO, NY	10.85	10.43	18.26
National all	All states	19.69	16.08	23.22
National ports of entry	CA, TX, NY	09.87	08.57	22.56
National population	CA, TX, FL, NY, PA, IL	11.85	09.10	19.80
National population Sans Florida	CA, TX, NY, PA, IL	09.62	08.96	20.68
National only	N/A	11.89	12.00	25.82

Table 4. Effect of metropolitan data on national forecast

Forecast	3 weeks SMAPE	7 weeks SMAPE	14 weeks SMAPE
National top 5 metros	11.02	12.72	26.39
National top 10 metros	10.87	10.33	19.47
National top 15 metros	12.67	09.89	23.77
National top 20 metros	12.27	11.06	23.73
National top 10 with states	11.56	10.23	21.47
National top 10 states only	10.31	10.08	21.33
National top 20 with states	15.07	10.46	25.62
National top 20 states only	10.60	12.01	20.22

Table 5. Effect of metropolitan data on state forecast

Forecast	SMAPE 3 week	SMAPE 7 week	SMAPE 14 week
California metro	14.34	16.07	20.84
California only	37.01	23.28	18.54
New York metro	20.43	22.79	33.35
New York only	38.42	13.03	29.32
Texas metro	19.85	19.40	41.37
Texas only	20.20	25.13	35.77

The 14 week forecasts also notably always show a higher level of SMAPE error than any of the earlier weeks. However, as can be seen in Fig. 5, a model's predictions can still be useful even when they do not follow the results of the outbreak perfectly. For the first outbreak in the testing data, the model is able to determine the peak week of the outbreak within one week of error, while keeping the number of cases comfortably within the confidence intervals. Although the

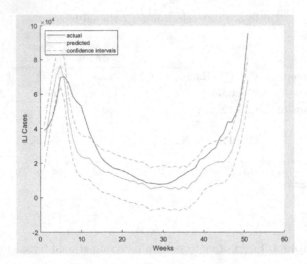

Fig. 5. National airports, 14 weeks

model performs more poorly after that point, it maps a general path of the virus in the off season, and more importantly, manages to keep the second outbreak at the end of the testing data close to its maximum confidence interval. Another consistent pattern is that the magnitude of the sharp, second outbreak is best captured by the 14 week forecasts.

The second point of note is that the no states added and all states added categories both performed worse than any of the curated state selections. As can be seen in Table 3 the all state model demonstrates the worst performance in the 3 and 7 week levels achieving 19.69% and 16.89% error rates respectively, far worse than any other model. While it does perform better in the 14 week forecast, it only does so by 2.6%. Furthermore, the accuracy with which the all state model predicts the magnitude and location of the peak week is worse than the no state model, which are the main benefits of the 14 week forecast to begin with.

The models based on largest ports of entry and highest population states, excluding Florida, are the only models that manage to break below 10% error in the 3 week forecast, and 9% error in the seven week forecast. Of the two, the model based on population performs best in the 3 week and 14 week forecast, but the ports of entry model achieves the lowest SMAPE score of only 8.57% error in the 7 week forecast. As can be seen in Fig. 6 the overall results are qualitatively similar, and it should be noted that the major difference between the two data sets is the inclusion of the states of Pennsylvania and Illinois in the population model.

Finally, the last major point of note can be seen in the effect that the inclusion of the state of Florida has in the population model compared to the one that excludes it. Similar to the no states/all states comparison, excluding Florida allowed the population model to perform better in the 3 and 7 week levels, but

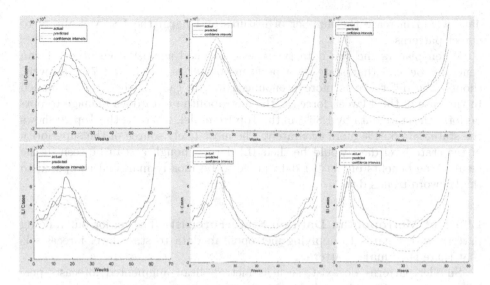

Fig. 6. Top: Ports of Entry (3, 7, 14 weeks) Bottom: Population sans FL (3, 7, 14 weeks)

in the 14 week level it performed 0.88% worse than the model containing Florida's ILI cases and keyword trends. In terms of the magnitude and peak week location measures, the two models also perform similarly, with only minor differences in the 3 week and 7 week forecasts where the Florida excluding model provides a better measure of the number of cases in the first outbreak in the testing data.

Effect of Metropolitan Data on National Forecast. For the models consisting of the top metropolitan areas, the results follow a pattern similar to state selection. The model performs worse both in the case of being provided with too little supporting data, and when provided with too many features. As each metropolitan data has four keywords to keep track of each as their own independent feature, the total number of metropolitan features can reach as many as 80 in the case of the Top 20 model.

Overall, the best performing model of the four was the Top 10 model as can be seen in Table 4. Achieving the best SMAPE scores for the 3 week and 14 week levels, and coming just 0.44% short of the best 7 week result, the model provides the most consistently accurate results across the three levels of forecast. With a total of 40 features added from the keyword trends, it has a higher feature count than most state selections, though only by ten.

Two additional models were created for the Top 10 and Top 20 data sets, adding the data for every state of the metropolitan areas as well as including a data set with only the state data. In all but a single case, the 7 week forecast for the Top 20 model, the models with both state and metropolitan data performed worse than either of the two data types alone. This was expected as adding state data would increase the number of features and harm the LSTM's ability to detect patterns.

When placing the two data types head to head against each other, it can generally be said that state data performs better at the 3 and 7 week levels, though the difference is more pronounced in the case of the Top 20 model. In the case of the 14 week forecast, the metropolitan data does manage to outperform the state data by 1.86% in the Top 10 model, where as the Top 20 shows the state data 3.51% more accurately. The most likely source of the superiority of the state level data would be their ILI data. Though as can be seen in the results, the benefits of the ILI data prove to be mostly marginal compared to the keyword trends data.

Effect of Metropolitan Data on State Forecast. The major outstanding pattern with regards to applying metropolitan data to state level forecasts is that there is no major pattern.

Smaller patterns do exist, such as metropolitan augmented forecasts performing worse at the 14 week forecast across all three states as can be seen in Table 5. But beyond that the results become more varied, such as the metropolitan data increasing accuracy in the 3 week forecasts, but with its improvements varying from highly significant in California (22.67%), to almost negligible in Texas (0.35%). In the case of the 7 week forecast, metropolitan data aids in the case of California and Texas, but adds even higher error in the case of New York. Furthermore, it should also be noted that this was not an exhaustive study of the effects of metropolitan data on state level forecasting. The states of California, New York, and Texas were examined as they were the states that appeared in every stat selection for national level predictions. The inconsistencies in the results here may suggest that the utility of metropolitan level forecasts may vary depending on the state in question. Further study will be required to draw serious conclusions, particularly in the case of low population states.

7   Future Work

7.1   Google Trends Data Ranges and Adjustments

As a result of the COVID-19 outbreak, a lot of the data has been skewed. Because of this, the model is currently trained on data predating the outbreak so that it would not be affected by this anomaly. However, the end goal of this software is for it to be practical for commercial use by pharmaceutical companies, which necessitates the creation of a solution to the current skewing of Google Trends data. This is because, in the future, there will likely still be a level of corruption in Google Trends data from COVID-19.

It may be possible to simply omit that data and work around it, but it is unknown how a missing chunk of data will affect the model's ability to make accurate predictions.

7.2   Influenza Strain-Level Predictions

The model is also expected to be able to predict the trends of influenza strains. There are four distinct strains of influenza: A, B, C, and D. Of these strains, influenza types A and B lead to the majority of influenza cases [5].

Ideally, predictions for different influenza strains would yield similar results as the influenza forecaster. However, this may need to be achieved through a different means than what is currently done. Types A and B do not have distinguishing symptoms [19], therefore symptoms of the strains cannot be used to predict the trends.

However, there are some general trends of the timing of the dominant strain, with type A being most prevalent at the start of the flu season and type B becoming more frequent in the latter half of the season [19]. Common trends of timing like this will be the starting point in helping the model determine a dominant strain during a given period of time.

7.3   Ease of Use

For future versions of eVision, there are hopes for a more uniform prediction process. Currently, there exists a multi-step prediction process involving running the Python scraper, acquiring the data, and running the MATLAB script that makes the prediction. There is the end goal of making the entirety of the model mostly autonomous by having the model run continually on a server. This will allow the model to make predictions more frequently and no longer require trained programmers to make edits to allow for said predictions.

There is also hope to incorporate a user-friendly and simplistic UI. The end goal for eVision has always been for it to be a tool used by pharmaceutical companies and healthcare providers to gauge the quantity of tester kits, vaccines, and medication they need to manufacture or resources they need to allocate in order to prevent and treat Influenza. Having a quality GUI for instance, will allow for its ease of use by even nontechnical staff at said organizations.

8   Conclusion

Through adding state level predictions in order to enhance national predictions and utilizing metropolitan area keyword trends to improve both state level and national predictions, eVision's success in making 3, 7, and 14 weeks in advance predictions were improved from 88.11%, 88%, and 74.18% accuracy to 90.38%, 91.43%, and 81.74% respectively. Furthermore, it was determined that the LSTM model is superior to the VAR model on all counts, and that generally speaking for national level forecasts state level data is superior to metropolitan data or a mixture of the two. Meaning, granularity in prediction is helpful in improving overall prediction as long as the grains are not selected to be too small, and not too many of them are selected such that the model is overwhelmed with features.

Acknowledgment. Many thanks are due to Ben Dorty, the New-Technology Senior Director at Cepheid Inc. for inspiring the project, and supporting it throughout development. Also to Prashanth Asuri, director of SCU's BioInnovation and Design Lab for obtaining financial support from Cepheid Inc. And to the School of Engineering's Frugal Innovation Hub as well as the Departments of Bio Engineering, Computer Science & Engineering, and Mathematics & Computer Science for their continued support of the eVision project. And lastly to other eVision team members: Yash Kamdar and Ron Huang, as well as past eVision team members: Yuhang Qian, Anika Shahi, Liying Liang, and Meghan McGinnis for their hard work on research, data collection, and software development in the earlier stages of the project.

References

1. Centers for Disease Control and Prevention (CDC): Preliminary in-season 2018–2019 burden estimates (2019). https://www.cdc.gov/flu/about/burden/preliminary-in-season-estimates.htm
2. Centers for Disease Control and Prevention (CDC): 2019–2020 U.S. flu season: Preliminary burden estimates (2020). https://www.cdc.gov/flu/about/burden/preliminary-in-season-estimates.htm
3. Chung, J.R., et al.: Effects of influenza vaccination in the United States during the 2018–2019 influenza season. Clin. Infect. Dis. **71**, e368–e376 (2020)
4. De Myttenaere, A., Golden, B., Le Grand, B., Rossi, F.: Mean absolute percentage error for regression models. Neurocomputing **192**, 38–48 (2016)
5. Centers for Disease Control and Prevention: Types of influenza viruses, 18 November 2019. https://www.cdc.gov/flu/about/viruses/types.htm
6. Dugas, A.F., et al.: Google flu trends: correlation with emergency department influenza rates and crowding metrics. Clin. Inf. Dis. **54**(4), 463–469 (2012)
7. Gada, D.: Country state city DB demo (2020). https://dr5hn.github.io/countries-states-cities-database
8. Ginsberg, J., Mohebbi, M.H., Patel, R.S., Brammer, L., Smolinski, M.S., Brilliant, L.: Detecting influenza epidemics using search engine query data. Nature **457**(7232), 1012–1014 (2009)
9. Google: Google flu trends (2019). https://www.google.org/flutrends/about
10. Google Trends Help: FAQ about google trends data (2020). https://support.google.com/trends/answer/4365533
11. Halbrooks, G.: What is a designated market area (DMA)?, 25 June 2019. https://www.thebalancecareers.com/what-is-a-designated-market-area-dma-2315180
12. Lee, V.J., et al.: Advances in measuring influenza burden of disease. Influenza Other Respir. Viruses **12**(1), 3–9 (2018)
13. Makridakis, S.: Accuracy measures: theoretical and practical concerns. Int. J. Forecast. **9**(4), 527–529 (1993)
14. MATLAB Help Center: Create vector autoregression (VAR) model (2020). https://www.mathworks.com/help/econ/varm.html
15. MDR ADC: 2014–2015 DMA's. https://www.mdreducation.com/pdfs/dma.pdf
16. Rolfes, M.A., et al.: Effects of influenza vaccination in the united states during the 2017–2018 influenza season. Clin. Inf. Dis. **69**(11), 1845–1853 (2019)
17. Santillana, M., Nguyen, A.T., Dredze, M., Paul, M.J., Nsoesie, E.O., Brownstein, J.S.: Combining search, social media, and traditional data sources to improve influenza surveillance. PLoS Comput. Biol. **11**(10), e1004513 (2015)

18. PennState Eberly College of Science: Vector autoregressive models VAR(p) models. https://online.stat.psu.edu/stat510/lesson/11/11.2
19. Seladi-Schulman, J.: How are influenza a and b different? 28 March 2020. https://www.healthline.com/health/cold-flu/influenza-a-vs-b#types
20. Shaghaghi, N., Calle, A., Kouretas, G.: eVision: influenza forecasting using CDC, who, and google trends data. In: 2020 IEEE Technology and Engineering Management Society (TEMS) 2020 International Conference on Artificial Intelligence for Good (AI4G). IEEE (2020)
21. Shaghaghi, N., Calle, A., Kouretas, G.: Expanding eVision's scope of influenza forecasting. In: 2020 IEEE Global Humanitarian Technology Conference (GHTC). IEEE (2020)
22. Shaghaghi, N., Calle, A., Kouretas, G.: Influenza forecasting. In: Proceedings of the 3rd ACM SIGCAS Conference on Computing and Sustainable Societies, COMPASS 2020, pp. 339–341. Association for Computing Machinery, New York (2020). https://doi.org/10.1145/3378393.3402286
23. Xie, W.: Spatial panel VAR and application to forecast influenza incidence rates of us states. Available at SSRN 2646870 (2015)

Explainable Deep Learning for Medical Time Series Data

Thomas Frick[1,3]($\boxtimes$), Stefan Glüge[2], Abbas Rahimi[3], Luca Benini[3],
and Thomas Brunschwiler[1]

[1] IBM Research Zurich, Smart System Integration, Zurich, Switzerland
{fri,tbr}@zurich.ibm.com
[2] Zurich University of Applied Sciences, Institute of Applied Simulation,
Zurich, Switzerland
stefan.gluege@zhaw.ch
[3] ETH Zurich, Integrated Systems Laboratory, Zurich, Switzerland
abbas@iis.ee.ethz.ch, lbenini@ethz.ch

Abstract. Neural Networks are powerful classifiers. However, they are black boxes and do not provide explicit explanations for their decisions. For many applications, particularly in health care, explanations are essential for building trust in the model. In the field of computer vision, a multitude of explainability methods have been developed to analyze Neural Networks by explaining what they have learned during training and what factors influence their decisions. This work provides an overview of these explanation methods in form of a taxonomy. We adapt and benchmark the different methods to time series data. Further, we introduce quantitative explanation metrics that enable us to build an objective benchmarking framework with which we extensively rate and compare explainability methods. As a result, we show that the Grad-CAM++ algorithm outperforms all other methods. Finally, we identify the limits of existing explanation methods for specific datasets, with feature values close to zero.

Keywords: Explainable deep learning · Convolutional Neural Network · Explanation quality metric · Medical time series data

1 Introduction

Neural Networks have become the state-of-the-art to model complex problems in computer vision [1], speech recognition [2], and many other areas [3]. Given enough data, they can be trained to be exceptionally accurate classifiers, sometimes even surpassing human performance. While some classical machine learning models such as Decision Trees are inherently interpretable, Neural Networks are unfortunately black boxes when it comes to understanding why a classification decision was made. However, for many applications, e.g. in autonomous driving or in healthcare, it is of uttermost importance that the decisions of

J. Ye et al. (Eds.): MobiHealth 2020, LNICST 362, pp. 244–256, 2021.
https://doi.org/10.1007/978-3-030-70569-5_15

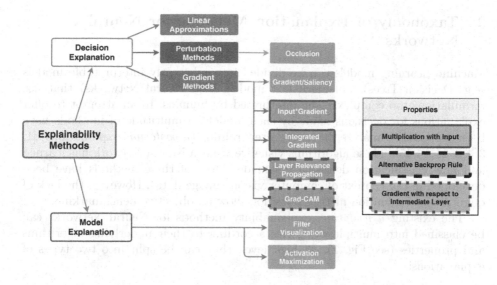

Fig. 1. Taxonomy of a few explanation methods for Neural Networks

machine learning models can be explained and therefore trusted. Decisions may
have severe consequences, especially in healthcare. Therefore, medical experts
need to be able to trust their models to make the right decisions for the right
reasons. Additionally, Neural Network explanations could be used to identify
new patterns in convoluted signals such as electroencephalography (EEG) and
therefore, advance scientific knowledge.

In the last few years, there has been an effort to develop different Neural
Network explanation methods [1,3–11]. Most of these methods have been proposed for computer vision tasks. They highlight the areas of the model input
that are most relevant to the decision process. These so-called attributions or
heat maps associate a relevance score with each individual input feature. Some
algorithms generate explanations in more complex feature spaces such as the
frequency domain. Ultimately, one could aim for explanations in a given expert
language - meaning that the explanation from a more complex feature space
is translated into terms that are familiar to the user (e.g. text book rules in
medicine).

In this study, our goal is to adapt and benchmark Neural Network explainability methods for medical time series data (Sect. 2). So far, researchers have
mainly compared explanation methods on image data, using a qualitative assessments of the resulting explanations by humans. There have been some theoretical
attempts at defining characteristics of good explanations [12,13]. In contrast, we
introduce and apply quantitative explanation metrics (Sect. 3). This allows us
to rate and compare the different methods objectively (Sect. 4). Additionally,
the metric demonstrates the strength and limitations of the various approaches.

2   Taxonomy of Explanation Methods for Neural Networks

Machine Learning models can be divided into inherently interpretable models (e.g. Decision Trees) and black box models (e.g. Neural Networks) that use formulations too complex to be interpreted by humans. In an attempt to offer explanations for decisions made by such models, a multitude of methods have been proposed to analyze the model after training (*a posteriori* explanations) [1, 3, 4, 6–11, 14, 15]. These algorithms visualize what a Neural Network has learned and how classification decisions are made. Most of these methods have been developed in the context of computer vision (image data). However, the lack of quantitative evaluation metrics does not allow an objective benchmarking.

The existing *a posteriori* explainability methods for Neural Networks can be classified into multiple categories according to their underlying algorithms and properties (see Fig. 1). At high level, they can be split into two types of explanations:

- **Model Explanations** are visualizations of the patterns and concepts that the network has learned during training.
- **Decision Explanations** highlight the most relevant parts of a given model input that led to a specific classification decision.

2.1   Model Explanations

Two kinds of model explanations are most relevant: *Filter Visualization* [7] and *Activation Maximization* [8]. The former depicts the kernel weights of the first few layers of Convolutional Neural Networks (CNN), indicating the patterns each filter is most susceptible to. The latter is based on the idea that each neuron is looking for a particular pattern in the input. If this pattern is present, the activation of the neuron is high, otherwise the activation is low or zero. This is achieved by optimizing the input to the network with the objective of maximizing the activation of a particular neuron. In the case of CNNs, there is the choice between optimizing the activation of a neuron, a layer, a channel, a class logit, or a class probability.

2.2   Decision Explanations

Decision explanations explain a specific classification decision, given a particular input sample, by attributing relevance scores to single pixels (for images) or time steps (for time series). The higher the relevance, the more impact a pixel or time step has on the classification decision. It is important to note that the terms saliency map, attribution map, heat map and relevance scores are used interchangeably to describe the same concept.

Decision explanations can be further divided into methods that linearly approximate the model, methods that use the internal gradient flow within the network, and perturbation based methods that alter the input while observing the change in output probabilities to calculate attribution:

1. **Linear approximation methods** (e.g. LIME [9]) construct a linear proxy model that serves as an approximation of a black box model by probing the output behavior around a given input sample.
2. **Perturbation-based methods** (e.g. Occlusion [16]) calculate attributions by removing or altering the input while observing how the classification probabilities change. The higher the change, the more relevant is the part of the input that has been altered.
3. **Gradient-based methods** (e.g. Saliency Maps [14], Gradient*Input [11] [6], Integrated Gradients [17], Epsilon Layer Relevance Propagation (Epsilon-LRP) [18], Grad-CAM [10], Grad-CAM++ [19]) make use of the partial derivative of the logits of the output class with respect to the input or with respect to the output of an intermediate layer as a measure of sensitivity, and thereby as a measure of attribution. Because gradient-based methods are computed with a single forward and backward pass, they are typically faster than occlusion or linear approximation methods. Additionally, Gradient-based methods can be classified using the following three characteristics as show in Fig. 1:
    - **Backpropagation:** Some methods (Epsilon-LRP) change the distribution of the gradients during backpropagation, to improve certain properties of the attribution map.
    - **Gradient:** Some methods either use the gradient with respect to the input (Gradient, Gradient*Input, Integrated Gradient, Epsilon-LRP) or the gradient with respect to an intermediate layer (Grad-CAM, Gad-CAM++).
    - **Multiplication with the Input:** Some methods (Gradient*Input, Integrated Gradient, Epsilon-LRP) use a multiplication with the input in their calculation of attribution.

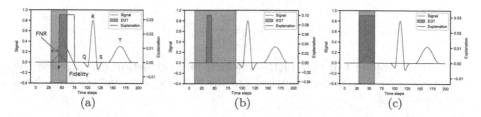

(a)   (b)   (c)

Fig. 2. Synthetic heartbeats (ECG) depicted as P, Q, R, S, T-complex with corresponding Explanation Ground Truth (EGT) and example explanations resulting in: (a) a Fidelity Score of 0.5 and a False Negative Rate of 0.5 for a normal sinus rhythm, (b) a Fidelity Score of 1.0 and a False Negative Rate of 0.8 for atrial fibrillation, (c) a Fidelity Score of 1.0 and a False Negative Rate of 0.0 for a normal sinus rhythm.

3   Explanation Ground Truth and Quality Metrics

To the best of our knowledge, no method exists to rate different explanation methods quantitatively with respect to a ground truth explanation. Most publications make use of qualitative comparisons. Alvarez-Melis et al. [20] proposed a quantitative metric to assess how *faithful* the generated explanation is with respect to the model. The basic idea is to observe the change in the model's predictions while removing pixels or time steps and correlating the attribution score of the explanation method with that change. This faithfulness metric is not a measure of how well the attributions correlate with a ground truth explanation of the input, but only indicates how *faithfully* the explanation represents what the model bases its decision on.

In order to asses the quality of generated explanations, we have to annotate the data with a "true" explanation, also called the **Explanation Ground Truth** (EGT). We can then assess individual explanations relative to this ground truth. It contains all pixels or time steps that provide distinctive information for the relevant class. The EGT does not contain features which are not distinct for the specific class and could appear in other classes as well. Figure 2 depicts an example of the EGT for a synthetic heartbeat as recorded by a ECG.

The P-Wave (first peak of the heartbeat waveform) is one of the distinctive factors to distinguish a sinus rhythm from atrial fibrillation. The patient is suffering from atrial fibrillation if the P-Wave is missing. Therefore, for the sinus rhythm class, we place the EGT on all time steps containing the P-Wave (see Fig. 2a). For the atrial fibrillation class, we define the EGT on all time steps where the P-Wave could be located if it would be present (see Fig. 2b).

We constructed our own synthetic time series datasets with distinct features, indicative for a specific class, to benchmark the explanation methods on controlled cases. Furthermore, this approach allowed us to identify strengths and limitations of the methods for time series data with different characteristics.

In order to benchmark an explanation, we defined **Scores** that allow to perform a quantitative comparison. First, the generated explanation $A = \{A_0, ..., A_N\}$ needs to be normalized to a total area of 1, for N time steps.

$$\bar{A}_i = \frac{A_i}{\sum_i A_i} \tag{1}$$

We then propose two new metrics, which in combination characterize the generated explanation under investigation: the Fidelity Score and the False Negative Rate.

– **Fidelity Score:** This metric measures how much of the explanation appears inside the actual "true" explanation. We define it as the total sum of all attribution values (area under the curve) inside the EGT. Due to the normalized total area, this corresponds to the precision metric in classification.

$$S_{Fidelity} = \sum_{i \in \mathcal{Z}} \bar{A}_i \qquad \text{where } i \in \mathcal{Z} \text{ if } EGT_i = 1 \qquad (2)$$

- **False Negative Rate (FNR):** This metric measures the completeness vs. narrowness of an explanation. We define it as the number of non-relevant pixels or time steps inside the EGT divided by the total number of pixels or time steps in the span of the EGT. Since the explanation values are almost never exactly zero, we use a threshold ϵ below which we consider the pixel or time step to have no relevance. This threshold is chosen to be equal to the explanation values of a perfectly distributed explanation (given a signal of length N): $\epsilon = 1/N$.

$$S_{\text{FNR}} = \frac{\sum_{i \in \mathcal{Z}} 1_{\{\bar{A}_i \leq \epsilon\}}}{\sum_i \text{EGT}_i} \qquad \text{where } i \in \mathcal{Z} \text{ if } EGT_i = 1 \qquad (3)$$

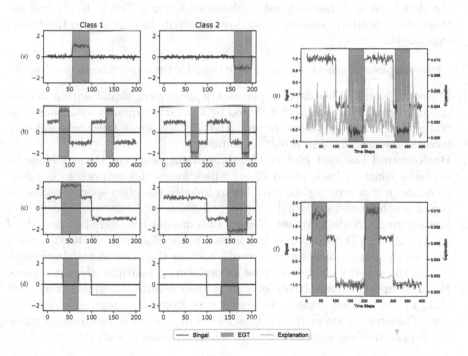

Fig. 3. Synthetic datasets (blue) generated for the benchmarking of the explanation methods: (a) Dataset Noise, (b) Background Dataset Noise, (c) Background Wide Dataset Noise, (d) Background Dataset Inverse; Example Explanations (green) for the Background Dataset Noise as resulted from: (e) Epsilon-LRP, (f) Grad-CAM++. EGT's are depicted in red for all cases. (Color figure online)

4   Experiments and Results

To evaluate our explanation score and the explanation methods, four synthetic datasets were designed and a Neural Network architecture was defined. Detailed results of the experiments are reported and discussed in this chapter. Each chosen explanation method was tested and analyzed. Finally, we show the limitations of existing explanation methods when applied to a carefully constructed dataset.

4.1   Datasets

The four synthetic datasets consist of uni-variate time series signals, with the following characteristics:

1. All generated datasets only contain clearly separable classes (1000 samples per class). There is no ambiguity about the class membership.
2. Each class must be characterizable by features present in a specific region of the signal. We call these regions Explanation Ground Truth (EGT) and use them to qualitatively measure how close an attribution map is to the "true" explanation.

The following four synthetic datasets were used for the experiments (see Fig. 3):

1. **Dataset Noise:** This dataset places a square wave signal within a class specific region. Class one is represented by a negative square wave, while class two is represented by a positive one. Additionally, white noise was added to increase the classification problem complexity.
2. **Background Dataset Noise:** This dataset augments the Dataset Noise by adding a constant background signal which forces the network to not only recognize a non zero region, but also to identify the class specific signal on top of another constant signal.
3. **Background Wide Dataset Noise:** This dataset considers two periods of the Background Dataset Noise. In contrast to the Background Dataset, there are two locations which simultaneously contain the class identifying signal, testing the network's ability to base its decision on multiple relevant regions.
4. **Background Dataset Inverse:** This dataset inverts the square wave such that, in the relevant region, the signal goes from the background value to zero. The explanation method is thus forced to cope with a zero signal where the explanation value should be high. Thus, no noise was added.

4.2   Models

For our experiments, we use a LeNet [4] and VGG [15] inspired Convolutional Neural Network (CNN): two convolutional layers and a MaxPooling layer make up a block that is repeated three times. This is followed by a single fully connected output layer.

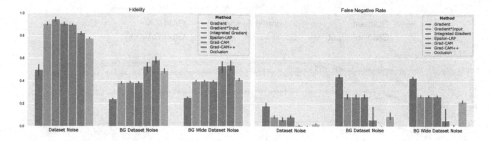

Fig. 4. Performance experiment results for three different datasets showing Grad-CAM++ outperforming all other methods.

4.3   Explanation Method Experiments

In our experiments, we investigated how well each method performs on a network that has been trained to perfect test accuracy. We then focused on the investigation of the convergence of explanation methods during training of the neural network.

Comparison of Converged Explanation Methods: In these experiments, we investigated the quality of the generated explanations using the proposed metrics. For every explanation we calculated the Fidelity Score and the FNR. As shown in Fig. 4, we observed that we can split the methods into four groups:

1. **Gradient** shows the lowest Fidelity Score and the highest FNR. This method clearly performs worse than any of the other explanation algorithms.
2. **Gradient*Input, Integrated Gradients and Epsilon-LRP** form a group of similarly performing methods. We attribute this to the shared property of these three methods: multiplication with the input resulting in attribution maps that are largely dominated by the input signal. Additionally, Ancona et al. [21] show that Gradient*Input and Epsilon-LRP are equivalent if the model under investigation exclusively uses ReLU activation functions. We therefore chose Epsilon-LRP as a representative for this group of the remaining experiments ($\epsilon = 10^{-7}$).
3. **Grad-CAM and Grad-CAM++** build a third group, outperforming all other methods in terms of Fidelity-Score and FNR. The improved Grad-CAM++ method slightly outperformed the original Grad-CAM algorithm. We used Grad-CAM++ as a representative of this group for the remaining experiments.
4. **Occlusion** performed slightly better than the second group but still worse than the third.

We note that Grad-CAM, Grad-CAM++ and Occlusion perform well, but show some artefacts, which result from the up-sampling of the embedding's attribution map, which in general is not aligned with changes in the signal. Therefore, we observe an attribution value that is an average of the attributions of either

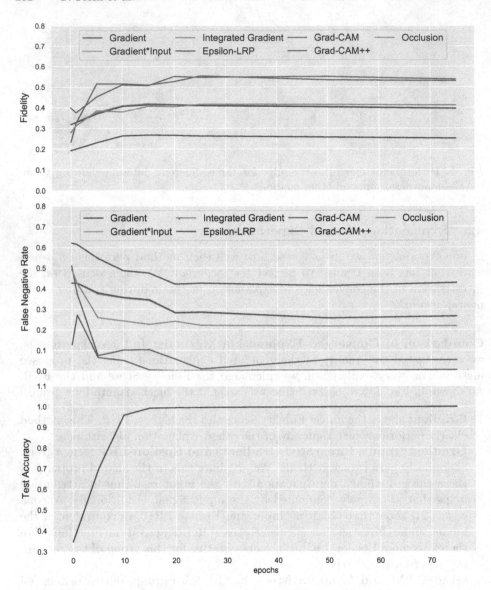

Fig. 5. Behavior of explanation methods during the training process of the Network. All methods converge to a steady state during training.

side of the input signal change. Figure 3e and 3f show two samples of generated explanations. We observe that methods which generate explanations using a partial derivative with respect to the input produce more noisy explanations as opposed to the Grad-CAM++ method. In summary, Grad-CAM++ outperformed all other methods with regard to Fidelity Score and FNR.

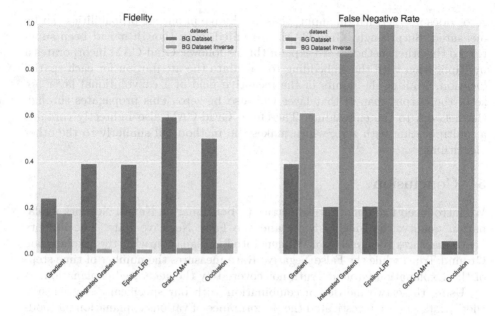

Fig. 6. Performance collapse of existing explanation methods on the inverse dataset due to an explicit or implicit multiplication with the input which is close to zero within the EGT.

Comparison of Explanation Methods During Training. In the next step, we investigated the evolution of explanations and their convergence during training of the Neural Network. We evaluated the performance of the explanation methods at different stages during training.

Figure 5 shows the change of the Fidelity Score and FNR during training. All methods improved the Fidelity Score and the FNR while the network was learning. Once the network converges to a state where the accuracy does not improve anymore (approximately after 20 epochs), the metrics converge to a steady state.

4.4   Limitations of Explanation Methods

We observed that the nature of the dataset influences the performance of the explanation methods. This is especially pronounced for methods that make use of a multiplication with the input signal. We push this to an extreme by constructing a dataset (Background Dataset Inverse 3(d)) for which these methods completely fail: The samples are constructed in such a way that the input signal is close to zero for time steps which belong to the EGT.

Figure 6 depicts the performance drop of methods that contain a multiplication with the input (i.e. Gradient*Input, Integrated Gradients, Epsilon-LRP) for the "Background Dataset Inverse" (Fig. 3(d)). The occlusion method also failed, since it replaces the original values of the input with zeros - replacing zeros with zeros does not perturb the input, thus no change in output probabilities can be measured. Surprisingly, Grad-CAM also failed, even though it had been superior to the other methods. We explain this as follows: Grad-CAM incorporates a multiplication with the embedding to calculate the attribution for each spatial location. If all of the inputs in the receptive field of a convolutional layer are zero, the output map of that layer will also be zero. This propagates through the network to the embedding. Therefore, Grad-CAM also indirectly contains a multiplication with zero, which makes the method fail similarly to the other algorithms.

5   Conclusion

We introduced two quantitative metrics to benchmark a Neural Network explanation quality: the Fidelity Score and the False Negative Rate. The Fidelity Score measures the overlap of the generated explanation with the Explanation Ground Truth while the False Negative Rate measures the number of time steps of the Explanation Ground Truth not covered by the generated explanation.

Using these two metrics in combination with our specifically crafted synthetic datasets, we investigated the performance of various explanation methods and concluded that the Grad-CAM++ algorithm outperforms all other methods (Saliency, Gradient*Input, Integrated Gradient, Layer Relevance Propagation and Occlusion).

Additionally, we demonstrated that existing explanation methods suffer from a performance collapse for input data with values close to zero within the Explanation Ground Truth.

5.1   Future Work

In Future work, the benchmarked explainability methods should be applied to actual ECG data. Additionally, the explanation methods described in this work produce explanations that indicate which locations of the input are responsible for the network's decision. However, location is not the only factor that influences a classification decision. There can also be frequency factors - the structure of an object - that are essential for discerning two classes. Existing explanation methods are not capable of communicating a reliance on frequency components (structural features). To fully explain a network's decision, an explanation algorithm should be developed that can visualize dependencies on a combination of location and frequency.

Acknowledgment. We would like to thank Anirban Das from the Rensselaer Polytechnic Institute and Adam Invankay from IBM Research Zurich for their valuable discussions and feedback on our work.

References

1. Krizhevsky, A., Sutskever, I., Hinton, G.E.: ImageNet classification with deep convolutional Neural Networks. Technical report. http://code.google.com/p/cuda-convnet/

2. Chiu, C.C., et al.: State-of-the-art speech recognition with sequence-to-sequence models, December 2017. http://arxiv.org/abs/1712.01769
3. Lecun, Y., Bengio, Y., Hinton, G.: Deep learning, May 2015. https://doi.org/10.1038/nature14539
4. Lecun, Y., Bottou, L., Bengio, Y., Haffner, P.: Gradient-based learning applied to document recognition. Proc. IEEE **86**(11), 2278–2324 (1998)
5. Gilpin, L.H., Bau, D., Yuan, B.Z., Bajwa, A., Specter, M., Kagal, L.: Explaining Explanations: An Overview of Interpretability of Machine Learning. Technical report (2019)
6. Kindermans, P.J., Schütt, K., Müller, K.R., Dähne, S.: Investigating the influence of noise and distractors on the interpretation of neural networks, November 2016. http://arxiv.org/abs/1611.07270
7. Krizhevsky, A., Sutskever, I., Hinton, G.E.: Imagenet classification with deep convolutional neural networks. In: Pereira, F., Burges, C.J.C., Bottou, L., Weinberger, K.Q. (eds.) Advances in Neural Information Processing Systems 25, pp. 1097–1105. Curran Associates, Inc. (2012). http://papers.nips.cc/paper/4824-imagenet-classification-with-deep-convolutional-neural-networks.pdf
8. Olah, C., Mordvintsev, A., Schubert, L.: Feature visualization. Distill **2**(11), e7 (2017). https://doi.org/10.23915/distill.00007. https://distill.pub/2017/feature-visualization
9. Ribeiro, M.T., Singh, S., Guestrin, C.: "why should I trust you?": explaining the predictions of any classifier. CoRR abs/1602.04938 (2016). http://arxiv.org/abs/1602.04938
10. Selvaraju, R.R., Cogswell, M., Das, A., Vedantam, R., Parikh, D., Batra, D.: Grad-CAM: visual explanations from Deep Networks via gradient-based localization, October 2016. http://arxiv.org/abs/1610.02391
11. Shrikumar, A., Greenside, P., Kundaje, A.: Learning Important Features Through Propagating Activation Differences. Technical report. http://goo.gl/qKb7pL
12. Hoffman, R.R., Mueller, S.T., Klein, G., Litman, J.: Metrics for explainable AI: challenges and prospects. CoRR abs/1812.04608 (2018). http://arxiv.org/abs/1812.04608
13. Holzinger, A., Carrington, A.M., Müller, H.: Measuring the quality of explanations: the system causability scale (SCS). comparing human and machine explanations. CoRR abs/1912.09024 (2019). http://arxiv.org/abs/1912.09024
14. Simonyan, K., Vedaldi, A., Zisserman, A.: Deep inside convolutional networks: visualising image classification models and saliency maps, December 2013. http://arxiv.org/abs/1312.6034
15. Simonyan, K., Zisserman, A.: Very deep convolutional networks for large-scale image recognition. In: International Conference on Learning Representations (2015)
16. Zeiler, M.D., Fergus, R.: Visualizing and Understanding Convolutional Networks. Technical report
17. Sundararajan, M., Taly, A., Yan, Q.: Axiomatic Attribution for Deep Networks. Technical report (2017)
18. Bach, S., Binder, A., Montavon, G., Klauschen, F., Müller, K.R., Samek, W.: On pixel-wise explanations for non-linear classifier decisions by layer-wise relevance propagation. PLoS ONE **10**(7), e0130140 (2015). https://doi.org/10.1371/journal.pone.0130140
19. Chattopadhyay, A., Sarkar, A., Howlader, P., Balasubramanian, V.N.: Grad-cam++: generalized gradient-based visual explanations for deep convolutional networks. CoRR abs/1710.11063 (2017). http://arxiv.org/abs/1710.11063

20. Alvarez-Melis, D., Jaakkola, T.S.: Towards robust interpretability with self-explaining Neural Networks, June 2018. http://arxiv.org/abs/1806.07538
21. Ancona, M., Ceolini, E., Öztireli, C., Gross, M.: Towards better understanding of gradient-based attribution methods for Deep Neural Networks, November 2017. http://arxiv.org/abs/1711.06104

The Effects of Masking in Melanoma Image Classification with CNNs Towards International Standards for Image Preprocessing

Fabrizio Nunnari[1,2]([envelope]), Abraham Ezema[1,2], and Daniel Sonntag[1,2]

[1] German Research Center of Artificial Intelligence, Kaiserslautern, Germany
{Fabrizio.Nunnari,Abraham_Obinwanne.Ezema,Daniel.Sonntag}@dfki.de
[2] Oldenburg University, Oldenburg, Germany
http://www.dfki.de/iml

Abstract. The classification of skin lesion images is known to be biased by artifacts of the surrounding skin, but it is still not clear to what extent masking out healthy skin pixels influences classification performances, and why. To better understand this phenomenon, we apply different strategies of image masking (rectangular masks, circular masks, full masking, and image cropping) to three datasets of skin lesion images (ISIC2016, ISIC2018, and MedNode). We train CNN-based classifiers, provide performance metrics through a 10-fold cross-validation, and analyse the behaviour of Grad-CAM saliency maps through an automated visual inspection. Our experiments show that cropping is the best strategy to maintain classification performance and to significantly reduce training times as well. Our analysis through visual inspection shows that CNNs have the tendency to focus on pixels of healthy skin when no malignant features can be identified. This suggests that CNNs have the tendency of "eagerly" looking for pixel areas to justify a classification choice, potentially leading to biased discriminators. To mitigate this effect, and to standardize image preprocessing, we suggest to crop images during dataset construction or before the learning step.

Keywords: Skin cancer · Convolutional neural networks · Masking · Reducing bias · AI standardization roadmap · Preprocessing

1 Introduction

As reported in the 2019 USA cancer statistics, skin diseases have been steadily increasing over the years, whereby skin cancer represents 7% of the total cancer cases. As of 2019, there were 104,350 expected cases of skin cancer, of which 96,480 were melanomas. The importance of promptly detecting skin cancer is evident from the high percentage of survival (92%) after surgery resulting from early detection [19].

© ICST Institute for Computer Sciences, Social Informatics and Telecommunications Engineering 2021
Published by Springer Nature Switzerland AG 2021. All Rights Reserved
J. Ye et al. (Eds.): MobiHealth 2020, LNICST 362, pp. 257–273, 2021.
https://doi.org/10.1007/978-3-030-70569-5_16

The classification of skin lesions using computer vision algorithms has been a subject of recent research [6,10,13]. One of the breakthroughs being the publication of Esteva et al. [8], reporting a better performance than expert dermatologists using transfer learning on a deep convolutional neural network (CNN). The network was first trained on a set of about one million diverse images, and then fine-tuned with more than 100k images of skin lesions.

Given the promising progress of computer vision algorithms in aiding skin lesion classification, the ISIC[1] (International Skin Imaging Collaboration) hosts a competition for the automated analysis of skin lesions. In the years 2016 [12], 2017 [5], and 2018 [4], the challenge included three tasks: segmentation, attribute extraction, and classification. These tasks replicate the procedure usually followed by dermatologists: to identify the contour of the skin lesion, highlight the areas in the lesion that suggest malignancy, and classify the specific type of lesion.

To accomplish these tasks, the ISIC challenge provides a public dataset that has grown from 900 images as of 2016 to more than 33,000 images for the 2020 edition. This is the largest publicly available dataset of dermoscopic images, and is widely used by many researchers throughout the world.

Masking skin lesion images, i.e., using segmentation to remove the pixels pertaining to the healthy skin and retaining the pixels belonging to the lesion, is an image pre-processing technique that is supposed to help the classification of skin lesions by removing unneeded, unwanted image artifacts.

In fact, Winkler et al. [23] found that the presence of *gentian violet* ink, often used by dermatologists to mark the skin in proximity to suspicious lesions, can disrupt the correct classification and lower the specificity of commercial DSS (Diagnosis Support Systems). Moreover, recently, Bissoto et al. [2] found a strong bias in the ISIC dataset; by completely removing 70% of the central part of the images (hence removing the totality of pixels containing the skin lesions), the CNN model was still able to reach 0.74 AUC (with respect to 0.88 AUC reached with full images). This suggests a strong bias of the dataset at its borders.

To date, while there seem to be clear advantages of masking out the skin surrounding the lesion area, it is not clear to what extent masking images influences (positively or negatively) the quality of classification (e.g., by removing bias). And what are other consequences for the process of training classifiers?

In this paper, we present a further investigation on image masking by, first, assessing the presence of biases at the dataset images' borders, and, second, comparing the classification performances when applying several types of masks. Third, we analyse the bias patterns through a visual inspection of Grad-CAM saliency maps [18]. This analysis employs four types of *masks* (see Fig. 1):

1. Rectangular Mask (RM) removes 30% of the image surface around the border. This is a direct contrast to the masking utilized by Bissotto et al. [2] to show the presence of bias at the borders and its influence on model performance. With this masking type, we verify whether removing the border affects the performance of a classifier.

---

[1] https://www.isic-archive.com/.

2. Circular Mask (CM) draws a circle at the middle of images. Here, we evaluate if removing the corners of the images and inspecting only its central part retains model performance.
3. Full Mask (M) reveals only the lesions and a fraction of the surrounding skin. It is used to reveal whether completely removing the skin surrounding a lesion improves prediction performance.
4. Finally, a rectangular cropping (CR) of the image is applied, which removes the image borders and increases the quantity of information passed to the classifiers.

In the rest of this paper, we conduct experiments on three popular skin lesion image datasets (ISIC 2016, ISIC 2018, and MedNode), each evaluated through a 10-fold cross validation approach to reduce biases by randomization. All the maskings were implemented using a dedicated U-NET (de-)convolutional neural network, following the procedure described in [14].

With the standardization roadmap for artificial intelligence, a comprehensive analysis of the current state of and need for international standards and specifications has been published [22]. Data bias and the bias of classifiers is a key factor. As a result of our experiments, we suggest to crop images during dataset construction or before the learning step, towards a process to standardize image preprocessing in CNN contexts.

Section 2 gives an overview of related work and on the importance of masking to avoid biases. Section 3 describes the method used to train and test the data material. Section 4 describes the experiments measuring the difference in performances among different masking conditions. Section 5 reports on the analysis of our results with the help of saliency extraction (visual explanation). Section 6 discusses the results, and Sect. 7 concludes the paper.

2 Related Work

The classification of skin lesions through the use of CNNs has increased in popularity since the publication of Esteva et al. [8]. Their CNN-based model matched the performance of experienced dermatologists. To this end, all performant neural-network-based solutions for skin lesion classification are based on a transfer learning approach [21]: a baseline deep CNN is pre-trained for example on the ImageNet dataset [7], and the transfer-learning steps consists of substituting the final fully-connect layers of the network with a few randomly initialized ones, then to continue training the model on skin lesion images. In our work, we perform transfer learning using pre-trained versions of VGG16 [20].

Rather than focusing on benchmarks [10], our goal in this contribution to investigate the change of performance between using plain images and segmented or normalized ones for the classification task. To train our reference classifier, we rely on three publicly available datasets: ISIC 2016 [12], ISIC 2018 [4], and MedNode [9]. All of them were used to train several models, each on a number masking methods, as later explained in Sect. 3.

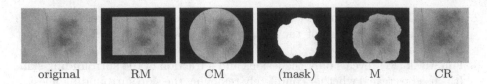

original   RM   CM   (mask)   M   CR

Fig. 1. Masking examples, from left to right: the original full image (ISIC_0024307), rectangular mask (RM), circular mask (CM), the segmentation mask, the segmented image (M), the image cropped on the mask bounding box (CR).

Burdick et al. [3] performed a systematic study on the importance of masking images used for training CNN models. They compared the performance of the CNN model using the full images compared to applying the masks on several levels: from fully masking out the surrounding skin to exposing some portion of the skin surrounding the lesion. Tests show best results when only a limited portion of the surrounding skin is kept for training. The hypothesis is that masking the healthy skin helps in classification while showing all the healthy skin in the image "confuses" the network, that is, it becomes more probable that the network learns image artefacts. Following the results in Burdick et al. [3], for each image, we also extend the lesion mask from segmentation to 110% of its original area, in order to expose a bit more of the surrounding skin areas during training than the original mask shows.

Binary masking of an image defines a black/white area within it, whereas white is associated with the pixels of interest, and black is associated with non-interesting or the confounding part of the image to be discarded in subsequent processing steps. This segmentation techniques have been significantly improved by the use of deep learning models. Ronneberger et al. [17] first proposed the application of the convolution-deconvolution network (U-Net) for medical image segmentation. The U-Net architecture applies stacks of convolutional layers with downsampling to extract latent image features and deconvolutional layers with upsampling within the network. This method of segmentation has been very successfully applied to medical image segmentation.

Variants of this model have shown to be very effective in the ISIC segmentation challenge in the past, with a Jaccard index score of 0.765 and 0.802 in the ISIC2017 and ISIC2018 editions, respectively, see [1,16]. In this paper, we implement a transparent segmentation model to show the effects of masking in melanoma images by using the approach described in [14] and using the data provided for Task 1 of the ISIC 2018 challenge [4].

3   Method Overview

Figure 2 illustrates the method we follow to test the effectiveness of the different masking conditions on prediction performance. The method is composed of three phases: preparation of the segmentation model, masked images construction, and training of the classification models. They are discussed in more detail in the following.

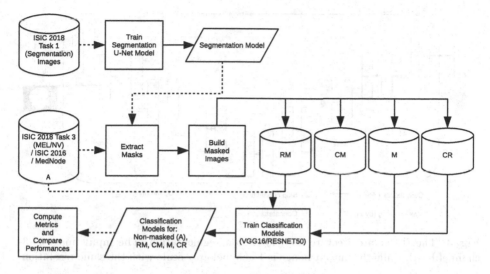

Fig. 2. Methodology overview. The top blocks depict the training of the segmentation model. The middle blocks are related to the preparation of the masked images, and the bottom blocks represents the training of the classification models.

3.1 Segmentation Model

We utilize the images from Task 1 of the ISIC 2018 to train a masking model based on the U-Net architecture [17]. This dataset comprised of 2594 RGB skin lesion images, and for each sample, the ground truth is a binary mask in the same resolution as the input image.

Figure 3 shows the U-Net architecture together with a sample input and output (binary mask). The architecture is composed of 9 convolution blocks, where each of them is a pair of 2D *same* convolution with a kernel size of 3 × 3 × 3. Downsamplig is the result of a max-pooling with size 2 × 2. Upsampling is the result of a 2 × 2 transposed 2D *same* convolution. After each upsampling step, the convolution is performed on the concatenation of the upsampling result and the output of the downsampling with corresponding resolution. The initial number of filters (32) doubles at each downsampling. For this work, we used an input/output resolution of 160 × 160 pixels.

3.2 Masked Image Datasets

The segmentation model described above is used to extract *masks* for Melanoma and Nevus images of the ISIC 2018 Task 3 [4], ISIC 2016 [12], and MedNode [9] datasets. From ISIC 2018 Task 3, we selected only nevus (NV) and melanoma (MEL) classes because these are the exactly the same classes which used as ground truth for the masks in Task 1. After an initial visual inspection, we realized that applying the mask prediction to any of the other 6 classes of the Task 3 dataset often leads to erroneous results due to the very different nature of the lesions.

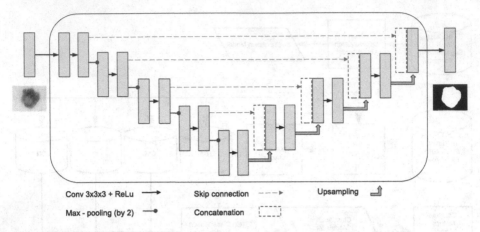

Fig. 3. The U-Net architecture used for lesion segmentation. The input image is 3-channel RGB, while the output image is 1-channel gray-scale with the same resolution.

In total we define five sets of pre-processed images: **A** (the full image, containing all of the pixels), and the four types already described in the introduction **RM**, **CM**, **M**, and **CR**. See Fig. 1.

The M and CR datasets are obtained through the composition between the original images and the extracted masks. For the M dataset, the mask is first scaled around its center by a factor of 1.1 to reveal a portion of the surrounding skin (as suggested by [3]). The composition setting converts all pixels outside the lesion mask to black. For the CR dataset, the mask is utilized to identify a rectangular cropping region containing the lesions contour.

The CR datasets contains a few less samples than the others, because an initial inspection revealed that the masks of samples with a thin lesion–foreground pixel variation result in very small (mostly inaccurate) lesion blobs. Hence, we automatically filtered these defective images from our samples based on an automated comparison between the area of the masks and the total image size. Images whose mask areas was less than $\frac{1}{8}$ of the picture were discarded.

3.3   Binary Classifiers

For each of the 3 datasets and 5 masking conditions, we trained 10 binary classification models using a 10-fold splitting strategy. Each fold was composed using 10% of the dataset for testing and another random 10% for validation. While splitting, we ensured to preserve the proportion between classes. In the rest of this paper, we report the mean and the standard deviation among the 10 folds.

The performance of the binary classifiers in discriminating *nevi* from *melanomas* are reported in terms of accuracy, specificity, sensitivity, and ROC AUC (Receiver Operating Curve - Area Under the Curve) on the test set, where the positive case is associated with the malignant melanoma.

```
1  ----------------------------------------------------------------------
2  Layer (type)                   Output Shape              Param #
3  ======================================================================
4  input_1 (InputLayer)           (None, 227, 227, 3)       0
5  ----------------------------------------------------------------------
6  block1_conv1 (Conv2D)          (None, 227, 227, 64)      1792
7  ----------------------------------------------------------------------
8  block1_conv2 (Conv2D)          (None, 227, 227, 64)      36928
9  ----------------------------------------------------------------------
10 block1_pool (MaxPooling2D)     (None, 113, 113, 64)      0
11 ----------------------------------------------------------------------
12 [... 13 more layers ...]
13 ----------------------------------------------------------------------
14 block5_conv3 (Conv2D)          (None, 14, 14, 512)       2359808
15 ----------------------------------------------------------------------
16 block5_pool (MaxPooling2D)     (None, 7, 7, 512)         0
17 ----------------------------------------------------------------------
18 flatten (Flatten)              (None, 25088)             0
19 ----------------------------------------------------------------------
20 fc1 (Dense)                    (None, 4096)              102764544
21 ----------------------------------------------------------------------
22 dropout_1 (Dropout)            (None, 4096)              0
23 ----------------------------------------------------------------------
24 fc2 (Dense)                    (None, 4096)              16781312
25 ----------------------------------------------------------------------
26 dropout_2 (Dropout)            (None, 4096)              0
27 ----------------------------------------------------------------------
28 predictions (Dense)            (None, 3047)              12483559
29 ======================================================================
30 Total params: 146,744,103
31 Trainable params: 146,744,103
32 Non-trainable params: 0
33 ----------------------------------------------------------------------
```

Listing 1.1. An excerpt of the VGG16 architecture used for the binary classification task.

As already successfully employed in previous research (e.g., [8]), all of the binary classifiers are based on the transfer learning approach [21] with CNNs. The base CNN model is the VGG16 [20] architecture pre-trained on ImageNet [11]. We then substituted the original three final fully connected layers with a sequence of two fully connected layers, each followed by a dropout of 0.5, and a final 2-class discrimination softmax layer. Listing 1.1 shows an excerpt of the architecture.

Each model was trained for a maximum of 100 epochs and optimized for accuracy. Input images were fed to the network with an $8\times$ augmentation factor, where each image was horizontally flipped and rotated by 0, 90, 180, and 270 degrees. To avoid the generation of black bands, images were rotated after scaling to the CNN input resolution. Class imbalance was taken into account using a compensation factor in the loss-function (parameter class_weight in the fit method of the Keras framework). For each model, we also report what epoch returned the most accurate model.

All training was performed on Linux workstations using our toolkit for Interactive Machine Learning (TIML)[2], which uses the Keras[3] (v2.2.4) framework with Tensorflow[4] (v1.13.1) as backend. Our reference Hardware is an 8-core Intel 9th-gen i7 CPU with 64 GB RAM and an NVIDIA RTX Titan 24 GB GPU.

4   Experiments

The following three sections report details on the analysis performed on the three datasets: ISIC2016, MedNode, and ISIC2018. For each dataset, the metrics of the binary classification are reported for each of the five masking conditions described before: A, RM, CM, M, and CR. The analysis focuses on determining a potential bias from the border of the images.

4.1   ISIC2018

Table 1 shows the distribution of the samples in the ISIC2018 dataset. Training a full model (6256 samples, 100 epochs) takes about 9 h on our reference hardware. Table 2 show the results of the tests.

Table 1. Distribution of the 7818 images from the ISIC2018 dataset.

conditions	samples	MEL	NV	train	val	test
A, RM, CM, M	7818	1113 (14.2%)	6705 (85.8%)	6256	781	781
CR	7645	1099 (14.3%)	6546 (85.9%)	6119	763	763

In order to measure the statistical significance of the metric among conditions, we run a set of t-tests for independent samples between the no-mask condition (A) against all the others. The results of the test are reported in Table 3. The tests compare the results across the 10 folds ($N = 10$). The table reports the compared conditions, followed by the different statistic metrics, their absolute and relative difference, and the significance code for the p-value (+: $p < .1$; *: $p < .05$; **: $p < .01$; ***: $p < 0.001$).

When applying a rectangular mask, the results show a significant reduction on almost all metrics. For example, accuracy drops by 2.99%. Also circular masks and full masking decrease accuracy by 2.85% and 4.37%, respectively. Only cropping shows some improvewd accuracy values. Although not significant, we report a positive tendency of 4.73% increase in sensitivity.

This results suggest that there is indeed a bias in the surrounding skin; the other explanation is that exposing a large portion of the surrounding skin helps

---

[2] https://github.com/DFKI-Interactive-Machine-Learning/TIML.

[3] https://keras.io/.

[4] https://www.tensorflow.org/.

Table 2. Results of the test on the ISIC2018 dataset.

set	testacc	testspec	testsens	testauc	epch
A	.909 (.014)	.933 (.017)	.763 (.062)	.948 (.010)	90.3 (6.7)
RM	.882 (.011)	.899 (.018)	.781 (.059)	.937 (.011)	41.8 (3.9)
CM	.883 (.017)	.899 (.021)	.789 (.066)	.938 (.012)	41.5 (6.1)
M	.870 (.013)	.884 (.014)	.785 (.034)	.930 (.011)	39.0 (10.7)
CR	.911 (.014)	.929 (.017)	.799 (.057)	.955 (.010)	40.7 (7.8)

Table 3. Significant differences between masking conditions in the ISIC2018 dataset.

Condition	Metric	Difference	Diff. pct	Signif.
A vs RM	ACC	−0.027	−2.99%	***
A vs RM	SPEC	−0.035	−3.73%	***
A vs RM	AUC	−0.011	−1.21%	*
A vs RM	EPOCH	−48.5	−53.71%	***
A vs CM	ACC	−0.026	−2.85%	**
A vs CM	AUC	−0.1	−1.11%	+
A vs CM	EPOCH	−48.8	−54.04%	***
A vs M	ACC	−0.04	−4.37%	***
A vs M	SPEC	−0.05	−5.33%	***
A vs M	AUC	−0.018	−1.90%	**
A vs M	EPOCH	−51.3	−56.81%	***
A vs CR	SENS	0.036	4.73%	0.2152
A vs CR	EPOCH	−49.6	−54.93%	***

in the classification to some extent. For the cropping condition, such deficiency might be compensated by higher quantity of information passed to the neural network. In fact, when the image is cropped, almost all of the 277×277 pixels of the image are covered by the lesion–hence increasing the quantity of detail attributed to the skin.

A common aspect across all our comparisons is the significant and consistent drop (more than 50%) of the number of epochs needed to train the model.

4.2   MedNode

Table 4 shows the distribution of the samples in the MedNode dataset. Training one fold of the full dataset (ca. 136 samples, 100 epochs) takes about 15 minutes on our reference hardware. Table 5 show the results.

In comparison to A, we observed a considerable decrease in the performance when applying a rectangular mask, e.g., accuracy −0.053 (−6.58%), and mild loss in performance for all other conditions. However, none of the differences is

Table 4. Distribution of the 170 images of the MedNode dataset.

conditions	samples	MEL	NV	train	val	test
A, RM, CM, M	170	70 (41.2%)	100 (58.8%)	136	17	17
CR	169	70 (41.4%)	99 (58.6%)	137	16	16

Table 5. Results of the test on the MedNode dataset.

set	testacc	testspec	testsens	testauc	epch
A	.806 (.123)	.870 (.100)	.714 (.181)	.869 (.131)	34.1 (12.9)
RM	.753 (.094)	.800 (.118)	.686 (.189)	.860 (.073)	36.1 (23.5)
CM	.818 (.140)	.830 (.135)	.800 (.194)	.890 (.114)	40.5 (21.3)
M	.806 (.112)	.830 (.090)	.771 (.214)	.880 (.111)	43.6 (24.7)
CR	.768 (.144)	.820 (.087)	.700 (.328)	.843 (.120)	55.9 (32.2)

significant according to our t-tests, likely because of the high variance in the measurements among the 10 folds from the limited number of samples.

4.3   ISIC 2016

Table 6 shows the distribution of the samples in the ISIC2016 dataset. Training one fold of the full dataset (722 samples, 100 epochs) takes about 1 h 30 m on our reference hardware. Table 7 show the results.

Table 6. Distribution of the 900 images of the ISIC2016 dataset. In the right columns, the mean of the number of samples among the 10 folds used for validation (standard deviation is ≤ 0.6).

conditions	samples	MEL	NV	train	val	test
A, RM, CM, M	900	173 (19.2%)	727 (80.8%)	722	89	89
CR	884	173 (19.6%)	711 (80.4%)	708	88	88

The only statistically significant difference stems from the specificity between the A and CM conditions (-0.026, -2.92%, $p < 0.1$). We can also observe a noticeable drop in sensitivity between A and CR conditions ($-0,092$, -22.18%), but it is not significant for our tests (p = 0.2352).

As for the MedNode dataset, the reduced number of samples led to a high variance during the cross-fold validation, making it thus impossible to validate the differences among conditions using our statistical method.

Table 7. Results of the on the ISIC2016 dataset.

set	testacc	testspec	testsens	testauc	epch
A	.806 (.028)	.898 (.031)	.416 (.163)	.773 (.074)	45.1 (38.4)
RM	.794 (.037)	.878 (.069)	.445 (.146)	.756 (.063)	49.2 (36.2)
CM	.788 (.026)	.872 (.030)	.432 (.151)	.790 (.059)	52.7 (26.9)
M	.784 (.035)	.866 (.065)	.445 (.181)	.774 (.066)	57.7 (28.7)
CR	.805 (.044)	.923 (.045)	.324 (.155)	.755 (.078)	46.3 (35.1)

5   Visual Inspection

In order to visually explain the characteristics that influenced model predictions, we leveraged the Grad-CAM method [18] to generate the saliency maps of *attention*. Figure 4 shows a nevus and a melanoma images from ISIC2018 and their relative attention maps on all masking conditions. All the saliency maps were extracted from the last convolutional layer of the VGG16 architecture (block5_conv3).

Two contrasting patterns emerge, thus giving additional details about the model's discrimination strategy. The saliency is higher on the skin lesion pixels (focused towards the center) for images correctly predicted as melanoma. In contrast, the saliency is higher on the skin pixels (towards the borders) in pictures correctly classified as nevus. The opposite happens when images are wrongly classified, with the attention for wrongly classified nevus towards the center and the attention for wrongly classified melanomas towards the border.

It is worth pointing out that the attention of the CNN moves towards the border regardless of the kind of masking strategy used. To systematically quantify this behaviour, we recorded the occurrence of this pattern in relation to the classification results, categorizing images according to whether the salient pixels are accumulated towards the (B)order or towards the (C) enter. The discrimination was made by a processing routine in terms of a pixel-level analysis. When the activation value for the pixel along the image borders (*left, top, bottom, right*) is very low (<0.1), then the image saliency map is considered as centered. For opposite cases, that is, when high activation values are present along the borders, an image-centred square patch covering $\frac{1}{16}th$ of the total image size is evaluated to confirm border images. As a result, when the patch is dominated by low activation values, a border case is recorded for the image, while a centered image is recorded for the opposite characteristic.

Table 8 shows the results on the ISIC2018 dataset. The observed behaviour (saliency is at the center for correct melanoma and wrong nevus, otherwise at the border) is prominent in the A, CM, and RM masking conditions, but less prominent for the M and CR conditions.

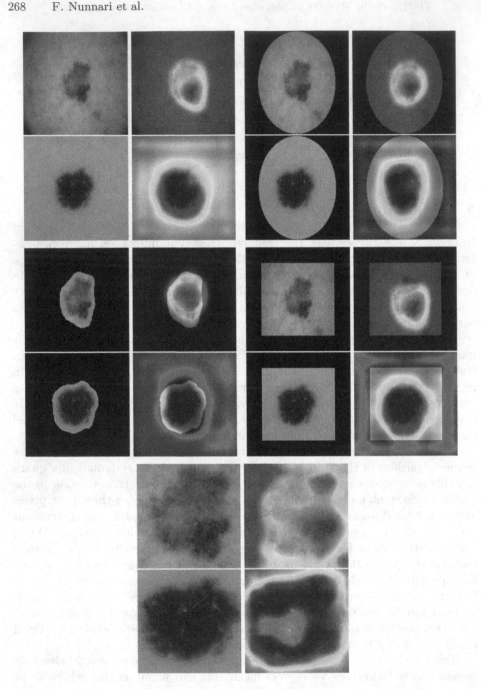

Fig. 4. ISIC 2018: colored saliency maps (aka heatmaps) extracted by Grad-CAM from the last convolution layer of the VGG16 model. The heatmaps are relative to one melanoma (top) and one nevus (bottom), both correctly classified. For each of the five masking conditions we show both the input image and its composition with the heatmap. Notice that for melanoma the heatmaps concentrate towards the center, while for nevus the model focuses on the border, regardless of the mask type.

Table 8. Results of the automatized saliency map inspection: counts of images with saliency map concentration at (B) order or (C), divided for Melanoma (MEL) and Nevus (NV), further split in (C)orrectly or (W)rongly classified.

ISIC 2018					
Mask	Concentration	MEL-C	MEL-W	NV-C	NV-W
A	B	54	258	5430	20
	C	795	6	830	425
CM	B	0	235	5974	0
	C	878	54	0	677
RM	B	0	244	6024	0
	C	869	0	2	679
M	B	163	219	2986	71
	C	711	20	2938	710
CR	B	325	185	3599	162
	C	554	36	2483	302

6   Discussion

Here we summarize our observations on the use of the different masking conditions arising from the classification results and from the visual inspections. As the low number of samples does not lead to statistically significant results for the MedNode and ISIC2016 datasets, we focus our analyses on the results obtained on the ISIC 2018 dataset.

From the classification results (Sect. 4.1) it is clear that masking the images affects the overall performance, likely because this eliminates any biases of the image borders. Moreover, we can notice a slight improvement in the sensitivity for images cropped to contain their lesions (hence, somehow zoomed), likely because of a increased quantity of details passed to the CNN model. We thus propose CR as the preferred condition which takes away potential biases in the data and forces the model to learn more from salient details (lesion area). We expect the models trained on CR to generalize better to unseen data and deviate from the learning process of models with high bias in data. This way, we can potentially improve data quality and reduce overfitting, although this means a slight drop in performance on the closed world test set.

It is worth noting that with all masking conditions, the number of epochs needed to converge to the best predicting model, decreases by over 50%. This happens not only when blackening out significant parts of the image, thus providing the CNN with flat-valued uniform color areas, but also when zooming into the image and maximizing the number of pixels belonging to lesions. This suggest that the network is indeed *learning faster* thanks to the high quantity of meaningful, focused, information.

From the visual inspection of the saliency maps (Sect. 5), it appears that when images are classified as melanoma, the network concentrates most of its "attention" in the central part of the image, as a human practitioner would do. In contrast, when images are classified as nevus, the saliency map is more spread towards the border. This last phenomenon is less regular in the M and CR conditions, where most of the healthy skin is absent, suggesting that the CNN (when classifiyng a nevus) tends to activate on the small areas of skin around the lesion. Notably, this happens regardless of the correctness of the prediction, showing that in fact the CNN learned to search for the features characterizing the positive case (melanoma) within the lesion area.

However, it seems that in absence of visual elements characterizing a melanoma, the network has the tendency to find a "reason" for the competing class (nevus) elsewhere in the image, either on blacked-out areas, which are surely non-discriminating, but also on healthy skin areas. This might in part question and refute the conclusions of Burdick et al. [3], who stated that extending the masks of a lesion allows us to take advantage of the contrast between the lesioned and healthy skin. Differently, it seems that CNNs really need an "area of alternative attention", which we could define as the portions of the image on which the CNN needs to concentrates the activation of its layers when predicting a negative case (nevus).

7   Conclusions

In this paper, we presented a comprehensive investigation on the effect of masking on the binary classification of skin lesions between nevus and melanoma towards international standards for image preprocessing to reduce bias and increase data quality.

We performed our analyses on three datasets (ISIC 2018, MedNode, and ISIC 2016) using a 10-fold cross validation procedure. Then, in order to discard shallow conclusions due to the intrinsic randomness of CNN training procedures, we considered only those differences that have been confirmed as significant through statistical tests.

Inspired by the work of Bisotto et al. [2], who discovered the possibility of classifying skin lesions still after covering 70% of the internal surface of the images, we verified that prediction power indeed diminishes when removing 30% around the border, thus confirming the existence of some kind of bias.

Further experiments, with other types of masking, confirmed the bias at the border, and also showed that the best non-biased performances can be achieved through automated cropping.

The cropping condition also leads to 50% shorter training times, suggesting that the presence of healthy skin is noisy information that slows the convergence of the training process.

Finally, an automated analysis of the saliency maps extracted from the CNN classifier via Grad-CAM led us to formulate an hypothesis of *area of alternative attention*. In fact, the analysis leads to the following informal argument: while it is true that one should better maximize the area of the image with visual features able to identify a (positive) class, at the same time some of the pixels should be left free for the network to "justify" the complementary (negative) class. Future work, with more fine-tuned masking along the border of the lesion, and on other datasets, should be conducted to confirm this hypothesis.

In fact, it is worth noticing that most of the research in image classification has been conducted on databases of images where the objects of interests occupy only a relatively small portion of an image. Consequently, visual explanation methods like GradCAM [18] and RISE [15] have been developed and tested with the goal of identifying the relatively small subset of pixels justifying a classification. Differently, in the domain of skin cancer detection very often the majority of the pixels of an image are associated to a single entity, and this case has been so far received very little attention.

In general, the outcome of this investigation supports the idea that the creation of systems for skin lesion classification should go through a cropping process, either automated or manual, for both the creation of training data and for samples classification. This would both increase prediction performances (at least on sensitivity) and would significantly reduce the computational power needed for training—towards a process to standardize image preprocessing in CNN contexts [22].

Acknowledgements. The research has been supported by the Ki-Para-Mi project (BMBF, 01IS19038B), the pAItient project (BMG, 2520DAT0P2), and the Endowed Chair of Applied Artificial Intelligence, Oldenburg University. We would like to thank all student assistants that contributed to the development of the platform (see https://iml.dfki.de/).

References

1. Berseth, M.: ISIC 2017 - skin lesion analysis towards melanoma detection. CoRR abs/1703.00523 (2017). http://arxiv.org/abs/1703.00523
2. Bissoto, A., Fornaciali, M., Valle, E., Avila, S.: (De)Constructing bias on skin lesion datasets. In: The IEEE Conference on Computer Vision and Pattern Recognition (CVPR) Workshops, June 2019
3. Burdick, J., Marques, O., Weinthal, J., Furht, B.: Rethinking skin lesion segmentation in a convolutional classifier. J. Digit. Imaging **31**(4), 435–440 (2017). https://doi.org/10.1007/s10278-017-0026-y
4. Codella, N., Rotemberg, V., Tschandl, P., Celebi, M.E., et al.: Skin Lesion Analysis Toward Melanoma Detection 2018, February 2019. http://arxiv.org/abs/1902.03368
5. Codella, N.C.F., Gutman, D., Celebi, M.E., Helba, B., et al.: Skin lesion analysis toward melanoma detection: a challenge at the 2017 International symposium on biomedical imaging. In: 2018 IEEE 15th International Symposium on Biomedical Imaging (ISBI 2018), Washington, DC, pp. 168–172. IEEE, April 2018. https://doi.org/10.1109/ISBI.2018.8363547

6. Curiel-Lewandrowski, C., Novoa, R.A., Berry, E., Celebi, M.E., et al.: Artificial intelligence approach in melanoma. In: Melanoma, pp. 1–31. Springer, New York, New York, NY (2019). https://doi.org/10.1007/978-1-4614-7322-0_43-1

7. Deng, J., Dong, W., Socher, R., Li, L.J., et al.: ImageNet: a large-scale hierarchical image database. In: 2009 IEEE Conference on Computer Vision and Pattern Recognition, Miami, FL, pp. 248–255. IEEE, June 2009. https://doi.org/10.1109/CVPR.2009.5206848

8. Esteva, A., Kuprel, B., Novoa, R.A., Ko, J., Swetter, S.M., et al.: Dermatologist-level classification of skin cancer with deep neural networks. Nature **542**, 115, January 2017. https://doi.org/10.1038/nature21056

9. Giotis, I., Molders, N., Land, S., Biehl, M., et al.: MED-NODE: A computer-assisted melanoma diagnosis system using non-dermoscopic images. Expert Syst. Appl. **42**(19), 6578–6585 (2015). https://doi.org/10.1016/j.eswa.2015.04.034

10. Kawahara, J., Hamarneh, G.: Visual Diagnosis of Dermatological Disorders: Human and Machine Performance, June 2019. http://arxiv.org/abs/1906.01256

11. Krizhevsky, A., Sutskever, I., Hinton, G.E.: ImageNet classification with deep convolutional neural networks. In: Advances in Neural Information Processing Systems, vol. 25, pp. 1097–1105, Curran Associates, Inc., (2012)

12. Marchetti, M.A., Codella, N.C., Dusza, S.W., Gutman, D.A., et al.: Results of the 2016 international skin imaging collaboration international symposium on biomedical imaging challenge. J. Am. Acad. Dermatol. **78**(2), 270–277.e1 (2018). https://doi.org/10.1016/j.jaad.2017.08.016

13. Masood, A., Ali Al-Jumaily, A.: Computer aided diagnostic support system for skin cancer: a review of techniques and algorithms. Int. J. Biomed. Imaging **2013**, 1–22 (2013). https://doi.org/10.1155/2013/323268

14. Nguyen, D.M.H., Ezema, A., Nunnari, F., Sonntag, D.: A visually explainable learning system for skin lesion detection using multiscale input with attention U-Net. In: Schmid, U., Klügl, F., Wolter, D. (eds.) KI 2020. LNCS (LNAI), vol. 12325, pp. 313–319. Springer, Cham (2020). https://doi.org/10.1007/978-3-030-58285-2_28

15. Petsiuk, V., Das, A., Saenko, K.: RISE: randomized input sampling for explanation of black-box models. In: Proceedings of the British Machine Vision Conference (BMVC) (2018)

16. Qian, C., Liu, T., Jiang, H., Wang, Z., et al.: A detection and segmentation architecture for skin lesion segmentation on dermoscopy images. CoRR abs/1809.03917 (2018). http://arxiv.org/abs/1809.03917

17. Ronneberger, O., Fischer, P., Brox, T.: U-Net: convolutional networks for biomedical image segmentation. In: Navab, N., Hornegger, J., Wells, W.M., Frangi, A.F. (eds.) MICCAI 2015. LNCS, vol. 9351, pp. 234–241. Springer, Cham (2015). https://doi.org/10.1007/978-3-319-24574-4_28

18. Selvaraju, R.R., Cogswell, M., Das, A., Vedantam, R., et al.: Grad-CAM: visual explanations from deep networks via gradient-based localization. In: The IEEE International Conference on Computer Vision (ICCV), October 2017

19. Siegel, R.L., Miller, K.D., Jemal, A.: Cancer statistics. CA: Cancer J. Clin. **69**(1), 7–34, January 2019. https://doi.org/10.3322/caac.21551

20. Simonyan, K., Zisserman, A.: Very Deep Convolutional Networks for Large-Scale Image Recognition, September 2014. http://arxiv.org/abs/1409.1556

21. Tan, C., Sun, F., Kong, T., Zhang, W., Yang, C., Liu, C.: A survey on deep transfer learning. In: Kůrková, V., Manolopoulos, Y., Hammer, B., Iliadis, L., Maglogiannis, I. (eds.) ICANN 2018. LNCS, vol. 11141, pp. 270–279. Springer, Cham (2018). https://doi.org/10.1007/978-3-030-01424-7_27

22. Wahlster, W., Winterhalter, C.: German Standardization Roadmap on Artificial Intelligence. Technical Report, DIN e.V. and German Commission for Electrical, Electronic and Information Technologies of DIN and VDE (2020)
23. Winkler, J.K., Fink, C., Toberer, F., Enk, A., et al.: Association between surgical skin markings in dermoscopic images and diagnostic performance of a deep learning convolutional neural network for melanoma recognition. JAMA Dermatol. **155**(10), 1135 (2019). https://doi.org/10.1001/jamadermatol.2019.1735

Robust and Markerfree *in vitro* Axon Segmentation with CNNs

Philipp Grüning[1]([⊠]) (ID), Alex Palumbo[2,3,4] (ID), Svenja Kim Landt[2,3] (ID),
Lara Heckmann[2,3] (ID), Leslie Brackhagen[1] (ID), Marietta Zille[2,3,4] (ID),
and Amir Madany Mamlouk[1] (ID)

[1] Institute for Neuro- and Bioinformatics, University of Lübeck, Lübeck, Germany
{gruening,madany}@inb.uni-luebeck.de
[2] Fraunhofer Research and Development Center for Marine and Cellular
Biotechnology, Lübeck, Germany
[3] Institute for Medical and Marine Biotechnology, University of Lübeck, Lübeck,
Germany
[4] Institute for Experimental and Clinical Pharmacology and Toxicology,
University of Lübeck, Lübeck, Germany

Abstract. The automated *in vitro* segmentation of axonal phase-contrast images to allow axonal tracing over time is highly desirable to understand axonal biology in the context of health and disease. While deep learning has become a powerful tool in biomedical image analysis for semantic segmentation tasks, segmentation performance has been limited so far since axons are long and thin objects that are sensitive to under- and/or over-segmentation. We here propose the use of an ensemble-based convolutional neural network (CNN) framework for the segmentation of axons on phase-contrast microscopic images. The mean ResNet-50 ensemble performed better than the max u-net ensemble on the axon segmentation task. We estimated an upper limit for the expected improvement using an oracle-machine. Additionally, we introduced a soft version of the Dice coefficient that describes the visually perceived quality of axon segmentation better than the standard Dice. Importantly, the mean ResNet-50 ensemble reached the performance level of human experts. Taken together, we developed a CNN to robustly segment axons in phase-contrast microscopy that will foster further investigations of axonal biology in health and disease.

Keywords: Axon segmentation · Microscopy · Ensembles · ResNet-50

1 Introduction

Axons are wire-like extensions from neuronal cell bodies that ensure the communication to neighboring neurons by building connections among them. Axonal morphology is highly complex, with varying lengths, diameters, and degrees of arborization [3] and studying the role of axons in health and disease is a major emphasis of current research [10].

© ICST Institute for Computer Sciences, Social Informatics and Telecommunications Engineering 2021
Published by Springer Nature Switzerland AG 2021. All Rights Reserved
J. Ye et al. (Eds.): MobiHealth 2020, LNICST 362, pp. 274–284, 2021.
https://doi.org/10.1007/978-3-030-70569-5_17

In cell culture, individual axonal structures can be followed over longer periods of time by time-lapse microscopy. The respective data analysis, however, requires dedicated software tools that allow for the precise identification of axonal structures. At the same time, these software tools need to cope with the large amount of data available from imaging where manual inspection is time consuming, prone to error, and impractical [1,12].

Over the past two decades, many software packages such as NeuronMetrics, NeuriteIQ, NeuriteTracer, and NeurphologyJ have been developed to trace axons [7,12]. All of these tools are able to trace axonal structures only semi-automatically and require high-contrast images that are only available in fluorescence and not in phase-contrast microscopy. Apart from bleaching issues, fluorescence imaging requires either fixation of the cells, which limits the observation to a single time point, or genetic modulation, which is less efficient in primary cells and may alter the behavior of the cells. Another tool, NeuronGrowth, is able to analyze live-cell imaging recordings, but also needs user intervention to select the starting point of the axonal structures to be traced [5]. Thus, automated software that allows for axonal tracing over time, based on phase-contrast images – as it is well-established for *in vitro* cell tracking [16] – is highly desirable and will greatly enhance our understanding of axonal function and morphology in health and disease.

Many approaches to automatically segment axons are based on traditional image processing algorithms, including global thresholding, Laplacian or Gaussian filters, and morphological operations [13]. These approaches come with a number of drawbacks: i) They are static and do not react robustly to changes in data collection or the hardware used, ii) most of these procedures are adapted to a particular application scenario and it is unlikely that they generalize well across a wide range of experimental setups and questions, and iii) they are therefore semi-autonomous, i.e., user interaction is required before the data can be collected and automatically evaluated. As axons display morphological variability, the complete segmentation of such an object is a highly demanding task.

In recent years, deep learning has expanded horizons in the field of image processing, ranging from image classification [8] to more intricate tasks such as detection or semantic segmentation with fully convolutional networks (FCNs) [11]. Especially in biomedical image analysis, a very common FCN architecture for segmentation tasks is the u-net [17]. In many cases, the segmentation performance of a network can be further increased using transfer learning [9], i.e., employing deeper architectures such as ResNets [6] that were previously trained on a demanding dataset, e.g., Imagenet [4].

There are few studies that have applied CNNs on axon segmentation in 2D [14,15,18] and 3D [20]. However, to our knowledge, there are no works on 2D phase-contrast microscopy images that enable the automated segmentation of axonal morphology over time.

In this work, we used CNNs to robustly and reliably segment axons on markerfree phase-contrast microscopic images in an automated manner. We employed an ensemble approach to improve the quality of the output and estimated an upper limit for the expected improvement using an oracle-machine. We introduced a soft version of the Dice coefficient that describes the visually perceived quality of axon segmentation better than the standard Dice. Finally, we demonstrate that our best model already reaches the performance level of human experts.

2   Data and Methods

Data. We used microfluidic devices to separate neuronal cell bodies from their axons [2]. We isolated murine primary cortical neurons from embryonic day 14.5 from Crl:CD1 (ICR) Swiss outbred mice (Charles River) as previously described [21] (under the prospective contingent animal license number 2017-07-06_Zille approved by the Schleswig-Holstein Ministry for Energy Transition, Agriculture, Environment, Nature and Digitalization). We seeded the cells to one compartment of the device, which extended their axons through the microgrooves to the other compartment due to the volume difference of the two compartments. We captured grayscale images of the axonal compartment using an Olympus IX2 inverted microscope from which 42 images were manually labeled using GIMP v.2.10.14 (GNU Image Manipulation Program, RRID:SCR_003182). Each image had a size of 1200 × 1000 pixels on average. Figure 1 shows an example of the data.

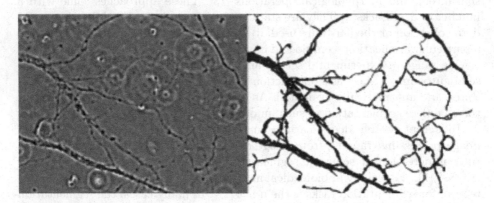

Fig. 1. Original image and binary label image: The left picture shows a pre-processed section of the original data, i.e., microscopic images of axons. The corresponding (manually drawn) binary mask can be seen on the right image, which denotes all pixels that are part of an axon in the left image.

Network Training and Ensembles. We compared two architectures: a standard u-net [17] and a u-net with a ResNet-50 encoder [6]. For each architecture, we trained 8 networks on 10 *splits*. For each split, we separated the dataset into 31 training images and tested on 11 images. Both architectures were trained for

90 epochs with stochastic gradient descent, a momentum of 0.9 and a learning rate of 0.1. Every 30 epochs, we decreased the learning rate by a factor of 10. We used a batch size of 4. For data augmentation, images were cropped randomly with an input size of 512×512 pixels. Different input sizes did not alter the performance and the size of 512 pixels exceeds the receptive field of both networks.

By training 8 networks per split, we generated 8 output maps for each test image. We compared the pixel-wise mean with the pixel-wise maximum and the best single model of each split (*mean-ensemble, max-ensemble, best model*).

Oracle Machine. To investigate the impact of different ensemble strategies, we used an oracle-machine. The max-ensemble achieved a much better recall than the mean-ensemble (0.900 versus 0.799 for ResNet-50). Therefore, we defined a max-mean-oracle for the two critical cases when both, max- and mean-ensemble disagreed in their decision: If the max-ensemble recognized an axon but the mean-ensemble did not (false negatives for the mean-ensemble) and - vice versa - if the max-ensemble was wrong (false positives for the mean-ensemble). As the oracle-machine can perfectly distinguish both cases, we used this oracle to estimate an upper limit on how good the performance would be when combining the information from both ensemble strategies.

ε-Dice Score. We based our evaluation on the standard Dice score. But even if the prediction-label pairs looked reasonable on visual inspection, the Dice score can be low. To test whether areas were just missed or simply not detected at all, we used a soft version of the Dice score, called ε-Dice: If a ground truth pixel was within the proximity of a false positive prediction (i.e., in a neighborhood of ε pixels), we defined this false positive as an over-segmented true positive. Thus, axon predictions that were slightly thicker than the ground truth mask were not counted as errors. False negatives were defined as under-segmented true positives, if there was another true positive in the given neighborhood.

Note that the ε-Dice requires explicit knowledge of the ground truth and thus did **not** improve the accuracy of the segmentation in any way. Rather, we used this measure to estimate how much of the error occurred in the immediate vicinity of the axons or whether there were completely undetected axon segments.

Comparison to Human Performance. To further test our assumption that a perfect Dice score is almost impossible to accomplish on this dataset, we compared it to the human performance level on this task using 7 images labeled by three experts, which we compared to each other and to our best model.

3   Results

The Mean ResNet-50 Ensemble Outperformed the U-Net Ensemble and All Single Networks. To identify the best performing CNN, we compared the mean- and max-ensembles as well as the best single models of each split for both u-net and ResNet-50 (see Table 1). We observed that the ResNet-50 was superior to the u-net with the mean ResNet-50 giving the best results (Dice = 0.827). To estimate the influence of the pixels for which max- and mean-ensemble would vote differently, we defined an oracle-ensemble, which would always make the right decision in these cases. The oracle improved the Dice score for both u-net and ResNet-50 by about 20 %.

Table 1. Dice score for 10 train and test splits with the u-net and ResNet-50. *bestmodel* was the best of the 8 single networks. *max* always used the highest output from the ensemble. *mean* was rated based on the average ensemble rating. With different ratings of *max* and *mean*, *oracle* always made the correct decision. The results are shown for u-net and ResNet-50 using normal Dice score ($\varepsilon = 0$) and a soft Dice ($\varepsilon = 1$).

Method	u-net		ResNet-50 ($\varepsilon = 0$)		ResNet-50 ($\varepsilon = 1$)	
	mean	std	mean	std	mean	std
bestmodel	0.757	0.042	0.815	0.023	0.939	0.018
max	**0.784**	**0.034**	0.805	0.029	0.927	0.028
mean	0.754	0.046	**0.827**	**0.021**	**0.942**	**0.016**
oracle	0.852	0.028	0.887	0.014	0.965	0.011

Segmentation Errors Occurred on the Object Border. Comparing the original mask (ground truth) and the resulting masks from the different approaches, the potential errors occurred at the edges of the object. Upon closer examination, we revealed that the critical pixels were located more or less randomly at the object edges (Fig. 2) and it was hardly ever the case that a whole section of an axon was not segmented (Fig. 3). We did not find any further scheme that was able to distinguish over- or under-segmentation here.

The ε-Dice Described Best the Visually Perceived Quality of Axon Segmentation. To test whether the observed segmentation error can be attributed to cumulative individual errors, we used the ε-Dice score that also includes the surrounding pixels in the evaluation. We observed that the ε-Dice exceeded 90 % for all examined approaches, with the ResNet-50 mean-ensemble achieving the best result with 94 % (Table 1). Also noteworthy is the reduction in the distance between our ensemble approach and the oracle to only 2 %, indicating that many of the critical pixels were located close to uncritical axon structures.

The Recall-Precision Trade-Off Can Be Altered by Linear Classification. We observed that the max-ensemble achieved a better recall than the mean-ensemble (0.900 vs. 0.799). Therefore, we investigated if combining the max-recall with the mean resulted in a better segmentation. When both approaches made the same decision, the performance did not improve. However, two cases are critical (Fig. 4): If the max-ensemble recognized an axon but the mean-ensemble did not (mean false negatives, case a) and - vice versa - if the max-ensemble is

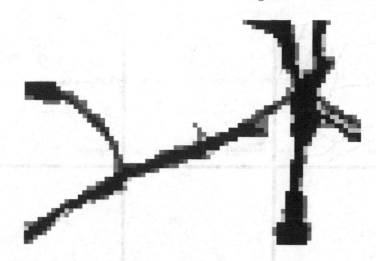

Fig. 2. Comparison of the mean- and max-ensemble and the oracle (best viewed in color). Black pixels show true positives correctly segmented by all approaches. Green and red pixels show false positives and false negatives of all approaches, respectively. The critical pixels that can further improve the result are shown in blue. Here, the max-ensemble yielded a true positive prediction, while the mean-ensemble predicted a false negative. However, the output of the max-ensemble increased the number of false positives (pink pixels). (Color figure online)

wrong (max false positives, case b). The distribution for case a) indicated that for many pixels, the max score was close to 1.0, the mean score was close to 0.5 but did not exceed it. In case b), however, the mean score was rather small (< 0.2) and the max-score was only slightly above 0.5.

Thus, we defined a 2-dimensional linear classifier that re-determined the output of the ensemble for those relevant pixels (Fig. 4). We evaluated the results for three linear classifiers, where each separating line was orthogonal to the manually determined line spanned between $p_0 = (0.05, 0.5)^T$ and $p_1 = (0.5, 1.0)^T$. The three classifiers had the same normal vector $n = (p_1 - p_0)/\|p_1 - p_0\|^2$, but differed in their bias value $b \in \{0.3, 0.5, 0.7\}$. Note that b can be seen as the percentage of the distance between p_0 and p_1. The decision is reached as follows:

$$f(x) = \begin{cases} 1 \ if \ (x - p_0)(n) \geq b \\ 0 \ else \end{cases}. \tag{1}$$

The first two approaches achieved a better recall than the mean-ensemble, but since the precision decreased similarly, the overall Dice-score did not change (Fig. 5). The third approach was almost identical to the mean-ensemble, and again, the quality of the segmentation did not improve.

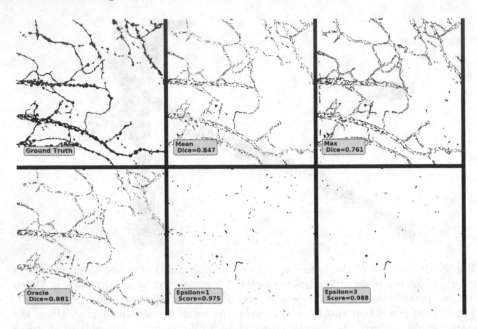

Fig. 3. Ground truth and error images of the different approaches and metrics: In all images except the ground truth image, a black pixel indicates a deviation from the label. The two images on the bottom middle and bottom right show the counted error pixels of the mean-ensemble when the ϵ-Dice score was used. Although, the max-ensemble increased the recall, a strong over-segmentation decreased the precision. The oracle further detected the few axon pixels that were correctly predicted by the max-ensemble but were neglected by the mean-ensemble. The ϵ-Dice images show that the majority of errors was due to over- and under-segmentation and only scarcely, small isolated regions were misclassified.

The Mean ResNet-50 Ensemble Reached Human Expert Performance. Finally, in addition to the expert that labeled the entire data set, we asked two more experts to re-label some of the images used here to examine the variance in their ratings (Table 2). Thus, we had the opinions of three experts for evaluation and the test segmentation results of a ResNet-50 ensemble. These experts among themselves hardly achieved a better result than the mean ResNet-50 ensemble. On the contrary, none of the other experts came as close to the masks of the author of the training data (Expert 02) as the CNN ensemble (Dice = 0.793, 0.766, and 0.833 for 01, 03, and mean ResNet-50 vs. 02). This highlights that our approach can sensitively and specifically segment axons on phase-contrast microscopic images at a level similar to manual labeling by experts and is thus suitable for further application.

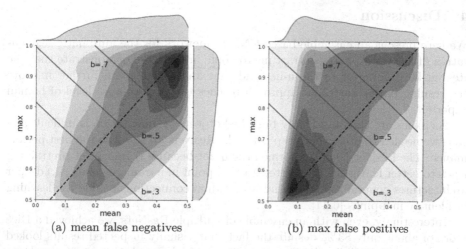

(a) mean false negatives   (b) max false positives

Fig. 4. Distribution of critical pixels on mean- and max-ensembles (darker shades indicating a higher point density). All pixels that were rated differently by the mean- and max-ensemble were considered critical. There were two cases: **(a)** the pixels that the mean-ensemble did not recognize as axons (mean false negatives) and **(b)** those that the max-ensemble incorrectly recognized as axons (max false positive).

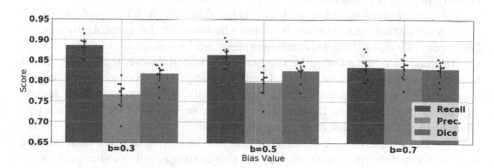

Fig. 5. Scores for different line values. For three different configurations, a linear classifier for the critical points was chosen and decided after its voting. The critical data was mixed and consequently, either recall or precision improved for each of the settings, but without improving the Dice score significantly.

Table 2. Dice score comparison of different human annotators and our best approach (mean ResNet-50). Note that 02 annotated the training data for the network.

Name	01	02	03	mean ResNet-50
01	1.000 ± 0.000	0.793 ± 0.016	0.773 ± 0.035	0.794 ± 0.026
02	0.793 ± 0.016	1.000 ± 0.000	0.766 ± 0.040	0.833 ± 0.033
03	0.773 ± 0.035	0.766 ± 0.040	1.000 ± 0.000	0.750 ± 0.043
mean ResNet-50	0.794 ± 0.026	0.833 ± 0.033	0.75 ± 0.043	1.000 ± 0.000

4   Discussion

We here present an ensemble-based CNN framework for the automatic segmentation of axons on phase-contrast microscopic images. We demonstrate that the ResNet-50 is superior to the u-net and that an ensemble can further improve the results. Importantly, our approach reaches the performance level of human experts.

As axons are thin and highly branched objects, segmentation is difficult and thus we needed to use a very deep network (ResNet-50) to reach the best performance. The ResNet-50 outperformed the u-net because i) ImageNet pretraining leads to better features and a better starting point in parameter space, ii.) deeper architectures generalize better, and iii) residual connections enable the learning of identity mappings [6,11].

Interestingly, even with an ensemble of multiple ResNets, we achieved a Dice score of about only 83 %, despite the fact that visually inspected results looked very convincing. While the Dice score is a widely used measure to evaluate segmentation results, here, the cumulative errors in the very close proximity of the axons induced a strong bias. Therefore, we proposed the soft Dice score and were able to demonstrate that 94 % of the ground truth within a 1-pixel radius were actually recognized by our ensemble, which we think better reflects the visually perceived performance.

We further demonstrated with the help of an oracle what perfect ensemble recombination can achieve. It would theoretically be possible to reach a Dice score of almost 89 % by combining max- and mean-ensemble. However, in practice and as demonstrated by the linear regression model, this seems almost impossible to achieve as we did not identify an approach to combine the knowledge of both ensembles in a usable way. Finally, a comparison with human experts revealed that our ResNet-50 ensemble can very well reach human performance level in the task of axon segmentation.

The dataset used here is relatively small due to the remarkably high labeling cost for these delicate structures, but the size is comparable to similar datasets such as the IOSTAR retina vessel segmentation set [19]. This further strengthens the contribution of our approach as using a network with a performance comparable to an expert can aid in labeling more images.

Taken together, the proposed ensemble CNN allows for the automated axon segmentation at a near-human performance level that makes the high-throughput analysis of the markerfree *in vitro* detection of axonal morphology, growth, and degeneration in health and disease a feasible task.

Acknowledgments. This work was supported by a Fraunhofer MEF grant (Project number 600199) to M.Z.

Contribution of Authors. P.G. developed the deep learning algorithms and performed the computational experiments and analyzed the data. A.P. performed the *in vitro* experiments. A.P., S.K.L., and L.H. labeled the images. P.G., M.Z., and A.M.M. wrote the manuscript. All authors discussed and commented on the final version of the manuscript.

Data Availability. The data and code are available upon reasonable request.

References

1. Acciai, L., Soda, P., Iannello, G.: Automated neuron tracing methods: an updated account. Neuroinformatics **14**(4), 353–367 (2016)
2. Darbinyan, A., Pozniak, P., Darbinian, N., White, M.K., Khalili, K.: Compartmentalized Neuronal Cultures, pp. 147–152. Humana Press, Totowa (2013)
3. Debanne, D., Campanac, E., Bialowas, A., Carlier, E., Alcaraz, G.: Axon physiology. Physiol. Rev. **91**(2), 555–602 (2011)
4. Deng, J., Dong, W., Socher, R., Li, L.J., Li, K., Fei-Fei, L.: ImageNet: a large-scale hierarchical image database. In: 2009 IEEE Conference on Computer Vision and Pattern Recognition, pp. 248–255. IEEE (2009)
5. Fanti, Z., Elena Martinez-Perez, M., De-Miguel, F.F.: Neurongrowth, a software for automatic quantification of neurite and filopodial dynamics from time-lapse sequences of digital images. Dev. Neurobiol. **71**(10), 870–881 (2011)
6. He, K., Zhang, X., Ren, S., Sun, J.: Deep residual learning for image recognition. In: Proceedings of the IEEE Conference on Computer Vision and Pattern Recognition, pp. 770–778 (2016)
7. Ho, S.Y., Chao, C.Y., Huang, H.L., Chiu, T.W., Charoenkwan, P., Hwang, E.: NeurphologyJ: an automatic neuronal morphology quantification method and its application in pharmacological discovery. BMC Bioinformatics **12**(1), 230 (2011)
8. Krizhevsky, A., Sutskever, I., Hinton, G.E.: ImageNet classification with deep convolutional neural networks. In: Pereira, F., Burges, C.J.C., Bottou, L., Weinberger, K.Q. (eds.) Advances in Neural Information Processing Systems, vol. 25, pp. 1097–1105. Curran Associates, Inc. (2012). http://papers.nips.cc/paper/4824-imagenet-classification-with-deep-convolutional-neural-networks.pdf
9. Lin, G., Milan, A., Shen, C., Reid, I.: RefineNet: multi-path refinement networks for high-resolution semantic segmentation. In: Proceedings of the IEEE Conference on Computer Vision and Pattern Recognition, pp. 1925–1934 (2017)
10. Lingor, P., Koch, J.C., Tönges, L., Bähr, M.: Axonal degeneration as a therapeutic target in the CNS. Cell Tissue Res. **349**(1), 289–311 (2012)
11. Long, J., Shelhamer, E., Darrell, T.: Fully convolutional networks for semantic segmentation. In: The IEEE Conference on Computer Vision and Pattern Recognition (CVPR), June 2015
12. Meijering, E.: Neuron tracing in perspective. Cytometry Part A **77**(7), 693–704 (2010)
13. Meijering, E.: Cell segmentation: 50 years down the road [life sciences]. IEEE Signal Process. Mag. **29**(5), 140–145 (2012)
14. Mesbah, R., McCane, B., Mills, S.: Deep convolutional encoder-decoder for myelin and axon segmentation. In: 2016 International Conference on Image and Vision Computing New Zealand (IVCNZ), pp. 1–6. IEEE (2016)
15. Naito, T., Nagashima, Y., Taira, K., Uchio, N., Tsuji, S., Shimizu, J.: Identification and segmentation of myelinated nerve fibers in a cross-sectional optical microscopic image using a deep learning model. J. Neurosci. Methods **291**, 141–149 (2017)
16. Rapoport, D.H., Becker, T., Madany Mamlouk, A., Schicktanz, S., Kruse, C.: A novel validation algorithm allows for automated cell tracking and the extraction of biologically meaningful parameters. PLoS ONE **6**(11), e27315 (2011)

17. Ronneberger, O., Fischer, P., Brox, T.: U-Net: convolutional networks for biomedical image segmentation. In: Navab, N., Hornegger, J., Wells, W.M., Frangi, A.F. (eds.) MICCAI 2015. LNCS, vol. 9351, pp. 234–241. Springer, Cham (2015). https://doi.org/10.1007/978-3-319-24574-4_28

18. Zaimi, A., Wabartha, M., Herman, V., Antonsanti, P.L., Perone, C.S., Cohen-Adad, J.: AxonDeepSeg: automatic axon and myelin segmentation from microscopy data using convolutional neural networks. Sci. Rep. **8**(1), 1–11 (2018)

19. Zhang, J., Dashtbozorg, B., Bekkers, E., Pluim, J.P.W., Duits, R., ter Haar Romeny, B.M.: Robust retinal vessel segmentation via locally adaptive derivative frames in orientation scores. IEEE Trans. Med. Imaging **35**(12), 2631–2644 (2016)

20. Zhou, Z., Kuo, H.C., Peng, H., Long, F.: DeepNeuron: an open deep learning toolbox for neuron tracing. Brain Inform. **5**(2), 1–9 (2018)

21. Zille, M., et al.: Ferroptosis in neurons and cancer cells is similar but differentially regulated by histone deacetylase inhibitors. eNeuro **6**(1), ENEURO.0263-18.2019 (2019). https://doi.org/10.1523/ENEURO.0263-18.2019

Using Bayesian Optimization to Effectively Tune Random Forest and XGBoost Hyperparameters for Early Alzheimer's Disease Diagnosis

Louise Bloch[1,2](✉) and Christoph M. Friedrich[1,2]

[1] Department of Computer Science, University of Applied Sciences and Arts
Dortmund, Emil-Figge-Str. 42, 44227 Dortmund, Germany
{louise.bloch,christoph.friedrich}@fh-dortmund.de
[2] Institute for Medical Informatics, Biometry and Epidemiology (IMIBE),
University Hospital Essen, Essen, Germany

Abstract. Many research articles used Machine Learning (ML) for early
detection of Alzheimer's Disease (AD) especially based on Magnetic Resonance Imaging (MRI). Most ML algorithms depend on a large number of hyperparameters. Those hyperparameters have a strong influence
on the model performance and thus choosing good hyperparameters is
important in ML. In this article, Bayesian Optimization (BO) was used
to time-efficiently find good hyperparameters for Random Forest (RF)
and eXtreme Gradient Boosting (XGBoost) models, which are based on
four and seven hyperparameters and promise good classification results.
Those models are applied to distinguish if mild cognitive impaired (MCI)
subjects from the Alzheimer's disease neuroimaging initiative (ADNI)
dataset will prospectively convert to AD. The results showed comparable cross-validation (CV) classification accuracies for models trained
using BO and grid-search, whereas BO has been less time-consuming.
The initial combinations for BO were set using Latin Hypercube Design
(LHD) and via Random Initialization (RI). Furthermore, many models
trained using BO achieved better classification results for the independent test dataset than the model based on the grid-search. The best
model achieved an accuracy of 73.43% for the independent test dataset.
This model was an XGBoost model trained with BO and RI.

Keywords: Bayesian optimization · Computer-aided diagnosis · Early
Alzheimer's Disease diagnosis · eXtreme Gradient Boosting · Random
Forests

1 Introduction

Alzheimer's Disease (AD) is a neurodegenerative disease [2] and the most frequent cause of dementia. The early identification of subjects at risk to develop
AD is important to recruit and monitor subjects for therapy studies, as there currently is no causal therapy [2]. Subjects with Mild Cognitive Impairment (MCI)

© ICST Institute for Computer Sciences, Social Informatics and Telecommunications Engineering 2021
Published by Springer Nature Switzerland AG 2021. All Rights Reserved
J. Ye et al. (Eds.): MobiHealth 2020, LNICST 362, pp. 285–299, 2021.
https://doi.org/10.1007/978-3-030-70569-5_18

have a higher risk to develop AD [8] than cognitively normal (CN) controls. Thus, the prediction of future conversion to AD is important for MCI subjects. There have been many articles that used Machine Learning (ML) to improve the identification of those subjects. Most of them use models with a large number of hyperparameters.

Finding good hyperparameters is one of the key problems in ML. Hyperparameter tuning can improve model performance and prevent overfitting. For real-world problems, like the prediction of AD, good hyperparameters often depend on the data [34, p. 305]. Thus, parameter tuning is a complex and time-consuming task. One possibility to find good hyperparameters are optimization methods, which have the advantage to time-efficiently find robust parameters.

1.1 Prior Work

Many articles used ML models with a large number of hyperparameters to predict different AD stages. Some approaches used the default hyperparameters [4, 20] to reduce the complexity of this problem. However, neither good performance nor high generalizability can be guaranteed. Other articles used grid-search [5, 19, 27], which is time-consuming for models with many hyperparameters. Some articles had no documentation about the hyperparameters at all. Only a few approaches used methods for time-efficient and stable hyperparameter optimization. In [18], Bayesian Optimization (BO) with Random Initialization (RI) was used to predict MCI conversion within three years. The hyperparameters of different ML models like Support Vector Machines (SVMs) [12] and Random Forests (RFs) [6] were tuned for 353 subjects with stable MCI (sMCI) and 193 with progressive MCI (pMCI) from the Alzheimer's Disease Neuroimaging Initiative (ADNI) [29] cohort. The feature set included sociodemographic and clinical characteristics, neuropsychological tests, and the baseline (BL) MCI type. The final ensemble model achieved an Area Under the Receiver Operating Characteristic (AUROC) of 0.88.

BO with RI has been also used in [28] to optimize the hyperparameters of a Deep Neural Network (DNN). Two datasets, which are available online (https:// github.com/ChihyunPark/DNN_for_ADprediction. Last accessed 8 Aug 2020), were used. The first one included large-scale gene expressions from 257 CN and 439 AD subjects and the second one contained Deoxyribonucleic Acid (DNA) methylation data of 68 CN and 74 AD subjects. The final model achieved an accuracy of 82.3% for the test dataset.

[32] used BO with RI to tune the parameters of a radial-basis SVM and classifies 17 subjects with Subjective Cognitive Impairment (SCI) vs. 53 MCI vs. 50 AD. The dataset was not publicly available. The feature set included neuropsychological tests and the results of a reaction test. Accuracies of 80.6% and 65.0% were reached for MCI vs. AD and SCI vs. MCI vs. AD classification.

This article aims to efficiently tune the parameters of RFs and eXtreme Gradient Boosting (XGBoost) models for early AD diagnosis. In addition to the previous articles, a Latin Hypercube Design (LHD) [25] was used to initialize the BO. The results of this method were compared to a RI, a grid-search and

Table 1. ADNI demographics at BL. p-values are calculated using Mann-Whitney-U-test for continuous variables and χ^2-test for frequency variables.

	sMCI	pMCI	Σ	p-value
n	401	319	720	
Age in years (mean ± sd)	73.2 ± 7.5	74.0 ± 7.1	73.5 ± 7.3	0.1156
Gender (proportion of males)	59.6%	59.9%	59.7%	1.000
MMSE (mean ± sd)	27.8 ± 1.8	27.0 ± 1.7	27.4 ± 1.8	<0.0001
CDR (mean ± sd)	0.5 ± 0.0	0.5 ± 0.0	0.5 ± 0.0	0.2634
ApoEε4 (count of ApoEε4 alleles): 0	56.9%	34.2%	46.8%	<0.0001
ApoEε4: 1	33.9%	49.5%	40.8%	
ApoEε4: 2	9.2%	16.3%	12.4%	
Time to final diagnosis in months (mean ± sd)	47.1 ± 32.4	30.6 ± 24.7	39.8 ± 30.4	<0.0001

the default parameters. Section 2 presents the dataset and methods. The ML workflow is described in Sect. 3. The experimental results are demonstrated in Section 4 and finally discussed in Sect. 5.

2 Materials and Methods

2.1 Dataset

Data used in the preparation of this article were obtained from the ADNI [29] cohort. 720 subjects of the study phases ADNI-1 (354 subjects), ADNIGO (92 subjects) and ADNI-2 (274 subjects) were selected. All subjects had a BL diagnosis of MCI and were classified as sMCI if all subsequent diagnoses correspond to MCI and as pMCI if they converted to AD at any visit and AD was the diagnosis for all subsequent visits. Subjects who reverted to CN or MCI were excluded from this study. The demographic data are summarized in Table 1. The time between the BL and the final diagnosis ranged between 4.7 and 156.2 months.

For each subject, one fully preprocessed [21] BL 1.5 T or 3 T T1-weighted Magnetization-Prepared Rapid Gradient-Echo (MP-RAGE) Magnetic Resonance Imaging (MRI) scan was selected. FreeSurfer v6.0 [15] extracted volumes of 34 cortical Regions of Interest (ROIs) per hemisphere, defined in Desikan-Killiany atlas [13], 34 subcortical ROIs [16], and the estimated Total Intracranial Volume (eTIV). The resulting 103 MRI features were normalized by eTIV [33].

Two different datasets were used for model training. *Dataset 1* included 106 features - MRI-features, age, gender and count of Apolipoprotein E ε4 (ApoEε4) alleles. *Dataset 2* added Mini-Mental State Examination (MMSE), a logical long-term (LDEL) and short-term memory test (LIMM) resulting in 109 features. Clinical Dementia Rating (CDR) was excluded due to small variance.

2.2   eXtreme Gradient Boosting

Boosting algorithms assume that the iterative combination of multiple weak classifiers leads to a strong classifier. Gradient boosting [17] meets this assumption by training the first classifier to learn the independent variable and the subsequent classifiers to learn the gradients of the previous classifiers. The gradients $l(y_i, \hat{y}_i^{(t-1)})$ are defined as the deviation between the additive classification $\hat{y}_i^{(t-1)}$ of the previous iteration $(t-1)$ and the correct classification y_i of observation i. The loss function $L^{(t)}$ at iteration t using n observations corresponds to Eq. 1. Here, f_t represents the weak classifier at iteration t and $\Omega(f_t)$ is a regularization term which controls the complexity of the classifier.

$$L^{(t)} = \sum_{i=1}^{n} l\big(y_i, \hat{y}_i^{(t-1)} + f_t(x_i)\big) + \Omega(f_t) \tag{1}$$

The additive combination of all weak classifiers f_k determines the final classification $\hat{y}_i$ for observation i, as can be seen in Eq. 2.

$$\hat{y}_i = \sum_{k=1}^{K} f_k(x_i) \tag{2}$$

eXtreme Gradient Boosting (XGBoost) [10] is an open-source software library and an implementation of gradient boosting with a high focus on scalability, parallelization and distributed execution. XGBoost with Classification and regression trees (CARTs) [7] as weak classifier depends on seven hyperparameters, summarized in Table 2. *nrounds* (*n*) determines the number of iterations in the training process. The learning rate *eta* (*η*) controls the influence of each weak classifier on the final model and thus prevents overfitting. The hyperparameter *gamma* (*γ*) determines the minimum loss reduction required to specialize leaf nodes. High values lead to preserving models. *max_depth* (*d_{max}*) specifies the maximum depth of a tree. Deep models are more complex and prone to overfitting. The parameter *min_child_weights* (*w_{min}*) sets the minimum number of weighted observations in a child node. High values for *min_child_weights* achieve more conservative models. *subsample* (*s*) sets the ratio of training instances randomly selected in each iteration. Small values prevent overfitting. *colsample_bytree* (*c*) is the ratio of randomly subsampled features in each iteration. Small values lead to robust models, but values near zero lead to poor results.

2.3   Random Forest

Random Forests (RFs) [6] are based on multiple CARTs and the majority voting is used to robustly predict an unknown observation. Table 3 summarizes the hyperparameters for the RF. n_{tree} sets the number of trees in the RF. Training only a few trees often leads to less accurate results. For each tree, a bootstrap sample [14] of the dataset is generated and for each split, a subset of *mtry* (*m_{try}*) features are randomly chosen to train the models. The higher *mtry*, the higher

Table 2. XGBoost parameters and intervals. The grid is a grid-search of length five.

Name	Minimum	Maximum	Grid
nrounds (n)	1	500	$\{1.00,\ 125.00,\ 250.00,\ 375.00,\ 500.00\}$
eta (η)	0	1	$\{0.00,\ 0.25,\ 0.50,\ 0.75,\ 1.00\}$
gamma (γ)	0	20	$\{0.00,\ 5.00,\ 10.00,\ 15.00,\ 20.00\}$
max_depth (d_{max})	1	20	$\{1.00,\ 5.00,\ 10.00,\ 15.00,\ 20.00\}$
min_child_weights (w_{min})	1	30	$\{1.00,\ 8.25,\ 15.50,\ 22.75,\ 30.00\}$
subsample (s)	0	1	$\{0.00,\ 0.25,\ 0.50,\ 0.75,\ 1.00\}$
colsample_bytree (c)	0	1	$\{0.00,\ 0.25,\ 0.50,\ 0.75,\ 1.00\}$

Table 3. RF parameters and intervals. The grid refers to a grid-search of length five.

Name	Minimum	Maximum	Grid
mtry (for *dataset 1*) (m_{try})	2	109	$\{2,\ 28,\ 55,\ 82,\ 109\}$
mtry (for *dataset 2*) (m_{try})	2	112	$\{2,\ 29,\ 57,\ 84,\ 112\}$
ntree (n_{tree})	250	1250	$\{250,\ 500,\ 750,\ 1000,\ 1250\}$
nodesize (s_{min})	1	20	$\{1,\ 5,\ 10,\ 15,\ 20\}$
maxnodes (nd_{max})	50	100	$\{50,\ 62,\ 75,\ 87,\ 100\}$

is the risk of overfitting. *nodesize* (s_{min}) sets the minimum size of terminal nodes for each tree. The smaller *nodesize*, the less robust the trained models are. Hyperparameter *maxnodes* (nd_{max}) specifies the maximum number of terminal nodes for each tree. Trees with many terminal nodes tend to overfit the dataset.

2.4 Latin Hypercube Design

Latin hypercube design (LHD) [25] is a method to generate a nearly random sample based on a multi-dimensional distribution. The objective is to select p samples from a q-dimensional space. To generate an LHD each dimension is split into p equidistant intervals. One value is randomly selected per interval, resulting in p parameters for each dimension. The parameters of the individual dimensions are randomly merged to p samples with q dimensions. LHD ensures complete coverage of the range for each variable.

2.5 Bayesian Optimization

Bayesian Optimization (BO) [26] is a global optimization method for black-box functions. In this research, hyperparameter tuning has been considered as the optimization of a black-box function. The model performance was maximized dependently on the hyperparameters. First, a set of initial parameter combinations were arranged. In this article, LHD and RI were used for this purpose. The models were evaluated for each combination to estimate their performance. A Gaussian Process (GP) was fitted to model the relationship between parameter combinations and model performances. This GP was optimized to find the next promising parameter combination. The optimization considered exploration and exploitation using an acquisition function, which depends on the expected model performance $\hat{\mu}_\Theta$ and the covariance $\hat{\Sigma}_\Theta$ at parameter combination Θ. The covariance $\hat{\Sigma}_\Theta$ was smaller the closer previously examined parameter combinations were. In this work, the upper confidence bounds (UCB) [1,22], given in Eq. 3, was used as the acquisition function. The parameter κ determines, the proportion between exploitation and exploration. For higher values of κ, exploration is preferred, whereas lower values favour exploitation.

$$UCB(\Theta) = \hat{\mu}_\Theta + \kappa \cdot \hat{\Sigma}_\Theta \tag{3}$$

The performance of the ML model was evaluated using the new parameter combination and added to the GP model. This process was repeated until previously determined criteria, e.g. a maximum number of iterations, were met.

3   Machine Learning Workflow

In this article, an ML workflow was implemented, using the programming language R v3.5.3 [30], to distinguish sMCI and pMCI subjects. Figure 1 gives an overview of the workflow. Subject selection and image processing are described in Sect. 2.1. The subjects of each diagnosis group were randomly split into a training and an independent test dataset. The test dataset contained 20% of the original dataset and the remaining 80% were used to train the model and tune the hyperparameters. LHD, implemented using the R package SPOT v2.0.3 [3], and RI were used to generate ten initial parameter combinations for the BO. After training the initial BO model, promising parameter combinations were successively determined and evaluated. 25 parameter combinations were generated by BO to tune the hyperparameters of RF and XGBoost models. BO, XGBoost and RF were implemented using the R packages rBayesianOptimization v1.1.0 [35], xgboost v0.82.1 [11] and randomForest v4.6-14 [24]. 10 × 10-fold Cross-Validation (CV) [31] was used as a resampling strategy and was implemented using the R package caret v6.0-82 [23], by splitting the training dataset into ten distinct folds. Ten iterations were performed with a different fold used as validation dataset in each iteration and the remaining nine folds were used to train the model. This procedure was repeated ten times, whereas the data was shuffled and stratified in each repetition. CV-accuracy was used as the metric for BO. The best parameters were selected to train the final model. The preprocessing, nested in the tuning workflow, included centering, scaling and median imputation. Synthetic Minority Over-sampling Technique (SMOTE) [9] compensated class imbalances during the parameter tuning. The final model was evaluated for the independent test dataset.

As a comparison, a grid-search was implemented using the R package caret v6.0-82 [23]. The grid contained the cartesian product with five values per parameter, which results in $5^7 = 78125$ XGBoost and $5^4 = 525$ RF combinations.

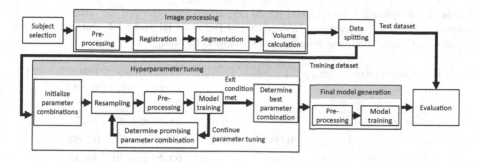

Fig. 1. Machine learning workflow.

4 Results

In the experiments, BO has been applied to optimize four hyperparameters of an RF classifier (Sect. 4.1) and seven hyperparameters of an XGBoost model (Sect. 4.2). This optimization has been demonstrated on two previously described AD datasets. *Dataset 1* included volumetric MRI features, demographics, and ApoEϵ4, and *dataset 2* added cognitive test results to *dataset 1*.

The experiments, that used BO, included ten initial parameter combinations and 25 combinations during optimization, resulting in 35 evaluations. The grid-search models used five values per hyperparameter m, resulting in 5^m and thus $5^4 = 625$ RF and $5^7 - 78125$ XGBoost grid combinations. Thus, the number of grid-search evaluations increased exponentially with the number of hyperparameters, while the number of evaluations was constant for BO. BO was applied using five different values for the parameter κ ($\kappa \in \{0.5, 1.0, 2.0, 5.0, 10.0\}$).

4.1 Bayesian Optimization for Random Forest Classifiers

Dataset 1. Table 4 summarizes the RF results for the different hyperparameter tuning methods on *dataset 1*. The best CV-results were 69.76% and achieved using BO with RI and $\kappa = 2.0$. The grid-search model performed 0.30% worse than the best model. The default parameter model reached the worst accuracy of 68.20%. The LHD BO models obtained CV-accuracies between those values. BO with RI outperformed the LHD initialization for this dataset and CV-results.

The best accuracy for the independent test dataset was 67.83%, achieved by the grid-search and the BO model with LHD initialization and $\kappa = 2.0$. All LHD BO models except the model with $\kappa = 2.0$ selected the same hyperparameters and thus obtained equal results. The worst accuracy for the independent test set was 62.94%, reached by the BO model with RI and $\kappa = 5.0$. The performances for the independent test dataset differed by 4.89% between the tuning methods.

The boxplots in Fig. 2 show the relations between grid-search parameters and the mean CV-accuracies. The best performances for the hyperparameter *mtry* were obtained for a value of 28. Consistently, all BO models selected *mtry* values between 25 and 35. Increasing values of *ntree* led to better model performances.

Table 4. Classification results and RF hyperparameters achieved for *dataset 1*. Comparison of default parameters, grid-search and BO with RI and LHD initialization for parameter tuning. The best results are highlighted in bold.

Hyperparameter optimization	m_{try}	n_{tree}	s_{min}	nd_{max}	CV-accuracy (mean ± sd) in %	Test accuracy in %
Default parameters	10	500	1	max	68.20 ± 6.47	65.73
Grid-search	28	1000	15	50	69.46 ± 6.53	**67.83**
BO RI $\kappa = 0.5$	25	1107	8	50	69.26 ± 6.30	66.43
BO RI $\kappa = 1.0$	30	615	8	50	69.28 ± 6.34	67.13
BO RI $\kappa = 2.0$	35	464	1	56	**69.76 ± 6.35**	65.73
BO RI $\kappa = 5.0$	30	1216	1	50	69.28 ± 6.54	62.94
BO RI $\kappa = 10.0$	33	647	3	81	69.10 ± 6.48	67.13
BO LHD $\kappa \in \{0.5, 1.0, 5.0, 10.0\}$	27	808	16	96	68.79 ± 5.99	65.73
BO LHD $\kappa = 2.0$	29	1250	3	68	68.96 ± 6.16	**67.83**

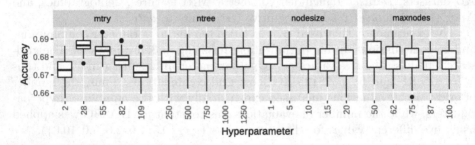

Fig. 2. Boxplots summarizing the mean CV-accuracies for RF grid-search hyperparameters and *dataset 1*.

A slight decrease was detected on the mean CV-accuracy for increasing values of *nodesize*. The hyperparameter *maxnodes* obtained better results for a value of 50 and the performance decreased for higher values. The observations were mainly reflected in the BO model with LHD initialization and $\kappa = 2.0$ and all RI models except for $\kappa = 10.0$. The other models selected deviating parameters.

Dataset 2. *Dataset 2* supplemented cognitive test results to *dataset 1*. However, the experiments executed on the datasets do not differ and the results are summarized in Table 5. CV-results of the RF models trained on *dataset 2* were between 70.01%, achieved by the default parameter model and 70.68% and thus differ by 0.67%. The BO model with LHD initialization and $\kappa = 2.0$ obtained the best results. The CV-results on *dataset 2* outperformed the results for *dataset 1*. The grid-search model reached a CV-accuracy of 70.61%.

The results for the independent test dataset were similar to the CV-results. The worst result of 67.13% for the independent test dataset was achieved for

Table 5. Classification results and RF hyperparameters achieved for *dataset 2*. Comparison of default parameters, grid-search and BO with RI and LHD initialization for parameter tuning. The best results are highlighted in bold.

Hyperparameter optimization	m_{try}	n_{tree}	s_{min}	nd_{max}	CV-accuracy (mean ± sd) in %	Test accuracy in %
Default parameters	10	500	1	max	70.01 ± 6.41	69.23
Grid-search	29	1000	10	100	70.61 ± 6.53	69.93
BO RI $\kappa = 0.5$	11	959	9	60	70.52 ± 5.93	69.23
BO RI $\kappa = 1.0$	21	1250	16	72	70.61 ± 5.78	70.63
BO RI $\kappa = 2.0$	13	756	5	74	70.42 ± 6.10	69.23
BO RI $\kappa = 5.0$	18	1250	1	95	70.42 ± 5.91	69.23
BO RI $\kappa = 10.0$	39	1250	1	100	70.19 ± 6.13	**71.33**
BO LHD $\kappa = 0.5$	13	1250	16	92	70.48 ± 5.92	69.23
BO LHD $\kappa = 1.0$	16	757	20	62	70.23 ± 5.80	68.53
BO LHD $\kappa = 2.0$	20	1250	11	85	**70.68 ± 6.01**	67.13
BO LHD $\kappa = 5.0$	16	808	16	96	70.21 ± 6.32	67.83
BO LHD $\kappa = 10.0$	23	1250	1	82	70.49 ± 6.02	**71.33**

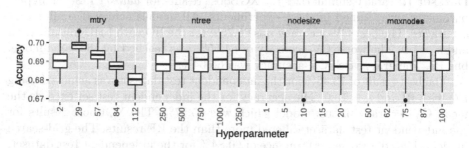

Fig. 3. Boxplots summarizing the mean CV-accuracies for RF grid-search hyperparameters and *dataset 2*.

the BO model with LHD initialization and $\kappa = 2.0$. This model achieved the best CV-results. The best accuracy for the independent test dataset of 71.33% has been reached for the BO models with $\kappa = 10.0$ and both LHD and RI. The grid-search model reached an accuracy of 69.93%.

The boxplots in Fig. 3 illustrate the mean CV-accuracies depending on the grid-search hyperparameters. The hyperparameters *mtry* and *ntree* showed similar relations as those observed for *dataset 1*. All BOs, except the model with RI and $\kappa = 10.0$, selected values between 11 and 23 for the *mtry* parameter. BO preferred high values for *ntree*. *nodesize* showed slightly worse results for a value of 20 in the boxplots, however, BO with LHD initialization and $\kappa = 1.0$ selected this value. *maxnodes* showed slightly increasing results for higher values. All BO models selected values higher than 62.

Table 6. Classification results and XGBoost hyperparameters for *dataset 1*. Using default parameters, grid-search and BO with RI and LHD initialization for parameter tuning. CV-accuracies are given as mean ± sd. The best results are highlighted in bold.

Hyperparameter optimization	n	d_{max}	η	γ	c	w_{min}	s	CV-accuracy in %	Test accuracy in %
Default parameters	100	6	0.300	0.000	1.000	1.000	1.000	65.29 ± 6.81	68.53
Grid-search	250	20	0.250	10.000	0.750	1.000	1.000	66.64 ± 6.46	60.84
BO RI $\kappa = 0.5$	490	7	0.020	10.263	0.190	2.580	0.924	66.26 ± 5.56	64.34
BO RI $\kappa = 1.0$	484	16	0.186	7.477	0.071	2.847	0.363	64.55 ± 5.67	62.24
BO RI $\kappa = 2.0$	483	14	0.095	19.642	0.283	17.813	0.200	66.44 ± 5.68	65.03
BO RI $\kappa = 5.0$	110	20	0.163	1.526	0.525	1.000	0.612	66.09 ± 5.69	71.33
BO RI $\kappa = 10.0$	500	20	0.200	0.000	0.439	1.000	0.935	65.57 ± 5.60	**73.43**
BO LHD $\kappa = 0.5$	149	6	0.010	11.364	0.781	8.062	0.817	66.59 ± 5.24	60.84
BO LHD $\kappa = 1.0$	452	2	0.085	20.000	1.000	1.000	1.000	**66.75 ± 4.97**	63.64
BO LHD $\kappa = 2.0$	426	1	0.120	0.371	0.349	17.080	0.746	65.14 ± 5.80	67.83
BO LHD $\kappa = 5.0$	50	1	0.171	20.000	0.994	19.490	0.654	66.54 ± 5.05	60.14
BO LHD $\kappa = 10.0$	193	1	0.045	0.000	1.000	29.822	1.000	66.66 ± 5.38	64.34

4.2 Bayesian Optimization for XGBoost Classifiers

Dataset 1. Table 6 summarizes the XGBoost results for *dataset 1*. Seven hyperparameters were tuned in these experiments. All models achieved similar CV-accuracies. The best CV-accuracy was 66.75% for the BO with LHD initialization and $\kappa = 1.0$. The worst CV-accuracy of 64.55% was reached by the same model but RI. The grid-search CV-accuracy was 66.64%.

The best result of 73.43% for the independent test dataset was achieved using BO with RI and $\kappa = 10.0$. The accuracy for the independent test set exceeds the mean CV-accuracy of this model which was 65.57%. The XGBoost results for the independent test dataset differed more than the RF results. The grid-search model achieved a worse performance of 60.84% for the independent test dataset. The BO model with $\kappa = 5.0$ reached the worst accuracy of 60.14%.

The boxplots in Fig. 4 summarize the relations between the grid-search hyperparameters and the mean CV-accuracies. All 28125 observations with a value of 0.00 for *eta* or *subsample* were excluded because a learning rate of 0.00 means that there is no learning effect and a subsampling of 0.00% led to a model training without any subjects. All excluded results achieved mean CV-accuracies less than 45.00%, which would distort the interpretability of the figure. All boxplots had a large number of outliers below the box. Small values for *eta* were associated with better results. Consistently, all BO models selected values between 0.010 and 0.200. The minimum value of 0.000 for hyperparameters *gamma* and *colsample_bytree* and 1 for *nrounds*, showed stronger variations in the results than the remaining values. Using only one boosting iteration led to worse results. Small differences were detected between using 125 and 500 boosting iterations. The BO selected values between 50 and 500 for this parameter.

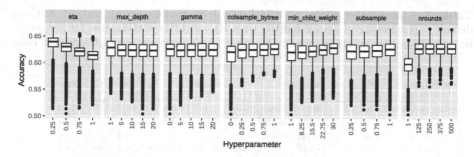

Fig. 4. Boxplots summarizing the mean CV-accuracies for XGBoost grid-search hyperparameters and *dataset 1*. All combinations with *eta* or *subsample* = 0.00 were excluded.

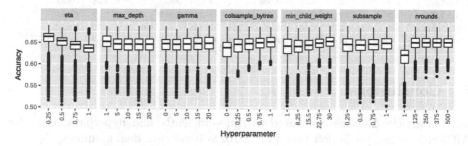

Fig. 5. Boxplots summarizing the mean CV-accuracies for XGBoost grid-search hyperparameters and *dataset 2*. All combinations with *eta* or *subsample*=0.00 were excluded.

Dataset 2. Table 7 shows the results achieved by training an XGBoost model with *dataset 2*. The achieved CV-accuracies exceed the results of *dataset 1*. The best CV-accuracy was 69.14% ± 5.48%, reached by the BO model with RI and $\kappa = 1.0$. The grid-search model achieved a CV-accuracy of 68.95% ± 6.25% and the default parameter model a CV-accuracy of 68.08% ± 6.61%.

The results for the independent test dataset were between 65.03%, for the BO with RI and $\kappa = 2.0$ and 71.33%, for the default parameter model and the BO model with LHD initialiation and $\kappa = 5.0$. The grid-search model achieved an accuracy of 69.93% for the independent test dataset.

The boxplots in Fig. 5 show the effects of the grid-search hyperparameters on the mean CV-results. Consistently with Fig. 4, all examinations with an *eta* or *subsample* value of 0.00 were excluded, as they represent random models. For the parameter *eta*, small values performed better than large ones. This observation is consistent with the BO parameter selection. The hyperparameters *gamma*, *colsample_bytree* and *min_child_weight* showed slightly better results the higher the parameter values. BO showed no clear focus for these parameters. However, all BO models with RI, except the model with $\kappa = 5.0$ selected values higher than 0.929 for *colsample_bytree*. The BO and the boxplots show, that using only one boosting iteration has a negative effect on the mean CV-accuracy.

Table 7. Classification results and XGBoost hyperparameters for *dataset 2*. Using default parameters, grid-search and BO with RI and LHD initialization for parameter tuning. CV-accuracies are given as mean ± sd. The best results are highlighted in bold.

Hyperparameter optimization	n	d_{max}	η	γ	c	w_{min}	s	CV-accuracy in %	Test accuracy in %
Default parameters	100	6	0.300	0.000	1.000	1.000	1.000	68.08 ± 6.61	**71.33**
Grid-search	250	20	0.250	20.000	0.250	30.000	0.250	68.95 ± 6.25	69.93
BO RI $\kappa = 0.5$	127	8	0.143	20.000	1.000	20.442	0.326	68.30 ± 5.42	67.83
BO RI $\kappa = 1.0$	359	14	0.146	3.037	1.000	30.000	0.174	**69.14 ± 5.48**	69.93
BO RI $\kappa = 2.0$	481	10	0.102	14.519	0.961	13.497	0.321	68.68 ± 5.53	65.03
BO RI $\kappa = 5.0$	418	3	0.134	14.849	0.280	23.008	0.316	68.20 ± 5.12	69.23
BO RI $\kappa = 10.0$	452	20	0.138	19.556	0.929	25.000	0.834	67.63 ± 5.55	65.73
BO LHD $\kappa = 0.5$	357	11	0.077	12.699	0.298	28.618	0.480	68.14 ± 5.32	70.63
BO LHD $\kappa = 1.0$	323	4	0.026	0.000	0.372	8.693	0.847	68.08 ± 6.04	69.23
BO LHD $\kappa = 2.0$	259	19	0.088	9.922	0.696	19.255	0.595	68.21 ± 5.92	67.83
BO LHD $\kappa = 5.0$	447	5	0.104	6.379	0.718	1.938	0.441	67.56 ± 5.95	**71.33**
BO LHD $\kappa = 10.0$	300	14	0.002	7.291	0.475	10.290	0.683	68.18 ± 6.03	66.43

5   Conclusions

In this article, BO has been used to time-efficiently find hyperparameters for MCI-conversion prediction based on MRI volumetrics, demographics, ApoEϵ4 features and cognitive test results. As a comparison, a time-consuming grid-search has been implemented. The XGBoost and RF models were evaluated using 10×10-fold-CV, a robust resampling method, and an additional evaluation for an independent test dataset. The outcomes showed that BO was able to find parameters which can keep up with the time-efficient grid-search and is thus most interesting for models with many hyperparameters. Some tendencies for good hyperparameter choices which were detected considering the grid-search models can be also recognized for the BO parameter selection. Thus, BO offered a trade-off between the time-efficiency and robust, reproducible models.

The approach was applied for two different AD datasets of the ADNI cohort. *Dataset 1* included MRI volumetric, demographic and ApoEϵ4 features and *dataset 2* additionally included BL cognitive test results. The results of the RF models showed better accuracies for models trained on *dataset 2*. The best result for the independent test dataset was achieved for *dataset 1* and an XGBoost model. The outcomes showed promising results for the models trained using BO for hyperparameter optimization. For both datasets and both ML techniques, the best CV-accuracies were achieved using BO. This observation could also be confirmed for the independent test dataset except for the RF models trained on *dataset 1*. In this case, BO and grid-search achieved the same accuracy. Comparing CV-accuracies of the XGBoost and RF models, better results were achieved by the RF models. The results for the independent test dataset showed a different observation because two XGBoost models achieved outstanding results. No major differences were detected between randomly initialized BO and BO with LHD initialization. Some of the model errors for pMCI subjects can be traced back to a large distance in time between BL diagnosis and conversion diagnosis. For these subjects, a classifier depending on longitudinal input data might be more expedient. Future studies should validate the results for different AD cohorts. Both classifiers in this article were tree-based models. Thus, it should be investigated in future research, how BO and LHD initialization works for different ML models. The use of alternative optimization methods such as Sequential Parameter Optimization (SPO) [3] might be another promising research approach.

Acknowledgment. Data used in the preparation of this article were obtained from the Alzheimer's Disease Neuroimaging Initiative (ADNI) database. We thank the patients and ADNI for the availability of the data.

The work of Louise Bloch was partially funded by a PhD grant from the University of Applied Sciences and Arts Dortmund, Germany.

References

1. Agrawal, R.: Sample mean based index policies with O(log n) regret for the multi-armed bandit problem. Adv. Appl. Prob. **27**(4), 1054–1078 (1995). https://doi.org/10.2307/1427934
2. Alzheimer's Association: 2020 Alzheimer's Disease facts and figures. Alzheimer's Dement. **16**(3), 391–460 (2020). https://doi.org/10.1002/alz.12068
3. Bartz-Beielstein, T., Lasarczyk, C., Preuss, M.: Sequential parameter optimization. In: Proceedings of the IEEE Congress on Evolutionary Computation, vol. 1, pp. 773–780 (2005). https://doi.org/10.1109/cec.2005.1554761
4. Benussi, A., et al.: Classification accuracy of transcranial magnetic stimulation for the diagnosis of neurodegenerative dementias. Ann. Neurol. **87**(3), 394–404 (2020). https://doi.org/10.1002/ana.25677
5. Bloch, L., Friedrich, C.M.: Classification of Alzheimer's disease using volumetric features of multiple MRI scans. In: Proceedings of the 41st Annual International Conference of the IEEE Engineering in Medicine and Biology Society (EMBC), pp. 2396–2401, July 2019. https://doi.org/10.1109/EMBC.2019.8857188
6. Breiman, L.: Random forests. Mach. Learn. **45**(1), 5–32 (2001). https://doi.org/10.1023/A:1010933404324
7. Breiman, L., Friedman, J., Stone, C.J., Olshen, R.A.: Classification and Regression Trees, 1st edn. CRC Press, Boca Raton (1984). https://doi.org/10.1201/9781315139470
8. Burns, A., Iliffe, S.: Alzheimer's disease. BMJ **338** (2009). https://doi.org/10.1136/bmj.b158
9. Chawla, N.V., Bowyer, K.W., Hall, L.O., Kegelmeyer, W.P.: SMOTE: synthetic minority over-sampling technique. J. Artif. Intell. Res. **16**(1), 321–357 (2002). https://doi.org/10.1613/jair.953
10. Chen, T., Guestrin, C.: XGBoost: a scalable tree boosting system. In: Proceedings of the 22nd ACM SIGKDD International Conference on Knowledge Discovery and Data Mining, pp. 785–794. New York, August 2016. https://doi.org/10.1145/2939672.2939785
11. Chen, T., et al.: XGBoost: eXtreme Gradient Boosting. R package v0.82.1 (2019). https://CRAN.R-project.org/package=xgboost. Accessed 5 Aug 2020

12. Cortes, C., Vapnik, V.: Support-vector networks. Mach. Learn. **20**(3), 273–297 (1995). https://doi.org/10.1007/BF00994018

13. Desikan, R.S., et al.: An automated labeling system for subdividing the human cerebral cortex on MRI scans into GYRAL based regions of interest. NeuroImage **31**(3), 968–980, August 2006. https://doi.org/10.1016/j.neuroimage.2006.01.021

14. Efron, B., Tibshirani, R.: Bootstrap methods for standard errors, confidence intervals, and other measures of statistical accuracy. Stat. Sci. **1**(1), 54–75 (1986). https://doi.org/10.1214/ss/1177013815

15. Fischl, B.: FreeSurfer. NeuroImage **62**(2), 774–781 (2012). https://doi.org/10.1016/j.neuroimage.2012.01.021

16. Fischl, B., et al.: Whole brain segmentation: automated labeling of neuroanatomical structures in the human brain. Neuron **33**(3), 341–355 (2002). https://doi.org/10.1016/S0896-6273(02)00569-X

17. Friedman, J.H.: Greedy function approximation: a gradient boosting machine. Ann. Stat. **29**(5), 1189–1232 (2001). https://doi.org/10.1214/aos/1013203451

18. Grassi, M., et al.: Alzheimer's disease neuroimaging initiative: a novel ensemble-based machine learning algorithm to predict the conversion from mild cognitive impairment to Alzheimer's disease using socio-demographic characteristics, clinical information, and neuropsychological measures. Front. Neurol. **10**, 756 (2019). https://doi.org/10.3389/fneur.2019.00756

19. Gupta, Y., Lama, R.K., Kwon, G.R., Alzheimer's disease neuroimaging initiative: prediction and classification of alzheimer's disease based on combined features from Apolipoprotein-E genotype, cerebrospinal fluid, MR, and FDG-PET imaging biomarkers. Front. Comput. Neurosci. **13**, 72 (2019). https://doi.org/10.3389/fncom.2019.00072

20. Hon, M., Khan, N.M.: Towards Alzheimer's disease classification through transfer learning. In: Proceedings of the IEEE International Conference on Bioinformatics and Biomedicine (BIBM), pp. 1166–1169, November 2017. https://doi.org/10.1109/BIBM.2017.8217822

21. Jack Jr., et al.: Magnetic resonance imaging in Alzheimer's disease neuroimaging initiative 2. Alzheimer's Dement. **11**(7), 740–756 (2015). https://doi.org/10.1016/j.jalz.2015.05.002

22. Katehakis, M.N., Robbins, H.: Sequential choice from several populations. Proc. Nat. Acad. Sci. **92**(19), 8584–8585 (1995). https://doi.org/10.1073/pnas.92.19.8584

23. Kuhn, M.: Caret: Classification and Regression Training. R package v6.0-82 (2019). https://CRAN.R-project.org/package=caret. Accessed 5 Aug 2020

24. Liaw, A., Wiener, M.: Classification and regression by random forest. R News vol. 2, no. 3, pp. 18–22 (2002). https://www.r-project.org/doc/Rnews/Rnews_2002-3.pdf. Accessed 12 Aug 2020

25. McKay, M.D., Beckman, R.J., Conover, W.J.: A comparison of three methods for selecting values of input variables in the analysis of output from a computer code. Technometrics **21**(2), 239–245 (1979). https://doi.org/10.2307/1268522

26. Močkus, J.: On Bayesian methods for seeking the extremum. In: Marchuk, G.I. (ed.) Optimization Techniques 1974. LNCS, vol. 27, pp. 400–404. Springer, Heidelberg (1975). https://doi.org/10.1007/3-540-07165-2_55

27. Oh, K., Chung, Y.C., Kim, K., Kim, W.S., Oh, I.S.: Classification and visualization of Alzheimer's disease using volumetric convolutional neural network and transfer learning. Sci. Rep. **9** (2019). https://doi.org/10.1038/s41598-019-54548-6

28. Park, C., Ha, J., Park, S.: Prediction of Alzheimer's disease based on deep neural network by integrating gene expression and DNA methylation dataset. Expert Syst. Appl. **140**, 112873 (2020). https://doi.org/10.1016/j.eswa.2019.112873
29. Petersen, R.C., et al.: Alzheimer's disease neuroimaging initiative (ADNI). Neurology **74**(3), 201–209 (2010). https://doi.org/10.1212/WNL.0b013e3181cb3e25
30. R Core Team: R: A Language and Environment for Statistical Computing. R Foundation for Statistical Computing, Vienna, Austria (2019). https://www.R-project. org/. Accessed 5 Aug 2020
31. Refaeilzadeh, P., Tang, L., Liu, H.: Cross-validation. In: Liu, L., Özsu, M.T. (eds.) Encyclopedia of Database Systems, pp. 532–538, Springer, US, Boston, MA (2009). https://doi.org/10.1007/978-0-387-39940-9_565
32. Wallert, J., Westman, E., Ulinder, J., Annerstedt, M., Terzis, B., Ekman, U.: Differentiating patients at the memory clinic with simple reaction time variables: a predictive modeling approach using support vector machines and Bayesian optimization. Front. Aging Neurosci. **10**, 144 (2018). https://doi.org/10.3389/fnagi. 2018.00144
33. Westman, E., Aguilar, C., Muehlboeck, J.S., Simmons, A.: Regional magnetic resonance imaging measures for multivariate analysis in alzheimer's disease and mild cognitive impairment. Brain Topogr. **26**(1), 9–23 (2012). https://doi.org/10.1007/ s10548-012-0246-x
34. Witten, I.H., Frank, E., Hall, M.A. (eds.): Data mining: practical machine learning tools and techniques. In: The Morgan Kaufmann Series in Data Management Systems, Morgan Kaufmann, Boston, 3rd edn. (2011). https://doi.org/10.1016/B978-0-12-374856-0.00023-7
35. Yan, Y.: rBayesianOptimization: Bayesian Optimization of Hyperparameters. R package v1.1.0 (2016). https://CRAN.R-project.org/package=rBayesianOptimization. Accessed 5 Aug 2020

A Proposal of Clinical Decision Support System Using Ensemble Learning for Coronary Artery Disease Diagnosis

Rawia Sammout[1]([✉]), Kais Ben Salah[2], Khaled Ghedira[3], Rania Abdelhedi[4], and Najla Kharrat[4]

[1] National School of Computer Sciences, Manouba, Tunisia
rawia.sammout@ensi-uma.tn
[2] Computing and Information Technology Faculty of Computing and Information Technology, Jeddah, South Africa
Kbensalah@uj.edu.sa
[3] SSOIE COSMOS National School of Computer Sciences, Manouba, Tunisia
khaledghedira3@gmail.com
[4] Laboratory of Molecular and Cellular Screening Processes Centre of Biotechnology of Sfax, Sfax, Tunisia
rania.abdelhedi@gmail.com, najla.kharrat@gmail.com

Abstract. Coronary Artery heart Disease (CAD) is the leading cause of mortality in the world. It is a complex and multifactorial disease resulting in several acute coronary syndromes and lead to death. In healthcare, an accurate clinical decision support system (CDSS) for CAD prediction has become increasingly important for making granted decisions at premature stage. Intensive research has been conducted on improving classification performance using machine learning techniques and metaheuristics algorithms. But most of these studies introduced the "classic risk factors" for CAD diagnosis i.e., demographic and clinical data. In this study, we present a novel CDSS based on ensemble learning for CAD prediction and we emphasize on adding other medical markers i.e., therapy data, some genetic polymorphisms along with classical factors. The new framework exploits the potential of three base classifiers including Support Vector Machines, Naïve Bayes and Decision Tree C4.5 to improve the prediction performance. Six experimental data used to build the proposed framework: the first one is collected from a Tunisian biotechnology center and the five other datasets from the University of California at Irvine repository. The analysis of the results shows that the proposed CDSS has the highest rate on classification accuracy, precision, recall and F1-measure when compared with CSGA Bagging and Adaptive boosting on the different datasets and proves that some medications and genetic polymorphisms such as Antivitamin K, Dose Beta Blocker, Proton pump inhibitor, CYP2C19*17, Clopidogrel active metabolite have an impact in CAD diagnosis.

Keywords: Coronary artery heart disease · Genetic factors · Medications · Ensemble learning

J. Ye et al. (Eds.): MobiHealth 2020, LNICST 362, pp. 300–314, 2021.
https://doi.org/10.1007/978-3-030-70569-5_19

1 Introduction

According to the World health organization report of 2017 [1], Coronary heart disease (CHD) represents the highest death rate among non-infectious diseases in the world. Various forms of cardiovascular disease exist such as stroke, rheumatic fever/rheumatic heart disease, high blood pressure, valvular heart disease and coronary heart disease on which our paper is focused. A blood clot resulting in a heart attack is typically the main cause of a sudden blockage of a coronary artery which leads to the reduction of blood and oxygen supply to the heart and to the coronary artery disease (CAD) [2]. Moreover, the atherosclerotic plaque growth model combines information from genetic and biological data of the patients. Therefore, it is essential to study the effect of certain genetic polymorphisms in the genes of patients with biological markers for CAD diagnosis. To the best of our knowledge, previous studies have used mainly different factors to diagnose CAD such as demographic, clinical, Electrocardiogram (ECG), symptoms and physical examination features [3, 4, 5]. Only a few of studies utilized some genetic polymorphisms in CAD diagnosis. Hence, it is still an active research in finding indicators for CAD diagnosis. However, Various techniques are used in CAD diagnosis such as ECG, Echocardiogram, Stress test, Cardiac catheterization and angiogram, Heart scan [3, 5] etc. But unfortunately, all these methods are expensive, protracted, and invasive. Moreover, the treatment cost for CAD is very expensive (estimated to US $ 14 billion per year) in the USA [6]. Therefore, new alternatives based on data mining (artificial neural networks, boosting, SVM) and soft computing (fuzzy logic, genetic algorithms) have been proposed to overcome time complexity, high diagnosis and treatment costs and adverse effects issues. Y. Niranjana Devi and S. Auto [7] used the decision tree algorithm to select significant attributes and then extract crisp if-then rules to constitute the fuzzy rule base for the fuzzy system. Finally, they applied genetic algorithm GA to optimize the fuzzy membership function. The results showed the performance of the system was significantly better than other systems. Next, Wiga Maulana Baihaqi et al. [8] examined the combination of datamining techniques (C4.5, CART, and RIPPER) and the fuzzy expert system to generate fuzzy rules to diagnose CAD. As a result, C4.5 and the fuzzy expert system outperforms studied classifiers with an accuracy of 81.82%. A recent research carried out by Kathleen H, Miao et al. [9] proposed for CAD diagnosis. An advanced ensemble machine learning model based on adaptive boosting (AdaBoost) algorithm was applied on four cardiac open datasets. The results indicated that the proposed ensemble achieves accuracy of 80.14% for Cleveland data, 89.12% for Hungarian data, 77.78% for Long beach data, and 96.72% for Switzerland data and outperforms existing models. Further, A new diagnosis model for CAD was introduced by N. Samadiani and S. Moameri [10]. The studied factors are extracted from SPECT heart disease images. Then a feature selection step was performed using Cuckoo Search CS and Genetic Algorithm GA to find the most significant features for CAD diagnosis. Then, the results are classified using the bagging classifier. The results of the proposed model (77,19%) are significantly better than GA or CS with a bagging classifier. Additionally, Kai Lei et al. [11] applied a weighted Naïve Bayes model on attribute relevancy for CAD diagnosis. The studied risk factors incorporated in this study are CAD symptoms. The improved Naïve Bayes model outperforms standard Naïve Bayes because of the studying of attributes relevance. While most of previous research yielded successful results for the diagnosis of CAD using single classifiers, ensemble classifiers also showed expected excellent results in CAD classification [9]. Therefore, research on using ensemble model for CAD diagnosis is still active. Even though several CDSS have been introduced for CAD diagnosis, most of them have incorporated specific risk factors with the studied population such as American, Indian, Indonesian, Chinese etc. But environmental factors, lifestyle, diet habits aren't the same. On the other hand, it might be other factors that may help to assess CAD disease in another community. The existing CDSSs are not able to incorporate new risk factors. These limitations are handled in this research by taking into consideration more heterogeneous factors (72 biomarkers) including four genetic features such as CYP2C19*2, CYP2C19*17, CYP2C9*2 (rs1799853) and CYP2C9*3 (rs1057910) polymorphisms and some medications plus demographic and clinical features to build a new CDSS for CAD diagnosis. The proposed framework aims to improve the prediction accuracy. This paper is organized as follows: Sect. 2 introduces the techniques used to build the proposed framework. Section 3 covers the experiment datasets, finding and a discussion of the results. Finally, Sect. 4 concludes this paper.

2   Materials and Methods

2.1   Design of the Proposed CDSS

The proposed CDSS for CAD diagnosis is presented in the following flowchart given in Fig. 1. It consists of three main phases detailed below: preprocessing, classification and prediction and evaluation.

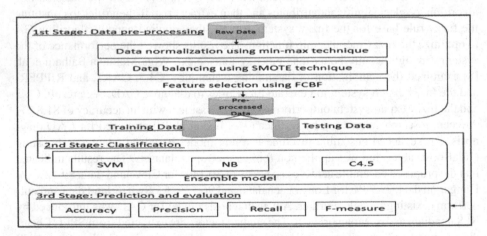

Fig. 1. General design of the proposed CDSS

2.2   Data Pre-processing Phase

A data preprocessing phase consists of three main steps: scale normalization, sampling, and feature selection, detailed below:

Normalization Using Min-Max Technique

Using data with different measurement units may have effect on the analysis and leads to different results. For example, using meters to measure the height instead of inches will lead to giving greater importance to the attributes with greater weight [12]. Therefore, normalization represents an essential step in preprocessing in order to give all attributes equal importance (weights). It aims to transform an original range of data to a new range. Also, it may be helpful to maintain the large variation in prediction or forecasting [13]. Min-max technique is widely used in the literature and known as a very simple method that provides a linear mapping of data from an unstructured range to new values of data. It also insures keeping relationship among original data values [14, 15]. Normalization is calculated using the following formula:

$$X' = \frac{X - X_{min}}{X_{max} - X_{min}} * (new_{max} - new_{min}) + new_{min}, \tag{1}$$

where X' *is the new value,* X_{min} is the minimum value and X_{max} is the maximum value in the attribute.

In the present study, the original data are mapping in the range [0, 1] (where new_{min} = 0 and new_{max} = 1) and the simplified following formula is used:

$$X' = \frac{X - X_{min}}{X_{max} - X_{min}}, \tag{2}$$

Sampling Using Smote Technique

Class imbalance ratio is high specifically in genomic dataset where the number of instances from one class is higher than the other class. The class having the higher number is called majority class, while the other one is known as minority class. Generally, classifiers are more sensitive to select majority class and less sensitive to detect minority class. Therefore, it may lead to a biased classification output. Hence, a combination between a classification algorithm and a sampling technique becomes mandatory. In this study, an oversampling technique known by synthetic minority oversampling technique (SMOTE) [16] is selected to handle this issue while the studied datasets are small. It has an ability to generate synthetically observations from the minority class samples to over-sample the minority distribution by joining any/all the k minority class nearest neighbors [17, 18]. It aims to balance a dataset with a binary target variable. Figure 2 below explains the process of this technique.

Fast Correlation-Based Feature Selection

A multivariate subset search technique called fast correlation-based filter selection (FCBF) [19] is used to select the subset of the most relevant and irredundant features among the full set of features. The attributes are ranked using an evaluation criterion called symmetric uncertainty (SU) [20]. Then, a threshold value of this latter is fixed and the attributes with values above this threshold (have highest dependency on the output variable) are selected to construct the model and the rest of attributes with values below the threshold (have low dependency) are removed. However, this technique has the ability of capturing non-linear correlation between features and modeling feature

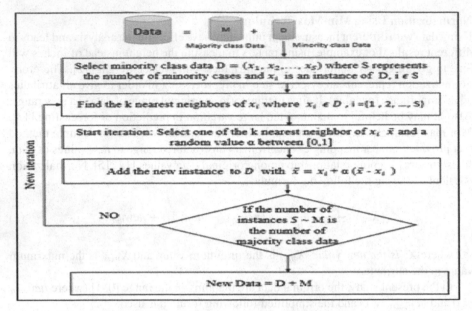

Fig. 2. Oversampling process using SMOTE technique

dependencies. Besides, it helps to reduce overfitting problem and time complexity and to improve the learner's performance [21]. The formula for calculating the SU measure is given below:

$$SU(X|Y) = 2\left[\frac{IG(X|Y)}{H(X) + H(Y)}\right] \tag{3}$$

Where $IG(X|Y)$ [22] is the information gain and represents the amount of the decrease of entropy of X provided as additional information by Y and calculating by the formula as follows:

$$IG(X|Y) = H(X) - H(X|Y) \tag{4}$$

With H(X) represents the uncertainty of a random variable X known by the entropy and is defined as:

$$H(X) = -\sum_i P(x_i) log_2(P(x_i)) \tag{5}$$

With $P(xi)$ is the probability of xi and H(X|Y) is the entropy of X after seeing values of Y and is calculated using (6) given by:

$$H(X|Y) = -\sum_j P(y_j) \sum_i P(x_i|y_j) log_2(P(x_i|y_j)) \tag{6}$$

With $P(yj)$ is the probability of yj and $P(xi|yj)$ is the conditional probability of xj given that yj has occurred.

$$P(x_i|y_j) = \frac{P(x_i \cap y_j)}{P(y_j)} \tag{7}$$

2.3 Classification Phase: Proposed Ensemble Learning Model

Ensemble Learning

Ensemble learning is a new concept that combines more than one model to predict a target output with more efficiency and accurate decisions than single model [23]. Thus, it leads to excellent classification results superior to those of a single classifier in many fields including cardiac arrhythmia [24], DNA microarray classification [25], and different heart diseases [26]. Diversity of ensemble members and different classification properties are required in ensemble learning in order to achieve high classification performance [27] with a good management of bias-variance errors [28]. A good ensemble strategy is ensured by the complementarity between its classifiers where the diversity between classifiers could be ensured by establishing sample techniques or training the classifiers by different training sets [27]. In this work, three techniques SVM, NB and DT are selected to build the ensemble learning, they will be discussed in the following subsections. The results of the analysis carried out by the discussed techniques are combined using a combination technique that will be explained below:

Support Vector Machines

As the sample studied in this review is a small dataset, support vector machines (SVM) is selected as a base classifier to be used in this study. It is recommended in the literature as an efficient classification technique for small-sample data [29]. Moreover, this classification model has been widely used to classify genomic datasets and yielded to excellent results. SVM is a supervised learning algorithm introduced by Vapnik (1998). It is a two-class classifier. It aims to design a N dimensional hyperplane that classify all training vectors (target variable/class label and feature variables) into two classes and leaves the maximum margin from both classes [30]. To maximize the margin, we have to solve a quadratic (nonlinear) optimization problem in order to maximum margin hyperplane as illustrated in Fig. 3 below:

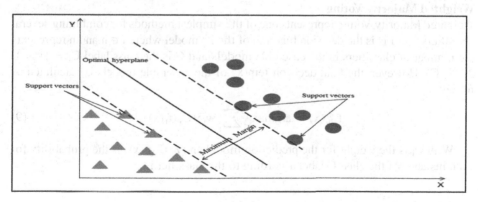

Fig. 3. Support Vector Machines

Naïve Bayes

Naive Bayes (NB) is a probability-based classification technique. It applies Bayes 'theorem with considering the independence assumption between all features [31]. The NB classifier calculates the probability that a given instance X belongs to a class label y. Given an instance X, characterized by a set of attributes $(x_1, x_2, ..., x_n)$, and a class output y, the Bayes theorem consists of calculating the posterior probability $P(y/X)$ using the following formula:

$$P(y/X) = \frac{P(y)P(X/y)}{P(X)} \tag{8}$$

Moreover, NB classifier yields generally to excellent classification results and surprisingly outperforms more sophisticated algorithms in classification even without considering the independence assumption [32].

Decision Tree C4.5

Decision trees have become one of the most powerful and popular classification approaches used in the literature. They have many advantages, such as being comprehensible, easy and they require low computational effort [33]. In this paper, we emphasize the study on C4.5 decision tree algorithm as it is one of the most popular algorithms which is widely used for genomic dataset analysis [34, 35]. C4.5 is a top-down tree growth algorithm proposed by Ross Quinlan in 1993 [36], and its algorithm starts by calculating entropy and equivalent information gain to measure the importance of the attributes. Feature with the highest information gain tends to be selected as the most influential attribute in the classification process. The set of examples will be splitted according to the possible values of the selected feature. This process will be repeated iteratively until the decision tree learns from the set of the training examples. The formula for measuring information gain IG and entropy H are described above in Eqs. (4) and (5) respectively.

Weighted Majority Voting

Weighted Majority Voting represents one of the simplest methods for combining several classifiers. Let f is is the decision function of the ith model where $i \in n$ and n represents the number of classifiers in the ensemble models and C is the class label $C_j = \{j = 1, 2, ..., C)$. However, the final decision fem(x) of the ensemble models is calculated as follow:

$$f_{em}(x) = \operatorname{argmax}_C \sum_i w_i \delta(C, f_i(x)) \tag{9}$$

With w_i is the weight for the prediction model and $\delta(C, f_i(x))$ is the probability for each instance of the class C label according to the classifier i.

2.4 Performance Evaluation Measurement

To evaluate the proposed CDSS performance with other models, we used the basic metrics such as precision, recall, classification accuracy and F-measure [37]. The main formulations of these metrics are:

$$Precision = \frac{T_p}{T_p + F_p} \tag{10}$$

$$Recall = \frac{T_p}{T_p + F_N} \tag{11}$$

$$Accuracy = \frac{T_N + T_p}{T_p + T_N + F_N + F_p} \tag{12}$$

$$F_{measure} = 2 * \frac{Precision * Recall}{Precision + Recall}, \tag{13}$$

With TP = True Positive, TN = True Negative, FN = False Negative, FP = False Positive. Indeed, accuracy represents the percentage of a correct CAD prediction (test is true) and a non-CAD prediction (test is false). Recall (sensitivity) is the true positive rate of CAD while precision is the positive predicted value of CAD. F-measure represents the weighted harmonic mean of precision and recall. In addition, a ten-fold cross validation (CV) has been successfully used for evaluating the performance of a machine learning algorithm(s) as it offers reliable approximates for the classification accuracy on each classification task [38]. Moreover, it is able to reduce the variability but increases the selection bias in case of feature selection or model parameters 'tuning. Thus, an external cross validation [39] is needed by holdout a testing set (30% of the sample) and applied 10-fold CV on the training (70%) and then evaluate model accuracy using the hold out testing set. This technique helps to reduce the selection bias and therefore guarantee the tradeoff between the bias and the variance.

3 Experimental Results and Discussion

3.1 Datasets

Based on a recent study of the National Public Health Institute 2018, heart diseases are the primary risk of death in Tunisia rather than infectious diseases. The studied population (see Table 1) consists of 213 patients from the south of Tunisia. The patients were admitted in the biotechnological Center in Sfax Tunisia for coronary artery disease diagnosis. The period of the study extends from January 1, 2010 to April 30, 2013. The dataset contains 72 categorical and numerical features considered for the prediction. The diagnosis result as the target variable. The studied features (see Table 2) represent clinical characteristics, genetic polymorphisms, and some medications for example. The target variable has a binary CAD diagnosis (1: diseased, 0: healthy). To ensure efficiency of the proposed CDSS, four majors most widely used cardiac databases from UCI repository are studied. They are Cleveland, Hungarian, Switzerland, and Long Beach [39]. These datasets consist of 76 attributes, but 14 of them are the mainly used. Furthermore, a cardiac Single Proton Emission Computed Tomography (SPECT) images dataset is studied for a comparison purpose. It is composed of 267 patient SPECT image records and 23 extracted binary features.

Table 1. Description of the experiment datasets

Dataset	Number of attributes	Number of classes	Number of positive cases	Number of negative cases	Total number of cases
Studied population	72	2	150	63	213
Cleveland	14	2	139	164	303
Hungarian	14	2	106	188	294
Switzerland	14	2	155	8	123
Long Beach	14	2	149	51	200
SPECT	23	2	212	55	267

Table 2. Description of the studied features in the Tunisian dataset

Variables	Description
Genetic polymorphisms	CYP2C19*2, CYP2C19*17, CYP2C9*2 (rs1799853), YP2C9*3 (rs1057910)
Biomarkers	Time of collection (Hours), Number of dilated arteries, Systolic blood pressure, Dyastolic blood pressure, Glycemia, Creatinine, Urea, CPK (creatine phosphokinase), Triglyceride, Cholesterol total, Na (sodium), CL (chlorine), K (potassium), Leukocytes, Hemoglobin, Platelets, Number of stents, Coronarography results, Event time (month), Event, Diagnosis (angina effort, SCA ST−, SCA ST+), INDICATION (TTT, PAC, ATL), Type of artery 1, Age, Sex, Non-insulinodependant diabetes, Insulin-dependent diabetes, Smoking, Dyslipidemia, HyperCT, HyperTG, Mixed dyslipidemia, Family history of CAD, Renal failure, Previous MI, Previous PCI, Previous CABG, Previous stroke, Alcohol
Medications	Clopidogrel loading dose, Clopidogrel maintenance dose, Clopidogrel treatment duration, Clopidogrel carboxylic acid (ng/ml), Clopidogrel (pg/ml), Clopidogrel acyl glucuronide (ng/ml), Clopidogrel active metabolite, Statins, Dose statins, Aspirin, Aspirin loading dose, AVK (Antivitamin K), ACE inhibitor, DOSE IEC, Angiotensin II receptor antagonist, Beta blockers, DOSE BB, Calcium channel blocker, Diuretic, DIURETIQ ARAII, proton pump inhibitor, Dose ipp, Nitrated derivatives, AGRASTAT, Reopro

3.2 Hyperparameters Setting

Hyperparameters represent parameters of the classifier that must be tuned before training to guarantee good classification results. In our case, SVM has two main parameters to optimize i.e., gamma, the coefficient C and the kernel, while DT has other parameters to tune such as number of features in each split, the minimum number of samples that must be in the leaf node, the minimum number of samples required in an internal node. Grid search algorithm (GS) is used in this study. It is a heuristic technique that aims to find the optimal parameters of a model among a given subset of hyperparameters space [40]. This algorithm is the most widely used algorithm because of its simplicity. The principle of this algorithm is to minimize a loss function using a combination of a tuple of parameters among the defined space. However, the grid search results must be evaluated using cross validation/boosting or hold-out test on the performance metrics to estimate the generalization performance. In this work, a ten-fold cross validation technique is used with grid search algorithm.

3.3 Results and Discussion

We applied the proposed CDSS to a Tunisian population dataset and four benchmark cardiac datasets to prove its Dataset Number of attributes Number of classes Number of positive cases Number of negative cases Total number of cases Studied population 72 2 150 63 213 Cleveland 14 2 139 164 303 Hungarian 14 2 106 188 294 Switzerland 14 2 155 8 123 Long Beach 14 2 149 51 200 SPECT 23 2 212 55 267 Variables Description Genetic polymorphisms CYP2C19*2, CYP2C19*17, CYP2C9*2 (rs1799853), CYP2C9*3 (rs1057910) Biomarkers Time of collection (Hours), Number of dilated arteries, Systolic blood pressure, Dyastolic blood pressure, Glycemia, Creatinine, Urea, CPK (creatine phosphokinase), Triglyceride, Cholesterol total, Na (sodium), CL (chlorine), K (potassium), Leukocytes, Hemoglobin, Platelets, Number of stents, Coronarography results, Event time (month), Event, Diagnosis (angina effort, SCA ST−, SCA ST+), INDICATION (TTT, PAC, ATL), Type of artery 1, Age, Sex, Non-insulinodependant diabetes, Insulin-dependent diabetes, Smoking, Dyslipidemia, HyperCT, HyperTG, Mixed dyslipidemia, Family history of CAD, Renal failure, Previous MI, Previous PCI, Previous CABG, Previous stroke, Alcohol Medications Clopidogrel loading dose, Clopidogrel maintenance dose, Clopidogrel treatment duration, Clopidogrel carboxylic acid (ng/ml), Clopidogrel (pg/ml), Clopidogrel acyl glucuronide (ng/ml), Clopidogrel active metabolite, Statins, Dose statins, Aspirin, Aspirin loading dose, AVK (vitamin K), ACE inhibitor, DOSE IEC, Angiotensin II receptor antagonist, Beta blockers, DOSE BB, Calcium channel blocker, Diuretic, DIURETIQ ARAII, proton pump inhibitor, Dose ipp, Nitrated derivatives, AGRASTAT, Reopro efficacity. The experiments conducted for evaluating the performance of the proposed ensemble learners and all the studied classifiers are performed using 10-fold CV strategy to alleviate the insufficiency of small studied samples. The proposed CDSS is implemented using 70% of a training set and testing splitting on 10-fold CV and a validation set of 30% and running on 100 different seeds to validate the results with the mean accuracy value. As described in Table 1 below, the skewed Tunisian dataset is composed of 163 CAD patients (as majority class) and 63 non-CAD patients as minority class. After applying SMOTE technique, a balanced dataset (BD) is generated with equal class sizes. Indeed, Table 3 compares results of DT classifier using 10-fold cross validation and grid search techniques before and after oversampling the data using different performance evaluation metrics. The results obtained when the data is imbalanced show that the positive class CAD has effective prediction results with high rates in precision 81%, recall 94% and F1-measure 87% while the negative class No CAD has low rates in precision 9%, recall 3% and F1 measure 4. However, after balancing the dataset we can see an increasingly prediction improvement for the negative class with 78% precision, 72% recall and 75% F1-measure. The sampling process is repeated for the four benchmark datasets while they have also imbalanced class distribution. Next, the numerical attributes of the balanced data are normalized using min_max normalization technique to avoid large variation in the prediction results and improve the prediction accuracy. Using the same classifier (DT) on the same data shows an improvement from 75,72% to 76,58% on accuracy rate and from 76% to 77% for other metrics.

Table 3. Performance evaluation before and after balancing the Tunisian dataset

	Imbalanced data		Balanced data	
Metrics/Class	CAD	No CAD	Metrics/Class	CAD
Precision	81%	9%	Precision	81%
Recall	94%	3%	Recall	94%
F1-measure	87%	4%	F1-measure	87%
Accuracy	77%		75,72%	

Then, this study has investigated the determination of CAD factors and emphasized on studying the impact of some genetic polymorphisms and medications which may help in the diagnosis of CAD. However, we performed a feature selection process using FCBF model to select the most significant attributes independently of the classifier. Then, we applied C4.5 algorithm to test the select features subset on prediction accuracy improvement as DT is simple and widely used in biology. Based on the results obtained in Table 4, we consider that the best subset of medical markers is sufficient to predict CAD with a high accuracy and provides less computational time than using all the features set. For example, the eight selected significant features from the Tunisian dataset represent one genetic feature (CYP2C19*17) among the four studied ones and five drugs (Antivitamins K (AVK), Dose Beta blockers, Proton pump inhibitor, Clopidogrel active metabolite) among all the studied medications and three other clinical markers (Event time/month, Previous stroke, Obesity). Hence, these results prove that the selected genetic factors and drugs are important indicators to diagnose CAD.

Furthermore, a classification stage is performed using the novel ensemble learners based on a weighted majority voting technique to aggregate the prediction results. The model weights are estimated according to their prediction accuracy (the model with the highest accuracy rate has the highest weight and so on). The proposed CDSS is examined on five different populations to prove its generalization ability and it yielded successful results. Table 5 lists the existing ensemble models including adaptive boosting (AdaBoost) [9] and CSGA Boosting [10] in the comparison. The results (Table 5) show that the new system achieved the best classification accuracies when comparing with the two existing ensembles. Indeed, comparing with AdaBoost on the five studied data, the new system yielded the highest prediction accuracies on the five studied populations i.e., Tunisian, Cleveland, Hungarian, Switzerland, and Long Beach respectively

Table 4. Performance evaluation before and after feature selection

Data	Attributes Number	Selected Features	DT Accuracy	Execution Time (s)
Tunisian	72	All the features	75,72%	3.73
Tunisian	8	Event time, AVK, Dose Beta Blockers, Proton pump inhibitor, Previous stroke, CYP2C19*17, Clopidogrel active metabolite, Obesity	78,85%	3.30
Cleveland	14	All	74,08%	3.44
Cleveland	8	Sex, cp, restecg, thalach, exang, old peak, ca, thal	78,66%	3.11
Hungarian	14	All	77,13%	3.61
Hungarian	8	Sex, cp, chol, fbs, exang, oldpeak, slope, thal	81,14%	3.04
Switzerland	14	All	86,09%	3.35
Switzerland	4	Sex, cp, fbs, exang	95,22%	3,12
Long beach	14	All	73,82%	3.541
Long beach	5	Age, sex, cp, exang, oldpeak	77.52%	3.28

with 79.41%, 82.27%, 89.48% and 97.45% compared with AdaBoost 71.15%, 80.14%, 89.12% and 96.72% and with CSGA Bagging 69.18%, 81,11%, 88,78%, 93,4%, 76,13%. Furthermore, Table 5 shows that the new framework achieved the highest accuracy rate of 79.72% on SPECT dataset while AdaBoost 76.41% and CSGA+ Bagging 77.19%. In conclusion, the proposed framework contributes efficiently to the prediction performance improvement due to its complementarity and diversity. However, the complementarity is ensured between the three used classifiers (SVM, DT and NB) by complementing the weaknesses between them and maximally improving the classification accuracy of the ensemble. Whereas the diversity is ensured by their different natures like probabilistic nature of NB and the complex nature of SVM and the tree-based nature of DT.

Table 5. Comparison of performance between the proposed CDSS and existing models

Dataset	Proposed ensemble	Adaptive boosting [9]	CSGA + Bagging [10]
Tunisian	79.41%	71.15%	69.18%
Cleveland	82.27%	80.14%	81,11%
Hungarian	89.48%	89.12%	88.78%
Switzerland	97.45%	96.72%	93.4%
Long beach	79.91%	77.78%	76.13%
SPECT	79.72%	76.41%	77.19%

4 Conclusion and Perspectives

In this study, we propose a new ensemble learning system based on three base classifiers SVM, NB and C4.5 DT in order to improve the prediction performance for CAD as a classification problem. The performance of the proposed CDSS is tested with 10-fold cross validation on different cardiac datasets from different populations such as Tunisian, Hungarian, Switzerland, etc. The original datasets have an uneven distribution which may affect the classification performance and lead to an overfitting. Hence, a SMOTE technique has been applied to balance the class distribution. Then, we applied a feature selection technique called FCBF in order to determine the most effective features needed in the diagnosis of CAD and reduce the classification time complexity. Further, it may eventually help to reduce the cost of CAD diagnosis by limiting clinical markers needed and administrate some specific medications for CAD. However, the results of this process prove that some medications and genetic polymorphisms such as Antivitamin K, Dose Beta Blockers, Proton pump inhibitor, CYP2C19*17, Clopidogrel active metabolite have an impact in CAD diagnosis. Finally, the reduced data are classified using the new proposed ensemble learning model and, as a result, we found that the proposed CDSS has the highest prediction rates comparing with the two existing ensemble models CSGA+ Bagging and Adaptive boosting on the different datasets. These results demonstrate the effectiveness of ensemble learning models in improving classification performance. For future work, several directions must be considered. First, we will examine the significance of the studied variables by using other feature selection techniques. Then, a fuzzification approach may be introduced to envisage information vagueness and decision-making uncertainty in engineering problems. Finally, we will focus to find way to reduce the computation time problem of the proposed system.

References

1. AHA Statistical Update.: Heart Disease and Stroke Statistics 2010 Update: Summary, A Report from the American Heart Association (2010)
2. Rajkumar, A., Reena, G.S.: Diagnosis of heart disease using datamining algorithm. Global J. Comput. Sci. Technol. **10**(10), 38 (2010)
3. Genders, T.S., Steyerberg, E.W., Alkadhi, H., et al.: A clinical prediction rule for the diagnosis of coronary artery disease: validation, updating, and extension. Eur. Heart J. **32**(11), 1316–1330 (2011)
4. Xu, H., Duan, Z., Miao, C., Geng, S., Jin, Y.: Development of a diagnosis model for coronary artery disease. Indian Heart J. **69**(5), 634–639 (2017)
5. AlHosani, A., AlShizawi, S., AlAli, S., Saleh, H., Assaf, T., Stouraitis, T.: Automatic detection of coronary artery disease (CAD) in an ECG signal. In: 24th IEEE International Conference on Electronics, Circuits and Systems (ICECS) (2017)
6. Martono, G.H., Adji, T.B.: Penggunaan Principal Component Analysis dan Pohon Keputusan untuk Mendeteksi Penyakit Jantung Koroner, Unpublished thesis, Dept. Elect. Eng., Universitas Gadjah Mada, Yogyakarta (2012)
7. Niranjana Devi, Y., Anto, S.: An evolutionary-fuzzy expert system for the diagnosis of coronary artery disease. Int. J. Adv. Res. Comput. Eng. Technol. (IJARCET) **34**) (2014)
8. Baihaqi, W.M., Setiawan, N.A., Ardiyanto, I.: Rule extraction for fuzzy expert system to diagnose coronary artery disease. In: 1st International Conference on Information Technology, Information Systems and Electrical Engineering (ICITISEE),Yogyakarta, Indonesia (2016)
9. Miao, K.H., Miao, J.H., Miao, G.J.: Diagnosing coronary heart disease using ensemble machine learning. Int. J. Adv. Comput. Sci. Appl. **7**(10), 30–39 (2016)
10. Samadiani, N., Moameri, S.: Diagnosis of coronary artery disease using cuckoo search and genetic algorithm in single photon emision computed tomography images. In: 7th International Conference on Computer and Knowledge Engineering (ICCKE 2017), 26–27 October 2017

11. Lei, K., Zhang, L., Shen, Y., Huang, X., Wu, J.: Syndromes diagnostic model for coronary artery disease (CAD): an improved naïve bayesian classification model based on attribute relevancy. In: IEEE 2nd International Conference on Big Data Analysis (ICBDA) (2017)

12. Han, J., Kamber, M., Pei, J.: Data Mining Concepts and Techniques. Morgan Kaufmann, Burlington (2011)

13. Shalabi, L.A., Shaaban, Z., Kasasbeh, B.: Data mining: a preprocessing engine. J. Comput. Sci. **2**(9), 735–739 (2006)

14. Gopal Krishna Patro, S., Parimita Sahoo, P., Panda, I., Sahu, K.K.: Technical analysis on financial forecasting. Int. J. Comput. Sci. Eng. **03**(01), 1–6. E-ISSN 2347-2693 (2015)

15. Panda, S.K., Nag, S., Jana, P.K.: A smoothing based task scheduling algorithm for heterogeneous multi-cloud environment. In: 3rd IEEE International Conference on Parallel, Distributed and Grid Computing (PDGC), Waknaghat. IEEE (2014)

16. Kotsiantis, S.B., Pintelas, P.E., Kanellopoulus, D.: Handling imbalanced datasets: a review. In: GESTS International Transactions on Computer Science and Engineering **30** (2006)

17. Wang, S., Yao, X.: Multiclass imbalance problems: analysis and potential solutions. IEEE Trans. Syst. Man Cybern. Part B: Cybern. **42**(4), 1119 (2012)

18. Chawla, N., Bowyer, K., Hall, L., Kegelmeyer, P.: SMOTE: synthetic minority over-sampling technique. J. Artif. Intell. Res. **16**, 321–357 (2002)

19. Wang, L., Ni, M., Zhu, L.: Correlation coefficient of dual hesitant fuzzy sets and its applications. Appl. Math. Model. **38**, 12 (2013).

20. Yu, L., Liu, H.: Efficient feature selection via analysis of relevance and redundancy. J. Mach. Learn. Res. **10**(5), 1205–1224 (2004)

21. Saeys, Y., Inza, I., Larranaga, P.: A review of feature selection techniques in bioinformatics. Bioinformatics Advance Access, 24 August 2007

22. Press, W.H., Flannery, B.P., Teukolsky, S.A., Vetterling, W.T.: Numerical Recipes in C. Cambridge University Press, Cambridge (1988)

23. Pradhan, D., Padhy, S., Sahoo, B.: Enzyme classification using multiclass support vector machine and feature subset selection. Comput. Biol. Chem. **70**, 211–219 (2017)

24. Bolón-Canedon, V., Sánchez-Maroño, N., Alonso-Betanzos, A.: Data classification using an ensemble of filters. Neurocomputing **135**, 13–20 (2014)

25. Bashir, S., Qamar, U., Khan, F.H.: IntelliHealth: a medical decision support application using a novel weighted multi-layer classifier ensemble framework. J. Biomed. Informatics **59**, 185–200 (2016)

26. Zhou, L., Lai, K.K., Yu, L.: Least squares support vector machines ensemble models for credit scoring. Expert Syst. Appl. **37**, 127–133 (2010)

27. Yu, L., Lai, K.K., Wang, S., Huang, W.: A bias-variance-complexity trade-off framework for complex system modeling. In: Gavrilova, M. (ed.) ICCSA 2006. LNCS, vol. 3980, pp. 518–527. Springer, Heidelberg (2006). https://doi.org/10.1007/11751540_55

28. Vapnik, V.N.: The Nature of Statistical Learning Theory, Springer, New York (2000). https://doi.org/10.1007/978-1-4757-3264-1

29. Cristianini, N., Shawe-Taylor, J.: An Introduction to Support Vector Machines. Cambridge University Press, Cambridge (2000)

30. Gunn, S.: Support Vector Machines for classification and Regression, Technical report, University of Southampton (1998)

31. Mitchell, T.M.: Machine Learning, 1st edn. McGrawHill, New York (1997)

32. Rokach, L.: Decision forest twenty years of research. Inf. Fusion **27**, 111–125 (2016)

33. Verma, L., Srivastava, S., Negi, P.C.: An intelligent noninvasive model for coronary artery disease detection. Complex Intell. Syst. **4**(1), 11–18 (2018)

34. Sharma, P., Saxena, K., Sharma, R.: Heart disease prediction system evaluation using C4.5 rules and partial tree. In: Behera, H.S., Mohapatra, D.P. (eds.) Computational Intelligence in

Data Mining—Volume 2. AISC, vol. 411, pp. 285–294. Springer, New Delhi (2016). https://doi.org/10.1007/978-81-322-2731-1_26

35. Kinaci, A.C., Yucebas, S.C.: Cost reduction in thyroid diagnosis: a hybrid model with SOM and C4.5 decision trees. In: Arik, S., Huang, T., Lai, W.K., Liu, Q. (eds.) ICONIP 2015. LNCS, vol. 9490, pp. 440–448. Springer, Cham (2015). https://doi.org/10.1007/978-3-319-26535-3_50

36. Quinlan, J.R.: C4.5: Programs for Machine Learning. Morgan Kaufmann Publishers Inc., Burlington (1993)

37. Özçift, A.: Random forests ensemble classifier trained with data resampling strategy to improve cardiac arrhythmia diagnosis. Comput. Biol. Med. **41**(5), 265–271 (2011)

38. Azar, A.T., Elshazly, H.I., Hassanien, A.E., Elkorany, A.M.: A random forest classifier for lymph diseases: Comput. Meth. Programs Biomed. **113**(2), 465–473 (2014)

39. Ambroise, C., McLachlan, G.J.: Selection bias in gene extraction on the basis of microarray gene-expression data. In: Proceedings of the National Academy of Sciences of the United States of America, vol. 99, no. 10, pp. 6562–6566 (2002)

40. Blake, B.K.-S.C., Merz, C.J.: UCI repository of machine learning databases: Dep. Inf. Comput. Sci. Univ. California, Irvine, CA (1998)

41. Cheung, B.K., Ng, A.C.: An efficient and reliable algorithm for non-smooth nonlinear optimization. Neural Parallel FJ Sci. Comput. **3**, 115–128 (1995)

Deep-Learning-Based Feature Encoding of Clinical Parameters for Patient Specific CTA Dose Optimization

Marja Fleitmann[1(✉)], Hristina Uzunova[1], Andreas Martin Stroth[2],
Jan Gerlach[2], Alexander Fürschke[2], Jörg Barkhausen[2], Arpad Bischof[2,3],
and Heinz Handels[1]

[1] Institute of Medical Informatics, University of Lübeck, Lübeck, Germany
fleitmann@imi.uni-luebeck.de
[2] Department of Radiology and Nuclear Medicine, UKSH Lübeck, Lübeck, Germany
[3] IMAGE Information Systems Europe, Rostock, Germany

Abstract. The use of contrast agents in CT angiography examinations holds a potential health risk for the patient. Despite this, often unintentionally an excessive contrast agent dose is administered. Our goal is to provide a support system for the medical practitioner that advises to adjust an individually adapted dose. We propose a comparison between different means of feature encoding techniques to gain a higher accuracy when recommending the dose adjustment. We apply advanced deep learning approaches and standard methods like principle component analysis to encode high dimensional parameter vectors in a low dimensional feature space. Our experiments showed that features encoded by a regression neural network provided the best results. Especially with a focus on the 90% precision for the "excessive dose" class meaning that if our system classified a case as "excessive dose" the ground truth is most likely accordingly. With that in mind a recommendation for a lower dose could be administered without the risk of insufficient contrast and therefore a repetition of the CT angiography examination. In conclusion we showed that Deep-Learning-based feature encoding on clinical parameters is advantageous for our aim to prevent excessive contrast agent doses.

Keywords: Feature encoding · Deep Learning · Case-based reasoning · Contrast agent

1 Introduction

Feature encoding is a preprocessing step used in many machine learning applications to reduce the dimension of the input feature vectors. The process of feature encoding removes redundant data so more meaningful or relevant features can be derived from the raw inputs. This can yield a higher accuracy of the given task.

© ICST Institute for Computer Sciences, Social Informatics and Telecommunications Engineering 2021
Published by Springer Nature Switzerland AG 2021. All Rights Reserved
J. Ye et al. (Eds.): MobiHealth 2020, LNICST 362, pp. 315–322, 2021.
https://doi.org/10.1007/978-3-030-70569-5_20

A well-known feature encoding technique is the principle component analysis (PCA) which represents the data as a linear combination of features with the greatest variance. In [14] the PCA is used to encode high dimensional genome expressions to predict the clinical outcome of breast cancer. Advancing to non-linear encoding techniques Deep Learning methods came in to focus. In [11] the authors implemented an autoencoder to encode surface meshes of segmented hippocampi to subsequently classify whether the patient suffers from Alzheimer's disease. This area of non-linear feature encoding also includes the variational autoencoder. The authors of [12] used this approach to extract features for the detection of pathologies while the authors of [10] trained a variational autoencoder to reduce the dimension of single tumor cells for differentiating between tumor subpopulations.

In this paper we propose a comparison between different means of feature encoding applied to clinical parameters for a classification task (Fig. 1). In this way a recommendation to reduce the standard dose can be made which is a part of the primary objective to adjust the dose of contrast agent (CA) used in CT angiographies (CTA) for each patient individually. This is based on the fact that CAs often contain in iodine that can cause harmful side effects including anaphylactic reactions and thyrotoxicosis [1,2]. It poses a risk especially to the renal system with contrast-induced renal nephropathy being the third leading cause of hospital acquired acute renal failure [9]. Unnecessarily high CA doses should therefore be avoided in order to minimize the health risk of the patient as well as saving expenses for CA. However, often a standard dose is administered in clinical practice. A previous method uses the body weight and a weight factor to compute an individualized CA dose [5]. Another approach tested a weight-based protocol incorporated with the tube potential selection to lower the CA dose [13].

In contrast, we considered a greater set of clinical parameters in addition to the body weight with the goal to give the medical practitioner an improved dose adjustment recommendation with respect to a standard dose. We compared different methods of Deep-Learning-based feature encoding including amongst others a variational autoencoder (VAE) and a regression neural network (RNN). As an already established feature encoding method we implemented a principal component analysis (PCA) to compare with the advanced techniques. For the evaluation of the influence of the encoded features on the dose prediction quality we used a k-Nearest-Neighbour (kNN) classification on the raw input features. Each method is used as a preprocessing step for kNN-based classification in one of two classes: 1) Non-excessive image contrast, 2) Excessive image contrast.

The determination of the classes and therefore the image contrast were previously executed. Based on Regions of Interest (ROI) set in CTA volumes a rule-based assessment was implemented. This assessment acts as the ground truth for the feature encoding classification.

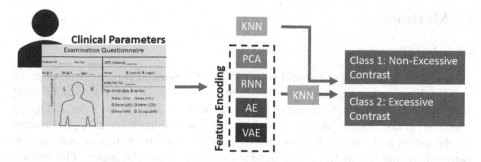

Fig. 1. Clinical parameters were encoded using the following methods: principle component analysis (PCA), regression neural network (RNN), autoencoder (AE) and variational autoencoder (VAE). The classification was implemented with k-Nearest-Neighbour (kNN). As a base comparison the kNN was used on the raw features.

2 Data

The clinical parameters and the corresponding CTA volumes were sourced from the radiology department of the UKSH Lübeck. All 76 CTA examinations were limited to the aorta area. The patients received a CA dose of 100 mL of the CA Imeron 300. Additionally, 20 clinical parameters were collected including body weight, height and blood pressure at rest among others.

To build the ground truth for the classification through feature encoding a quality assessment of the image contrast was executed. An overview of the assessment is displayed in Fig. 2. Experts placed three ROIs at predefined locations in axial CTA slices. The ROIs were defined to lie equally spaced across the CTA volume in order to encompass the entire contrast-enhanced area. Taking the mean HU values of each ROIs rules were applied resulting in the two aforementioned contrast classes.

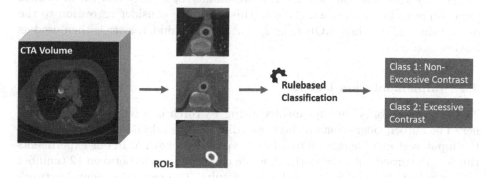

Fig. 2. ROIs are placed in axial slices of a CTA volume. Through a rule-based classification the image contrast class is determined.

3   Methods

3.1   Autoencoders

Autoencoders (AEs) [7] are neural networks, that consist of two parts: an encoder $Q(X)$, which maps the input X to a latent vector $\mathbf{z} \in \mathrm{R}^m$ and a decoder $P(\mathbf{z})$ that tries to reconstruct the input X given only $\mathbf{z}$. To ensure $X \approx P(Q(X))$ a reconstruction loss is applied, e.g. L1-loss. The latent space mapping makes autoencoders suitable for feature encoding, since the latent representation $\mathbf{z}$ is assumed to contain all the important information about the input. The feature encoding can be established by directly inputting an unseen vector in the trained encoder and considering its latent encoding.

3.2   Variational Autoencoders

Variational autoencoders (VAEs) [7] are an extension of conventional autoencoders assuming a prior distribution of the latent space. Typically a normal distribution $\mathbf{z} \sim \mathcal{N}(0,1)$ is enforced by using an additional loss function D_{KL} (Kullback-Leibler Divergence), which measures the distance between the predicted latent space distribution and the chosen a-priori distribution. To assure a normal distribution, the encoder predicts a mean μ and a standard deviation σ and the latent vector is calculated $\mathbf{z} = \mu + \epsilon\sigma$, where $\epsilon \sim \mathcal{N}(0,1)$.

3.3   Regression Neural Network

Regression or classification neural networks are frequently used as feature extractors by considering the outputs of intermediate layers [8]. While AEs and principle component analysis generate rather general features describing the most important properties of an input, the intermediate outputs of networks solving particular tasks rather concentrate on features that are problem-specific. In order to generate features that describe the probability of a particular set of clinical parameters to fit in a certain class, in this work, we consider regression to the mean values of the three ROIs (Fig. 2) [6]. The last hidden layer is then used as feature extractor.

3.4   Implementation Details

The neural networks are implemented using PyTorch in a fully-connected manner. The autoencoders contain three encoding and two decoding layers and map the input vectors of length 20 to a latent vector of length 5. In our experiments this length turned out to be optimal, while choosing lengths between 12 (number of modes in PCA) and 5 delivered worse results. The regression neural network features 4 fully-connected layers, whereas the last hidden layer maps the input to a feature length of 5 in a similar manner. An important detail is the augmentation of the inputs and regressed values by adding noise sampled from a normal distribution with standard deviation 0.3. Also, the input parameter vectors were standardized for all experiments. For linear feature encoding principle component analysis is also applied as reference method and to compare it with Deep-Learning-based feature encoding methods (Fig. 3).

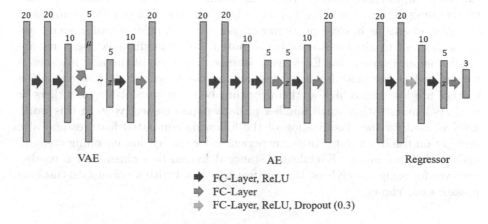

Fig. 3. Architectures of the neural networks. From left to right: VAE, AE, regression network. z denotes the feature encoding layer. For details see the legend on the bottom.

3.5 PCA

In this work, inspired by statistical shape models (SSMs) [3], principal component analysis (PCA) is used for dimensionality reduction and feature encoding of the clinical parameters. PCA is typically applied on discrete shape representations $X_1 \ldots X_n$ of a training dataset, where each representation consists of landmark positions. However, here every X_i is represented by a vector of clinical parameters. The main steps for the feature encoding are the following: 1) Compute the mean vector over all shapes $X_\mu = 1/n \sum_{i=1}^{n} X_i$. 2) Apply PCA: Build a covariance matrix $\mathbf{C} = 1/n \sum_{i=1}^{n} (X_i - X_\mu)(X_i - X_\mu)^T$ and compute its eigenvectors u_p and corresponding eigenvalues λ_p: $X u_p = \lambda_p u_p$. Since the eigenvectors corresponding to the largest eigenvalues describe the main variation in the data, only the first m eigenvectors are used in the following and the rest is omitted. Here, m is chosen to cover 95% of the variability of the training dataset resulting in 12 modes. New forms can now be described using this model as follows $X_{new} = X_\mu + \mathbf{U}c$, where $\mathbf{U} = [u_1 \ldots u_m]$, $c = [c_1 \ldots c_m]^T$ and c_j are coefficients for each eigenvector that can be varied. However, to reconstruct an unseen form X' using $X' = X_\mu + \mathbf{U}c'$, a coefficient vector $c' = \mathbf{U}^T(X' - X_\mu)$ needs to be found. Since those coefficients describe the input vector in an unambiguous dimensionality-reduced manner, they can be used as feature encodings of the clinical parameters.

3.6 KNN Contrast Classification

For the classification of the individual contrast class for CA dose adjustment recommendations the kNN classification was used. The k-Nearest-Neighbour method [4] is an intuitive way to classify previously unseen data. kNN is considered as an instance-based learning algorithm as its learning consist of storing the training data in the feature space. The algorithm assumes that samples of the same classes lie in close proximity of each other. To classify an unseen sample a distance to all stored data is computed. Different distance measures are applicable for example the Euclidean distance. The class of the new instance is determined as the most frequent class among the k nearest data. k should be neither too low or too high as the algorithm becomes susceptible to outliers or neglects classes with a small number of data points respectively. In this work, kNN is used for the classification of the following computed features and also directly on the input data. In our experience, for the feature encoding scenario kNN with $k = 5$ and an Euclidean distance delivered best classification results, however for using the kNN on the raw features $k = 3$ with a correlation distance measure was chosen.

4 Results

The results for the classification are shown in Table 1. All experiments are conducted in a leave-one-out manner and the values are averaged over the different training sets. For evaluation different values are calculated, that take into account the number of true positive (TP), false positive (FP), false negative (FN) and true negative (TN) classifications per class (excessive vs. non-excessive contrast agent).

$$Precision = \frac{TP}{TP+FP}$$

$$Recall = \frac{TP}{TP+FN}$$

$$Accuracy = \frac{TP+TN}{TP+TN+FP+FN}$$

$$F1\text{-}Score = 2\frac{Precision \times Recall}{Precision + Recall}$$

Note that the accuracy measure is the only one considering true negative values (patients are correctly classified as not class-related). For this reason the values for the accuracy might be high even if the precision and recall are considerably poor, e.g. PCA, AE and VAE feature encoding (Table 1). The best feature-encoding results are achieved with the regression method, since this method is more task-related, compared to the autoencoding methods. Interestingly, when using the regression-based features for classification better accuracy and F1-score are achieved compared to applying the rule-based classification to the regressed values. This is due to the fact, that features contain more abstract information and are less affected by noise or other small artifacts and errors.

Overall, the regression-based feature encoding delivers high accuracy and recall with an accent especially on the precision for class 2 (excessive contrast). With a precision of 0.9 the system is in a large proportion of cases capable to rightfully assign class 2, meaning that a recommendation to lower the CA dose can be given without risking a repeated scan due to insufficient image contrast.

Table 1. Comparison of classification results using different feature encoding techniques. From top to bottom: **raw data** - kNN directly on the raw input data vectors; **PCA** - kNN on PCA-extracted features; **Reg-Features** - kNN on features extracted with a regression network; **Reg-Class** - classification of HU values predicted by a regression network; **AE** -kNN on features extracted from the z-space of an autoencoder; **VAE** - kNN on features extracted from the z-space if a variational autoencoder. The measurements are calculated per class (class 1: non-excessive contrast; class 2: excessive contrast).

Method	Accuracy		Precision		Recall		F1-score	
	Class 1	Class 2	Class 1	Class 2	Class 1	Class 2	Class 1	Class 2
Raw data	0.78	0.78	1	0.77	0.15	1	0.26	0.86
PCA	0.73	0.73	0	0.73	0	1	0	0.84
Reg-Features	**0.89**	**0.89**	0.87	**0.90**	**0.72**	0.96	**0.79**	**0.93**
Reg-Class	0.88	0.88	0.92	0.87	0.61	0.98	0.73	0.92
AE	0.73	0.73	0.5	0.75	0.17	0.94	0.30	0.82
VAE	0.70	0.70	0	0.72	0	0.96	0	0.84

5 Discussion and Conclusion

In this work, we aim to establish a case-based reasoning for CTA contrast agent dose based on sets of clinical parameters. We presented different machine learning methods for feature encoding from clinical parameters. Encoded features are used in a kNN-based classification for determining whether a recommendation for using less contrast agent than the standard dose should be made. The feature encoding methods feature (variational) autoencoders a regression neural network and a PCA compared to directly classifying the raw data. Since the regression-based feature encoding is task-based, it delivers the best accuracy (0.89). Autoencoding and PCA-based methods deliver more general features, that cannot be classified with such high accuracy. Even though the used approaches are rather naive, a reliable recommendation can be made based on the regression method. However, the methods of this work will be adapted and improved in future work to enhance the result even more. We will consider a variety of architectural decisions and also a more sophisticated classification method as well as experiments with subsequent feature selection techniques. Future work will also include the exact dose determination based on this first recommendation to adapt the CA dose.

References

1. Andreucci, M., Solomon, R., Tasanarong, A.: Side effects of radiographic contrast media: pathogenesis, risk factors, and prevention. BioMed Res. Int. **2014**, 20 p. (2014). Article number: 741018
2. Becker, C.: Radiologisch praxisrelevante Prophylaxe und Therapie von Nebenwirkungen jodhaltiger Kontrastmittel. Der Radiologe **47**(9) (2007). Article number: 768. https://doi.org/10.1007/s00117-007-1550-4
3. Cootes, T.F., Taylor, C.J., Cooper, D.H., Graham, J.: Active shape models-their training and application. Comput. Vis. Image Underst. **61**(1), 38–59 (1995). https://doi.org/10.1006/cviu.1995.1004
4. Cover, T., Hart, P.: Nearest neighbor pattern classification. IEEE Trans. Inf. Theory **13**(1), 21–27 (1967)
5. Feng, S.T., et al.: An individually optimized protocol of contrast medium injection in enhanced CT scan for liver imaging. Contrast Media Mol. Imaging **2017**, 8 p. (2017). Article number: 7350429
6. Hannan, S.A., Manza, R.R., Ramteke, R.J.: Generalized regression neural network and radial basis function for heart disease diagnosis. Int. J. Comput. Appl. **7**(13), 7–13 (2010). https://doi.org/10.5120/1325-1799
7. Kingma, D., Welling, M.: Auto-encoding variational Bayes, December 2014
8. Lai, Z., Deng, H.: Medical image classification based on deep features extracted by deep model and statistic feature fusion with multilayer perceptron. Comput. Intell. Neurosci. **2018** (2018). https://doi.org/10.1155/2018/2061516
9. Pannu, N., Wiebe, N., Tonelli, M., Network, A.K.D., et al.: Prophylaxis strategies for contrast-induced nephropathy. JAMA **295**(23), 2765–2779 (2006)
10. Rashid, S., Shah, S., Bar-Joseph, Z., Pandya, R.: Dhaka: variational autoencoder for unmasking tumor heterogeneity from single cell genomic data. Bioinformatics (2019)
11. Shakeri, M., Lombaert, H., Tripathi, S., Kadoury, S.: Deep spectral-based shape features for Alzheimer's disease classification. In: Reuter, M., Wachinger, C., Lombaert, H. (eds.) SeSAMI 2016. LNCS, vol. 10126, pp. 15–24. Springer, Cham (2016). https://doi.org/10.1007/978-3-319-51237-2_2
12. Uzunova, H., Schultz, S., Handels, H., Ehrhardt, J.: Unsupervised pathology detection in medical images using conditional variational autoencoders. Int. J. Comput. Assist. Radiol. Surg. **14**(3), 451–461 (2018). https://doi.org/10.1007/s11548-018-1898-0
13. Vasconcelos, R., et al.: Reducing iodine contrast volume in CT angiography of the abdominal aorta using integrated tube potential selection and weight-based method without compromising image quality. Am. J. Roentgenol. **208**(3), 552–563 (2017)
14. Zhang, D., Zou, L., Zhou, X., He, F.: Integrating feature selection and feature extraction methods with deep learning to predict clinical outcome of breast cancer. IEEE Access **6**, 28936–28944 (2018)

COVID-19 Patient Outcome Prediction Using Selected Features from Emergency Department Data and Feed-Forward Neural Networks

Sophie Peacock[1], Mattia Cinelli[1], Frank S. Heldt[1]([✉]),
Lachlan McLachlan[1], Marcela P. Vizcaychipi[2,3], Alex McCarthy[2],
Nadezda Lipunova[1], Robert A. Fletcher[1], Anne Hancock[1], Robert Dürichen[1],
Fernando Andreotti[1], and Rabia T. Khan[1]

[1] Sensyne Health plc, Schrodinger Building, Heatley Road, Oxford Science Park,
Oxford OX4 4GE, UK
stefan.heldt@sensynehealth.com
[2] Chelsea and Westminster Hospital NHS Foundation Trust, 369 Fulham Road,
London SW10 9NH, UK
[3] Academic Department of Anaesthesia and Intensive Care Medicine,
Imperial College London, Chelsea and Westminster Campus, 369 Fulham Road,
London SW10 9NH, UK

Abstract. The severity of COVID-19 varies dramatically, ranging from asymptomatic infection to severe respiratory failure and death. Currently, few prognostic markers for disease outcomes exist, impairing patient triaging and treatment. Here, we train feed-forward neural networks on electronic health records of 819 confirmed SARS-CoV-2 positive patients admitted to a two-site NHS Trust hospital in London, England. To allow early risk assessment, the models ingest data collected in the emergency department (ED) to predict subsequent admission to intensive care, need for mechanical ventilation and in-hospital mortality. We apply univariate selection and recursive feature elimination to find the minimal subset of clinical variables needed for accurate prediction. Our models achieve AUC-ROC scores of 0.78 to 0.87, outperforming standard clinical risk scores. This accuracy is reached with as few as 13% of clinical variables routinely collected within the ED, which increases the practical applicability of such algorithms. Hence, state-of-the-art neural networks can predict severe COVID-19 accurately and early from a small subset of clinical variables.

Keywords: Machine learning · COVID-19 · Electronic health records

J. Ye et al. (Eds.): MobiHealth 2020, LNICST 362, pp. 323–335, 2021.
https://doi.org/10.1007/978-3-030-70569-5_21

1   Introduction

The novel severe acute respiratory syndrome virus 2 (SARS-CoV-2) has caused a pandemic outbreak of COVID-19 and a worldwide public health emergency. As of November 2020, the pandemic has led to more than 60 million confirmed cases and 1.5 million deaths [2]. While most COVID-19 patients have an asymptomatic infection or only suffer mild upper respiratory tract illness, the disease can progress to severe viral pneumonia with acute respiratory distress, respiratory failure and thromboembolic events that can lead to death [17,25,29]. Currently, few predictors for the transition to severe disease are known. However, an early identification of patients at-risk of severe outcomes may allow for faster intervention, improving treatment and therapy success.

The combination of state-of-the-art machine learning (ML) methods with electronic health records (EHRs) promises to predict patient deterioration with high precision [11,26]. Due to the scarcity of COVID-19 EHR data in the public domain, the majority of previous work has focused on statistical analyses or classical ML algorithms. Initial reports noted that factors such as age and underlying comorbidities can have an adverse effect on disease progression [7]. Zhou et al. used logistic regression on data of 191 COVID-19 positive patients to explore the risk factors for acute respiratory distress syndrome [31]. Similarly, Xie et al. applied logistic regression to the data of 299 COVID-19 positive patients to predict mortality [27]. Yan et al. [28] utilised XGBoost and EHR data of 375 COVID-19 patients in Wuhan, China to predict deterioration to a critical condition. While such studies provide insights into potential risk factors for severe COVID-19, most were conducted with limited patient numbers and data taken from both the patient's historical record and from throughout the current hospital admission [16,20,31]. The latter impairs an application to early patient triaging since, at the time of hospital presentation, the full EHR is rarely available. This problem is addressed by Jiang et al. [15] who applied ML methods to data available at the point of admission to hospital. However, with a sample size of just 53 patients the power of this study was limited.

Already prior to the COVID-19 pandemic, traditional risk scores were widely used in clinical practise to assess patient deterioration. Jones et al. explored the use of the sequential organ failure assessment (SOFA) score in combination with ML methods to forecast poor patient outcomes [16]. Using data collected from 248 patients over 2 years, they were able to predict in-hospital mortality by applying logistic regression to SOFA scores. Similarly, Scott et al. [21] have adopted the national early warning score (NEWS2) to predict the clinical outcome of patients. Yet, it remains unclear whether SOFA, NEWS2 or other similar clinical risk scores can be applied to COVID-19 patients.

A major obstacle to early patient triaging is the minimum number of clinical variables and, hence physiological tests, required to assess whether a patient is at risk. Feature selection methods, routinely applied in ML model development [4], can provide such a reduced feature set, retaining only the most informative clinical variables. Guyon and Elisseeff [12] introduce a number of methods which can be used to retain relevant information in a data set while reducing the number of features. These methods can be split into filter, wrapper and embedded methods. Both filter and wrapper methods were previously used by Pourhomayoun and Shakibi [20] when predicting mortality in COVID-19 patients. In addition, Yan et al. used simple feature importance metrics to perform feature selection for predicting deterioration to a critical condition in COVID-19 patients [28].

We propose to use feed-forward neural networks to extract non-linear interactions between clinical variables and predict whether patients will deteriorate to severe COVID-19. We define deterioration to severe COVID-19 by three endpoints: admission to an adult intensive care unit (AICU), a need for mechanical ventilation, and in-hospital mortality. We perform feature selection to identify a minimal subset of clinical features that allows patient stratification and compare these subsets between endpoints. To facilitate early risk assessment, we focus our analysis on data available during a patient's emergency department (ED) visit at a hospital. Hence, the main contributions of this work are three-fold: 1. Early prediction of COVID-19 patients' risk to deteriorate to one of three clinical endpoints using neural networks; 2. evaluation of prediction performance over classical clinical risk scores; and 3. exploration of the minimal set of clinical features required for accurate patient stratification.

2 Methods

2.1 Data

Anonymised patient EHRs have been collected from a two-site NHS Trust hospital in London between January 1st and April 23rd 2020. All data were supplied according to internal information governance review, NHS Trust information governance approval, and General Data Protection Regulation (GDPR) procedures outlined under the Strategic Research Agreement (SRA) and relative Data Sharing Agreements (DSAs) signed by the NHS Trust and ourselves on 25th July 2018.

We analysed data from adult patients aged 18 to 100 and confirmed SARS-CoV-2 positive, as determined by quantitative reverse-transcription PCR (qRT-PCR). A total of 96 clinical features have been collected in the study, including patient demographics, vital signs, laboratory measurements and clinical observations. Of these 96 features, those with a coverage of at least 5% were retained. These 64 features are listed in the appendix in Table 3. Observations with multiple values were aggregated using the minimum, maximum, mean and last observation values to avoid biasing models on the number of test results. However, for blood test results typically only a single measurement is available within the ED stay of a patient, such that there is no distinction between the four aggregated values.

2.2 Cohort Definition

Study parameters included EHRs of 3229 patients. The data were filtered to include patients with confirmed SARS-CoV-2 infection (1158 patients), recorded emergency department admission and subsequent ward stay, and their latest hospital admission being in 2020.

The patients were assigned in three cohorts (see Table 1): *Cohort A* was used to predict AICU admission. This cohort was divided into target patients who were admitted to an AICU at any time during their hospital stay, and control patients who were not. In the mechanical ventilation *Cohort B*, patients without clear information on oxygen supply were excluded; target patients required invasive mechanical ventilation, while control patients are those who required no or only minimal breathing assistance. For the mortality *Cohort C*, patients deceased during hospitalisation were considered target and discharged patients are included in the control group. Patients still hospitalised at the moment of study or deceased after hospitalisation were not considered.

Table 1. Patient numbers in study cohorts.

	COHORT A (AICU)	COHORT B (VENTILATION)	COHORT C (MORTALITY)
PATIENTS	819	818	508
TARGET	126 (15%)	62 (8%)	170 (33%)
CONTROL	693 (85%)	756 (92%)	338 (67%)

2.3   Prediction Algorithms

EHR data from ED visits were used as inputs to a feed-forward neural network to predict patient outcomes. Hyper-parameter optimisation was carried out using Bayesian optimisation with Gaussian process as surrogate model using Keras Tuner [19]. Optimisation parameters included the number of fully connected hidden layers ($n_{layers} \in [0,5]$) with ReLU activation functions containing a number of neurons per layer ($n_{neurons} \in [2,96]$), before a single-neuron output layer with sigmoid activation. Batch normalisation with a batch size of six and dropout rate ($d \in [0,0.5]$) were used after each hidden layer. Training used an Adam optimiser with binary cross-entropy loss and optimised learning rate ($n_{lr} \in [1e^{-4}, 1e^{-2}]$), for 100 epochs with early stopping. Optimisation was performed using the loss on the validation set from a nested stratified 80%/20% training/validation split derived from the training set of a 3-fold cross validation and the mean configuration was chosen (Table 4).

Prior to model training, features with less than 5% coverage were removed, missing values were imputed with a fixed value of -1 and the data were normalised using standard normalisation. Due to the large class imbalance, the minority class was oversampled using SMOTE [5].

The performance of ML algorithms was measured against the performance of the SOFA [18,23] and NEWS2 [1] scores, which are commonly used in clinical practice. The SOFA score was developed to evaluate morbidity in relation to organ dysfunction in critically ill patients [18,22]. Successive analyses have shown that SOFA scores are good indicators of prognosis [9,23]. The NEWS2 score aims to be a valid indicator of the patient's well-being at an early stage of their hospitalisation. Less frequently it is used as predictor of patient outcome [8]. In our analysis we use the maximum SOFA and NEWS2 score for each patient while in the Emergency Department. Where data are missing, zero points are added to each score.

2.4   Model Validation

Stratified 3-fold cross validation was used in the training and evaluation of the neural network models. Performance of the models is reported as area under the curve (AUC) of the receiver operating characteristic (ROC). The variability across folds provides a measure of model stability. Since the SOFA and NEWS2 scores are deterministic, 3-fold cross validation was not carried out. For these models we measure performance by the AUC-ROC.

2.5   Feature Selection

Due to the large number of features, such as laboratory results, we expect a large amount of redundant information. We therefore apply feature selection methods to find the minimal subset of clinical features that reliably predicts each endpoint. This feature subset allows accurate predictions and easy application in real-world settings where data may be sparse. Dimensionality reduction techniques similar to Principal Components Analysis were not implemented. Although these methods would create a smaller set of features, measurements from all parameters would still be required and therefore these techniques are not beneficial in practice.

Two feature selection methods were considered [12]. First, we applied univariate selection, a filter method in which the number of features to keep is specified. The dependency between each feature and the target output was calculated using mutual information [3]. The most important features according to mutual information were retained. We also considered recursive feature elimination (RFE), a wrapper method which starts with all of the features and repeats a process of eliminating the least informative features until only a set number of features remains [13]. A neural network was trained on each data set and permutation feature importances were used to determine which features to discard in each round [10].

Feature selection was performed on the training set of each of the cross validation folds in order to obtain a feature list containing a specified number of features. For each feature selection method a grid-search was carried out to determine the optimal number of features to keep within the folds. The feature list was then used to train a model and make predictions. The feature lists presented in the appendix in Table 5 contain the union of the three feature lists obtained from each cross validation fold. Optimality was determined by AUC of ROC curve of the models obtained from the three cross validation folds for each endpoint.

3 Results

In the following, we first present baseline model performance when predicting three clinical endpoints for COVID-19 patients. The minimal subset of features for each endpoint is shown in the appendix (Table 5).

3.1 Neural Network Performance

Figure 1 and Table 2 show that the neural network with no feature selection outperforms both the SOFA and NEWS2 scores by a large margin when predicting AICU admission and mechanical ventilation. This is expected as the network is able to model complex relationships between multiple features and non-linear interactions. The difference in performance between our neural network and traditional scores is most pronounced when predicting a need for mechanical ventilation. In predicting mortality, the SOFA score performance shows a significant increase, while that of the neural network does not. Since the SOFA score was developed to evaluate morbidity this is to be expected [23]. The neural network model reaches an AUC of 0.73 when predicting mortality. While the model outperforms the NEWS2 score, it is not able to achieve a better result than prediction based on SOFA, which has an AUC of 0.75.

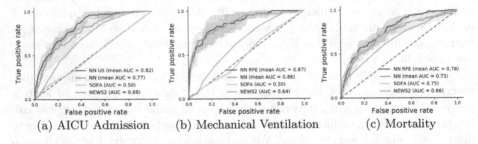

(a) AICU Admission   (b) Mechanical Ventilation   (c) Mortality

Fig. 1. Prediction performance for clinical endpoints. ROC curves of the neural network without (NN) and with feature elimination (NN RFE/NN US) and for SOFA and NEWS2. Solid lines and shaded areas indicate the mean and standard deviation across cross-validation folds, respectively. Dashed line indicates a random classifier.

3.2 Performance with Feature Selection

Next, we use feature selection to identify the minimal subset of clinical variables required for accurate predictions. Overall, univariate feature selection performs best for predicting AICU admission, while RFE is best for predicting a need for mechanical ventilation and in-hospital mortality (see Table 2). Figure 2 shows the model performance over successively reduced feature sets, using univariate selection for AICU admission and RFE for the other two endpoints.

When predicting AICU admission the optimal number of features to keep is 10 in each cross validation fold (see Fig. 2a); the list of retained features across

Table 2. Predictive performance (AUC) for all endpoints. NN, neural network; US, univariate selection; RFE, recursive feature elimination. Standard deviation across cross validation folds is shown in brackets for NN models.

	COHORT A (AICU)	COHORT B (VENTILATION)	COHORT C (MORTALITY)
SOFA	0.50	0.50	0.75
NEWS2	0.68	0.64	0.66
NN	0.77 (0.060)	0.86 (0.056)	0.73 (0.057)
NN + US	**0.82 (0.032)**	0.84 (0.047)	0.77 (0.035)
NN + RFE	0.78 (0.053)	**0.87 (0.054)**	**0.78 (0.035)**

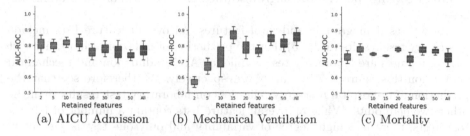

(a) AICU Admission   (b) Mechanical Ventilation   (c) Mortality

Fig. 2. Prediction performance for feature sets of varying size. Boxes indicate AUC-ROC over cross-validation folds using univariate selection (a) and RFE (b, c), with the median marked by the orange lines and interquartile range by box edges.

all folds is included in the appendix in Table 5. By using univariate selection we achieve a significant increase in AUC of 5%.

As can be seen in Fig. 2b, for Cohort B the best performance is achieved by RFE using 15 features in each cross validation fold. The features used across all folds are listed in Table 5. This model achieves an AUC of 0.87, an improvement of just 1% over the neural network with no feature selection, potentially due to the baseline performance without feature selection already being high for this endpoint.

For prediction of in-hospital mortality, predictive performance of 0.78 AUC is attained using RFE with 5 features in each fold. The features used across all folds for predicting in-hospital mortality are shown in Table 5. The ROC curve for this model (Fig. 1c) shows an improvement in the AUC of 5%. This increase in performance allows the neural network with RFE to outperform the SOFA score by 3%.

The number of features in the optimal feature subset varies across the endpoints. When predicting AICU admission a large improvement in performance is gained by using a small feature list of just 10 features in each cross validation fold (25 unique features across all folds). Using 15 features per fold (36 overall) when predicting a need for mechanical ventilation leads to an improvement in predictive performance of just 1%. An improvement of 5% is also achieved through the retention of just 5 features per fold (10 overall) for predicting in-hospital mortality. This improvement is especially significant as it enables the neural network model to outperform the SOFA score.

For all endpoints the overall feature list includes age and respiratory rate (Table 5). Markers of ethnicity are present for the prediction of a need for mechanical ventilation and in-hospital mortality. Vital sign measurements concerning temperature and fraction of inspired oxygen (FiO_2) are present for prediction of AICU admission and mechanical ventilation, while heart rate is retained for mechanical ventilation and in-hospital mortality. Although most of these features have very high coverage (both temperature and heart rate are above 99%), they are not consistently retained for all endpoints. A feature which has 100% coverage but is surprisingly discarded for prediction of AICU admission is sex.

As well as demographic and vital features, all overall feature lists include laboratory test results (Table 5). For the prediction of in-hospital mortality just 30% of features are laboratory tests, while for AICU admission and mechanical ventilation this figure is 72% and 61% respectively. We therefore see that the prediction of in-hospital mortality relies less on laboratory test results than the other two endpoints. While all overall feature lists contain a number of laboratory tests, there is a high degree of variability and only one test is present in all three feature lists - blood amylase. Various other laboratory tests are present for prediction of both AICU admission and mechanical ventilation; bicarbonate, creatinine, blood lactate, oxygen partial pressure, blood potassium and different forms of haemoglobin. Some of these laboratory tests, such as bicarbonate, oxygen partial pressure and blood lactate, have coverage of around 27%, but are retained over tests such as blood white cells or blood monocyte count, which have coverage of 84% but are not included in any of the three overall feature lists.

4   Discussion

This work was motivated by the need to predict whether patients deteriorate to severe COVID-19 early during their hospital stay and to provide clinicians with a minimal subset of clinical features which allow risk prediction. To address these points, we trained neural network models which use EHR data from COVID-19 patients' ED admissions to predict one of three endpoints: admission to AICU, need for mechanical ventilation, and in-hospital mortality. We have shown that feed-forward neural networks can achieve better predictive performance on the first two endpoints than traditional risk scores. Neural networks without feature selection were not able to outperform the SOFA score for predicting in-hospital mortality, possibly due to the SOFA score being developed to predict morbidity. Implementing feature selection using univariate selection and RFE enabled us to identify the minimal subset of clinical features required for early risk assessment of COVID-19 patients. For AICU admission, need for mechanical ventilation and in-hospital mortality, performance was improved by 5%, 1% and 5% respectively. For predicting in-hospital mortality, feature selection allowed us to achieve a predictive performance 3% higher than that of the SOFA score.

Aside from an improvement in predictive performance, a model requiring fewer features is extremely beneficial in its applicability to real-world scenarios. A significantly reduced set of required inputs means that the model can be applied in settings where data may be sparse and not all of the original features are available. Having to collect fewer data points in order to make a prediction increases the accessibility of the model and allows clinicians to prioritise testing.

The predictive performance achieved by our neural network models is comparable to previous work using an XGBoost model [14]. Feature selection methods are employed by Pourhomayoun and Shakibi [20] to reduce their feature set from 112 to 42 features, although they do not also present results for models trained using the entire feature set. Our findings that age and indicators of oxygenation status always remain in the final feature set are consistent with this work. Age in particular is consistently found to be an important feature in previous works [27,31]. Conversely, our finding that sex is not retained for prediction of AICU admission differs from previous works [24,30].

While laboratory test results are included in the feature list for all endpoints, there is not a large degree of consensus regarding which tests are most informative. Our finding that features relating to haemoglobin are retained for two out of three endpoints are consistent with those of Jiang et al. [15]. A surprising finding of this work which may invite further analysis is the absence of heart rate in the overall feature list for prediction of AICU admission, and of FiO_2 and temperature for predicting in-hospital mortality. Temperature in particular is a common indicator for severe viral infection [6].

Taken together, our analysis and previous studies suggest that patient age, demographic information and measures of oxygenation status, such as respiratory rate and FiO_2 level, are primary indicators of poor outcomes in COVID-19 patients. Prioritising the measurement and clinical assessment of these variables may improve early patient triaging.

This work uses EHR data captured during a patient's ED visit. While this more accurately reflects the data available in practice, it may well limit the performance of our models. Augmenting the data set with patients' medical history may be beneficial, particularly in predicting mortality where a patient's chance of survival may be heavily influenced by their comorbidities and other medical history. While our data set is comparatively large in relation to previous COVID-19 studies [27,29], further improvements could be made with access to more data. Longitudinal data from other hospitals in different locations could improve the generalisability of our models. A significantly larger data set would also make it feasible to train more complex, deeper neural networks which may achieve higher prediction performance. One future approach to overcome data availability issues is the use of transfer learning on other respiratory diseases or multi-task learning on several clinical endpoints simultaneously.

In conclusion, our models show that state-of-the-art neural networks can predict severe COVID-19 accurately from sparse, clinical data. Importantly, we are able to produce a minimal subset of clinical variables required for early risk assessment of COVID-19 patients. Models trained on this minimal subset of features can be used by clinicians with limited data available to them to stratify patients into risk groups.

Acknowledgments. This work uses data collected from patients by the NHS as part of their care and support. Thus, we would like to thank all those involved for their contribution. Special thanks are due to the Chelsea and Westminster NHS Foundation Trust COVID-19 AICU Consortium, comprising all critical care personnel who were part of the delivery of care during the COVID-19 pandemic.

A   Clinical Features

Table 3 contains all clinical features with over 5% coverage.

Table 3. All clinical features with at least 5% coverage

Age	Blood Glucose
Ethnicity	Blood Haematocrit
Sex	Blood Haemoglobin
FiO$_2$ level POC	Blood Lactate
Heart Rate	Blood Lactate Dehydrogenase Level
Respiratory Rate	Blood Lymphocyte Count
Temperature	Blood Magnesium
Blood Activated Partial Thromboplastin Time	Blood Mean Corpuscular Haemoglobin Concentration
Blood Adjusted Calcium	Blood Mean Corpuscular Haemoglobin
Blood Alanine Aminotransferase	Blood Mean Corpuscular Volume
Blood Albumin	Blood Mean Platelet Volume
Blood Alkaline Phosphatase	Blood Methaemoglobin
Blood Amylase	Blood Monocyte Count
Blood Anion Gap	Blood Neutrophil Count
Blood Base Excess	Blood Nucleated Red Blood Cell Count
Blood Basophil Count	Blood Oxygen PO$_2$ Partial Pressure
Blood Bicarbonate	Blood Oxyhaemoglobin
Blood Bilirubin Total	Blood pH
Blood C Reactive Protein	Blood Phosphate
Blood Calcium	Blood Platelet Count
Blood Calcium Ionised	Blood Potassium
Blood Carboxyhaemoglobin	Blood Prothrombin Time
Blood Chloride	Blood Red Blood Cell Count
Blood Cortisol	Blood Red Cell Distribution Width
Blood Creatine Kinase	Blood Sodium
Blood Creatinine	Blood Thyroid Stimulating Hormone
Blood D Dimer	Blood Thyroxine T4
Blood Deoxyhaemoglobin	Blood Total Protein
Blood Eosinophil Count	Blood Troponin T
Blood Ferritin	Blood Urea
Blood Fibrinogen	Blood White Cells
Blood Globulin	Brain Natriuretic Peptide

B   Model Hyper-parameters

Table 4 contains the optimal model hyper-parameters for each endpoint.

Table 4. Optimal model hyper-parameters for each endpoint.

	COHORT A (AICU)	COHORT B (VENTILATION)	COHORT C (MORTALITY)
HIDDEN LAYERS	2	3	2
NEURONS PER LAYER	31	35	28
DROPOUT RATE	0.12	0.30	0.26
LEARNING RATE	0.002	0.005	0.002

C   Feature Lists

Table 5 contains the features retained in the final trained models for predicting each endpoint. This list is the union of the features retained over the three cross validation folds for each endpoint.

Table 5. Overall features retained for each endpoint

AICU admission	Mechanical ventilation	Mortality
Age	Age	Age
Last alanine aminotransferase	Eth black african	Eth asian indian
Last amylase	Eth black caribbean	Eth asian pakistani
Last bicarbonate	Eth other chinese	Eth black other
Last blood ldh level	Eth unknown	Max amylase
Last nucleated red blood cell count	Eth white other	Max heart rate
Last oxyhaemoglobin	Last amylase	Mean blood ferritin
Last respiratory rate	Last blood lactate	Mean respiratory rate
Max anion gap	Last blood potassium	Min blood bilirubin total
Max blood ldh level	Last blood mean corpuscular haemoglobin mch	Sex
Max blood phosphate	Last deoxyhaemoglobin	
Max creatinine	Last FiO$_2$ level	
Max FiO$_2$ level	Last haemoglobin	
Max oxygen partial pressure	Last MCHC	
Max red blood cell width	Last mean platelet volume	
Max respiratory rate	Last respiratory rate	
Max temperature	Max amylase	
Mean alanine aminotransferase	Max carboxyhaemoglobin	
Mean blood lactate	Max FiO$_2$ level	
Mean blood ldh level	Max mean platelet volume	
Mean blood potassium	Max respiratory rate	
Mean fibrinogen	Max temperature	
Mean FiO$_2$ level	Mean blood magnesium	
Mean respiratory rate	Mean blood urea	
Min blood ldh level	Mean blood total protein	
	Mean FiO$_2$ level	
	Mean lymphocyte count	
	Mean MCHC	
	Min bicarbonate	
	Min creatinine	
	Min deoxyhaemoglobin	
	Min haemoglobin	
	Min heart rate	
	Min mean platelet volume	
	Min oxygen partial pressure	
	Sex	

References

1. National early warning score (news) 2, April 2020. https://www.rcplondon.ac.uk/projects/outputs/national-early-warning-score-news-2
2. Situation update worldwide, as of 16 July 2020 (2020). https://www.ecdc.europa.eu/en/geographical-distribution-2019-ncov-cases. Accessed 16 July 2020
3. Blum, A., Langley, P.: Selection of relevant features and examples in machine learning. Artif. Intell. **97**, 245–271 (1997)
4. Chandrashekar, G., Sahin, F.: A survey on feature selection methods. Comput. Electr. Eng. **40**(1), 16–28 (2014)
5. Chawla, N.V., Bowyer, K.W., Hall, L.O., Kegelmeyer, W.P.: SMOTE: synthetic minority over-sampling technique. J. Artif. Intell. Res. **16**, 321–357 (2002)
6. Chen, J., et al.: Clinical progression of patients with COVID-19 in Shanghai, China. J. Infect. **80**(5), e1–e6 (2020)
7. Chen, T., et al.: Clinical characteristics of 113 deceased patients with coronavirus disease 2019: retrospective study. BMJ **368**, m1091 (2020)
8. Churpek, M.M., et al.: Quick sepsis-related organ failure assessment, systemic inflammatory response syndrome, and early warning scores for detecting clinical deterioration in infected patients outside the intensive care unit. Am. J. Respir. Crit. Care Med. **195**(7), 906–911 (2017)
9. Ferreira, F.L., Bota, D.P., Bross, A., Mélot, C., Vincent, J.L.: Serial evaluation of the SOFA score to predict outcome in critically ill patients. JAMA **286**(14), 1754–1758 (2001)
10. Fisher, A., Rudin, C., Dominici, F.: All models are wrong, but many are useful: learning a variable's importance by studying an entire class of prediction models simultaneously. J. Mach. Learn. Res. **20**(177), 1–81 (2019)
11. Goldstein, B.A., Navar, A.M., Pencina, M.J., Ioannidis, J.: Opportunities and challenges in developing risk prediction models with electronic health records data: a systematic review. J. Am. Med. Inform. Assoc. **24**(1), 198–208 (2017)
12. Guyon, I.: An introduction to variable and feature selection. J. Mach. Learn. Res. **3**, 1157–1182 (2003)
13. Guyon, I., Weston, J., Barnhill, S., Vapnik, V.: Gene selection for cancer classification using support vector machines. Mach. Learn. **46**(1–3), 389–422 (2002). https://doi.org/10.1023/A:1012487302797
14. Heldt, F.S., et al.: Early risk assessment for COVID-19 patients from emergency department data using machine learning. medRxiv (2020)
15. Jiang, X., et al.: Towards an artificial intelligence framework for data-driven prediction of coronavirus clinical severity. Comput. Mater. Continua **63**(1), 537–551 (2020)
16. Jones, A.E., Trzeciak, S., Kline, J.A.: The Sequential Organ Failure Assessment score for predicting outcome in patients with severe sepsis and evidence of hypoperfusion at the time of emergency department presentation. Crit. Care Med. **37**(5), 1649–1654 (2009)
17. Klok, F.A., et al.: Incidence of thrombotic complications in critically ill ICU patients with COVID-19. Thromb. Res. **191**, 145–147 (2020)
18. Lambden, S., Laterre, P.F., Levy, M.M., Francois, B.: The SOFA score-development, utility and challenges of accurate assessment in clinical trials. Crit. Care **23**(1) (2019). Article number: 374
19. O'Malley, T., Bursztein, E., Long, J., Chollet, F., Jin, H., Invernizzi, L., et al.: Keras Tuner (2019). https://github.com/keras-team/keras-tuner

20. Pourhomayoun, M., Shakibi, M.: Predicting mortality risk in patients with COVID-19 using artificial intelligence to help medical decision-making. medRxiv (2020)
21. Scott, L.J., Redmond, N.M., Tavaré, A., Little, H., Srivastava, S., Pullyblank, A.: Association between national early warning scores in primary care and clinical outcomes: an observational study in UK primary and secondary care. Br. J. Gen. Pract. **70**(695), e374–e380 (2020)
22. Soo, A., et al.: Describing organ dysfunction in the intensive care unit: a cohort study of 20,000 patients. Crit. Care **23**(1), 186 (2019)
23. Vincent, J.L., et al.: The SOFA (Sepsis-related Organ Failure Assessment) score to describe organ dysfunction/failure. Intensive Care Med. **22**(7), 707–710 (1996). On behalf of the Working Group on Sepsis-Related Problems of the European Society of Intensive Care Medicine
24. Wang, D., et al.: Clinical characteristics of 138 hospitalized patients with 2019 novel coronavirus-infected pneumonia in Wuhan, China. JAMA **323**(11), 1061–1069 (2020)
25. Wu, Z., McGoogan, J.M.: Characteristics of and important lessons from the coronavirus disease 2019 (COVID-19) outbreak in China: summary of a report of 72 314 cases from the Chinese center for disease control and prevention. JAMA **323**(13), 1239–1242 (2020)
26. Wynants, L., et al.: Prediction models for diagnosis and prognosis of COVID-19 infection: systematic review and critical appraisal. BMJ **369**, m1328 (2020)
27. Xie, J., et al.: Development and external validation of a prognostic multivariable model on admission for hospitalized patients with COVID-19 (2020)
28. Yan, L., et al.: Prediction of criticality in patients with severe COVID-19 infection using three clinical features: a machine learning-based prognostic model with clinical data in Wuhan. MedRxiv (2020)
29. Yang, X., et al.: Clinical course and outcomes of critically ill patients with SARS-CoV-2 pneumonia in Wuhan, China: a single-centered, retrospective, observational study. Lancet Respir. Med. **8**(5), 475–481 (2020)
30. Zheng, Z., et al.: Risk factors of critical & mortal COVID-19 cases: a systematic literature review and meta-analysis. J. Infect. **81**(2), e16–e25 (2020)
31. Zhou, F., et al.: Clinical course and risk factors for mortality of adult inpatients with COVID-19 in Wuhan, China: a retrospective cohort study. The Lancet **395**, 1054–1062 (2020)

EAI International Workshop on Digital Healthcare Technologies for the Global South

Validation of Omron Wearable Blood Pressure Monitor HeartGuide™ in Free-Living Environments

Zilu Liang[1](✉)[ID] and Mario Alberto Chapa-Martell[2][ID]

[1] Kyoto University of Advanced Science (KUAS), Kyoto 615-8577, Japan
liang.zilu@kuas.ac.jp
[2] Silver Egg Technology, Osaka, Japan
mchapam0300@gmail.com

Abstract. Hypertension is one of the most common health conditions in modern society. Accurate blood pressure monitoring in free-living conditions is important for the precise diagnosis and management of hypertension. In tandem with the advances in wearable and ubiquitous technologies, a medical-grade wearable blood pressure monitor–Omron HeartGuide™ wristwatch–has recently entered the consumer market. It uses the same mechanism as the upper arm blood pressure monitors and has been calibrated in laboratory settings. Nevertheless, its accuracy "in the wild" has not been investigated. This study aims to investigate the accuracy of the HeartGuide™ against a medical-grade upper arm blood pressure monitor HEM-1022 in free-living environments. Analysis results suggest that the HeartGuide™ significantly underestimated systolic pressure and diastolic pressure by an average of 16 mmHg and 6 mmHg respectively. Lower discrepancy between the two devices on diastolic pressure was observed when diastolic pressure increased. In addition, the two devices agreed well on heart rate readings. We also found that device accuracy was related to systolic pressure, heart rate, body temperature and ambient temperature, but was not related salivary cortisol level, diastolic pressure, ambient humidity and air pressure.

Keywords: Personal informatics · Consumer wearables · Blood pressure · Quantified self

1 Introduction

Hypertension is the biggest risk factor for cardiovascular diseases and other health conditions from kidney problems to respiratory disorders [1,2]. The rate of hypertension rose substantially in the past three decades and deaths associated with hypertension also increased [3]. The American Heart Association recommends self-monitoring for all people with high blood pressure. Previous meta-analyses have shown that self-monitoring can improve blood pressure control and is an increasing common part of hypertension management [4,5].

© ICST Institute for Computer Sciences, Social Informatics and Telecommunications Engineering 2021
Published by Springer Nature Switzerland AG 2021. All Rights Reserved
J. Ye et al. (Eds.): MobiHealth 2020, LNICST 362, pp. 339–350, 2021.
https://doi.org/10.1007/978-3-030-70569-5_22

Such monitoring can help the healthcare provider determine the effectiveness of treatment and can be accompanied by additional support from doctors [6].

Self-monitoring on blood pressure can also enable more precise diagnosis of hypertension. Blood pressure fluctuate during the course of a day [7]. Office blood pressure–the one blood pressure measurement when people visit a clinic–is a snapshot that only tells the blood pressure at the moment of the measurement. Such snapshots may lead to false positive (e.g., "white coat hypertension" [8]) and false negative (e.g., "masked hypertension" [9]) in diagnosis. On the flip side, a record of readings taken over time provides a "time-lapse" picture of blood pressure fluctuations. Such information, with clinical accuracy, can generate powerful insights into heart health, help predict the onset of cardiovascular diseases and guide proper medication on hypertension [10,11]. Hence, the 2015 U.S. Preventive Services Task Force (USPSTF) report recommended around-the-clock blood pressure monitoring as the preferred method for screening hypertension and predicting cardiovascular disease risk [12].

To this end, accurate monitoring of blood pressure in free-living environment is critical for hypertension diagnosis and management. Many digital home blood pressure monitors have been developed in recent years. These devices leverage the oscillometric method for measuring systolic and diastolic blood pressure, and can be either worn on wrist or upper arm. Despite of their affordability and convenience, the portability of these devices is still limited. For example, a user will not be able to measure blood pressure using her home digital upper arm monitor when she is in workplace or during outdoor activities. It was not until last year the first medical-grade wearable blood pressure monitor–the Omron HeartGuide™ wristwatch–entered the consumer market. The HeartGuide™ combines oscillometric method and wearable technology to achieve both accuracy and convenience.

The HeartGuide™ has been validated in laboratory settings and achieved good agreement with sphygmomanometer (deviation within ±5 mmHg). Nevertheless, its accuracy in free-living environment is yet unclear. Previous validation studies on consumer wearable wristbands indicate that device accuracy is often compromised in free-living environment where users operation on the device is unconstrained. Therefore, the objective of this study is to investigate the accuracy of the HeartGuide™ against medical-grade upper arm blood pressure monitor. We also explore what factors may be associated to device accuracy.

2   Related Work

2.1   Blood Pressure Monitoring

Blood pressure refers to the pressure of circulating blood against the walls of the large arteries and is usually expressed in the terms of the systolic pressure over diastolic pressure. Blood pressure can vary throughout a day and normally shows a circadian rhythm over a 24-h period [7]. Blood pressure also changes in response to stress, diet, exercise, changes in posture, and smoking [7]. Hypertension occurs when the force against blood vessel walls becomes too high.

High blood pressure may come with no perceivable symptoms and is thus called "the silent killer". However, in the long run, chronic hypertension may can lead to serious health problems like heart attack and stroke [1,13,14]. In addition, blood pressure variability also has prognostic significance for cardiovascular complications [10,11].

Conventional blood pressure measurement in clinical settings uses a sphygmomanometer. A cuff fits over the upper arm and inflates, constricting the arteries. When the air is released, the first sound detected with a stethoscope is the systolic pressure. The silence that follows marks the diastolic pressure. Blood pressure readings obtained in clinics or hospitals are called office blood pressure. These readings only represent snapshots of blood pressure at the time of the clinic visits and are not sufficient to provide a holistic view of how blood pressure may fluctuate at different time of a day. For example, morning hypertension may not be diagnosed using office blood pressure. Moreover, in some cases high office blood pressure may not be pathological but rather due to nervousness during clinic visits. The likelihood of false positive and false negative of office blood pressure demands alternative ambulatory blood pressure measuring technologies that can be used in free-living environment.

Many portable and affordable consumer blood pressure monitors have been developed for home use. These devices largely fall into two categories: upper arm monitors and wrist monitors. An upper arm blood pressure monitor usually consists of a pre-formed cuffs and a digital screen. The measurement process is automated and users only need to press a start button. The advantage of upper arm type is that the cuff naturally rests at the same level as heart, saving the trouble of adjusting device placement and the posture during measuring. Wrist blood pressure monitors are devices that worn on the wrist. Wrist monitors are less bulk and more portable, and they are also ideal for people with arm mobility limitations. Many of these devices use the oscillometric method for simplicity and reliability, but motion artifact is considered a major drawback of this method [15,16].

2.2   Quantified Self and Consumer Wearables

The Quantified Self has become a popular everyday practice where people use digital devices and smartphone apps to gather real-time physiological, behavioral and emotional data from themselves [26]. The purpose of the self-tracking practices ranges from obtaining self-knowledge [17,18], improving productivity [19], preventing diseases [20], to managing health condition [21].

The Quantified Self phenomenon has attracted burgeoning interdisciplinary research interest. An extensive range of digital devices and apps have been developed to support self-tracking on physical fitness (e.g., Fitbit activity tracker), mental status (e.g., MUSE medication headband, Happify app), sleep (e.g., Neuroon eye mask, SleepAsAndroid app) and other dimensions of their bodies and lives. A growing body of research has investigated the accuracy of self-tracking technologies [22,23], how people interact with these technologies [24], and how people make sense of their data [18], and the obstacles for self-tracking technologies to make real-world impact [25].

A variety of wearable activity and sleep tracking devices have exist in the consumer market for a while. The development of wearable blood pressure monitor has somewhat lagged behind other types of wearable. It was not until last year that the first wearable blood pressure monitor–the Omron HeartGuide^{TM}– entered the consumer market. The HeartGuide^{TM} is a medical-grade blood pressure monitor in the shape of a wristwatch. It miniaturizes the components of traditional oscillometric measurement and uses an inflatable cuff within the watch band to take blood pressure readings. HeartGuide^{TM} also has the functions of tracking steps, distance, calories burned and sleep as well as setting daily reminders and getting notifications, so that it allows users to explore how lifestyle directly may be associated to heart health. Nevertheless, the device is more bulky compared to activity tracker that offer the same set of lifestyle tracking functions (e.g., Fitbit, Mi Band). Despite of being validated in laboratory settings, it remains unclear whether the HeartGuide^{TM} can produce accurate readings in the wild. Hence, this paper set out to validate HeartGuide^{TM} in free-living environments.

3   Methodology

3.1   Devices

To validate the accuracy of the HeartGuide^{TM} wristwatch, we compare its readings with a medical-grade upper arm blood pressure monitor Omron HEM-1022. Both devices uses the clinically validated oscillometric method to measure blood pressure.

The appearance of an HeartGuide^{TM} is depicted in Fig. 1. The major difference between HeartGuide^{TM} and other smart watches or activity tracker is the cuff below the wristband. One measurement takes 30 s. After completing the measurement, users can view the latest reading on the display of the HeartGuide^{TM} watch. The battery lasts for approximately 2 days after a full charge. The device can store up to 100 blood pressure readings. The HeartGuide^{TM} can be used in tandem with the HeartAdviser smartphone app. Figure 2 shows two screenshots HeartAdviser's dashboard. The blood pressure values are color-coded, with green and red representing safe and high blood pressure respectively. Users can compare the latest readings with previous readings or observe patterns and trends in historical data.

3.2   Data Collection Protocol

We measure blood pressure simultaneously using an HeartGuide^{TM} and an upper arm blood pressure monitor HEM-1022. All devices were made available in participants' homes. Participants were instructed to use both devices correctly.

The HeartGuide^{TM} wristwatch is worn on the left wrist, while the upper arm blood pressure monitor is used on the right arm. Participants were asked

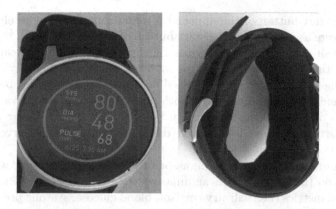

Fig. 1. An Omron wearable blood pressure monitor HeartGuide™. Left: blood pressure and heart rate readings on the display. Right: the wristband contains a cuff that will be inflated during a measurement.

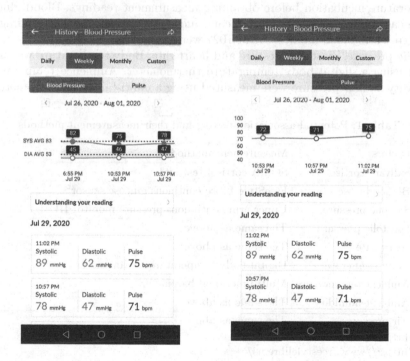

Fig. 2. Screenshots of the HeartAdviser smartphone app. Left: a weekly history of blood pressure. Right: a weekly history of heart rate.

to press the start button of the upper arm monitor first. Immediately following that, they were asked to press the start button of the HeartGuide™. They were required to sit still until both devices finish measuring, since HeartGuide™ takes more time than the upper arm monitor. In case either device requires re-measurement, participants were asked to adjust their postures before doing another round of measurement using both devices. Blood pressure was measured four times a day: right after waking up, before lunch, before dinner and before bedtime. Participants just follow their daily routine, and no intervention task was given.

To explore what factors may be associated to device accuracy, we also collected data on the list of factors summarized in Table 1. These factors include physiological metrics (i.e., salivary cortisol, blood glucose, systolic pressure, diastolic pressure, heart rate, and body temperature) and ambient conditions (i.e., ambient temperature, ambient humidity, and air pressure). Salivary cortisol was a reliable indicator of stress level. In this study, salivary cortisol was measured using the real-time SOMA cortisol test kit that only requires 10 min of room temperature incubation before obtaining measurement readings. Blood glucose was measured using FreeStyle Libre continuous glucose sensors. The readings of the upper arm blood monitor HEM-1022 were considered as the ground truth of systolic pressure, diastolic pressure and heart rate. Body temperature was measured using a digital body temperature thermometer. Ambience temperature, humidity and air pressure were measured using a multi-functional barometer.

Table 1. Potential association factors and their measurement methods

Factors	Measurement method
Salivary cortisol	SOMA cortisol test kit[a]
Blood glucose	FreeStyle Libre continous glucose sensor[b]
Systolic pressure	Upper arm continuous pressure monitor HEM-1022
Diastolic pressure	The same as above
Heart rate	The same as above
Body temperature	Digital body temperature thermometer
Ambient temperature	Multi-functional barometer
Ambient humidity	The same as above
Air pressure	The same as above

[a] http://somabioscience.com/.
[b] https://www.freestylelibre.us/.

3.3   Performance Measures

We compared the readings obtained using an HeartGuide™ with the those obtained using an upper arm blood pressure monitor HEM-1022. The metrics of our interest include systolic pressure, diastolic pressure and heart rate.

We adopted the following performance measures to quantify the agreement between the two devices.

- *Paired sample t-test* [29]. This test was used to determine if the means of the readings from two devices are significantly different from each other.
- *Scatter plots and the Pearson's correlation coefficient* [30]. The scatter plot visualizes the relationship between the two devices. The Pearson's correlation coefficient quantifies the linear relationship between the two devices.
- *Bland-Altman plots and mean differences* (95% confidence interval) [27]. The Bland-Altman plot visualizes the level off agreement between the two devices. In clinical settings, if the bias between two devices are not clinically important, then the two devices will be considered as equivalent and interchangeable [28].

We also investigate the associations between the Absolute Percent Error (APE) and a list of factors summarized in Table 1. The APE of the i-th pair of measurements is calculated using the equation below, where $\hat{x}_i$ and x_i denote the reading of the HeartGuide^{TM} and the upper arm blood pressure monitor respectively. Pairwise Pearson's correlation coefficient was calculated between APE and each factor.

$$APE_i = \frac{|\hat{x}_i - x_i|}{x_i} \tag{1}$$

4   Results

A total of 210 pairs of readings were obtained using both devices. Compared to the upper arm monitor, HeartGuide^{TM} showed lower value for systolic pressure (HeartGuide^{TM}: 87 ± 11 mmHg; upper arm monitor: 104 ± 12 mmHg; $t = 14.83$, $p < 0.001$), diastolic pressure (HeartGuide^{TM}: 54 ± 9 mmHg; upper arm monitor: 61 ± 8 mmHg; $t = 7.80$, $p < 0.001$).

Figure 3 shows the Bland-Altman plot and scatter plot on the readings of systolic pressure from two devices. The HeartGuide underestimated systolic pressure compared to HEM-1022 by an average of 16 mmHg (95% CI = [15, 18]). The scatter plot demonstrates positive strong correlation between the readings of two devices ($r = 0.70$, $p < 0.001$). Figure 4 shows the Bland-Altman plot and scatter plot on the readings of diastolic pressure from two devices. The Heart-Guide underestimated diastolic pressure compared to HEM-1022 by an average of 6 mmHg (95% CI = [5, 7]). The Bland-Altman plot for also demonstrated a trend in device difference as a function of the diastolic pressure: the difference between the two devices diminishes as the diastolic pressure increases. The scatter plot demonstrates positive strong correlation between the readings of two devices ($r = 0.69$, $p < 0.001$). Figure 5 shows the Bland-Altman plot and scatter plot on the readings of heart rate from two devices. The Bland-Altman plot indicates good agreement between two devices. The scatter plot demonstrates positive strong correlation between the readings of two devices ($r = 0.85$, $p < 0.001$).

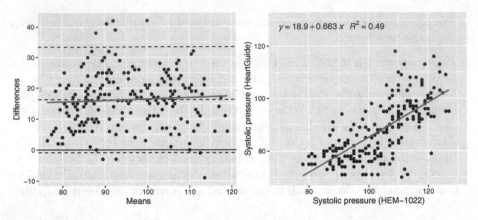

Fig. 3. Comparison between HeartGuide™ and digital upper arm blood pressure monitor on systolic pressure. Left: Bland-Altman plot demonstrates a systematic bias of 16 mmHg (95% CI = [15, 18]). Right: scatter plot shows a correlation coefficient of 0.70 ($p < 0.001$).

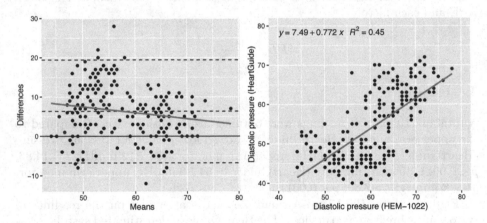

Fig. 4. Comparison between HeartGuide™ and digital upper arm blood pressure monitor on diastolic pressure. Left: Bland-Altman plot demonstrates a systematic bias of 6 mmHg (95% CI = [5, 7]), and the level of agreement between two devices increases with diastolic pressure. Right: scatter plot shows a correlation coefficient of 0.69 ($p < 0.001$).

Table 2 gives a summary of the Pearson correlation analysis between the APE of HeartGuide™ and the association factors. First, the APE of systolic pressure is weakly and positively correlated to the true systolic pressure, and weakly and negatively correlated to the heart rate and ambient temperature. Second, the APE of the diastolic pressure is weakly and negatively correlated to the systolic pressure, body temperature, and ambient temperature, and is

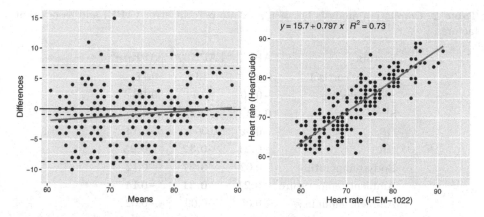

Fig. 5. Comparison between HeartGuide™ and digital upper arm blood pressure monitor on heart rate. Left: Bland-Altman plot demonstrates good agreement between two devices on heart rate readings. Right: scatter plot shows a correlation coefficient of 0.85 ($p < 0.001$).

moderately and negatively correlated to the true heart rate. Last but not the least, the APE of heart rate is weakly and positively correlated to blood glucose level, and is weakly and negatively correlated to the heart rate.

5 Discussion

This study has shown a quantitative comparison between the first consumer wearable blood pressure monitor HeartGuide™ and a medical-grade upper arm blood pressure monitor. We found that the HeartGuide™ systematically underestimated both systolic pressure and diastolic pressure when compared to the upper arm blood pressure monitor HEM-1022, but both devices agreed well on heart rate readings. Moreover, the difference between HeartGuide™ and the upper arm monitor on diastolic pressure diminishes as the diastolic pressure increased.

In clinical settings, two blood pressure monitoring methods are considered interchangable if their difference is within 5 mmHg [31]. Based on this criterion, the HeartGuide™ and HEM-1022 can be considered identical in measuring diastolic pressure and heart rate. The deviation of HeartGuide™ on systolic pressure should not be overlooked. Nevertheless, the mean difference of the two devices on systolic pressure is comparable to inter-observer differences among specialists using sphygmomanometer [32]. To this end, the HeartGuide™ is a plausible alternative to sphygmomanometer and upper arm cuff for ubiquitous blood pressure monitoring.

There are several factors that may play a role in the measurement accuracy of the HeartGuide™. The absolute percent error (APE) of systolic pressure slightly increases as the true systolic pressure increases, but slightly decreases as the true heart rate and ambient temperature increases. The APE of the diastolic

Table 2. Correlation analysis between absolute percent error (APE) and association factors.

Factors	APE$_{SP}$[a]	APE$_{DP}$[b]	APE$_{HR}$[c]
Salivary cortisol	0.09	0.13	0.17
Blood glucose	−0.10	−0.14	**0.28**[*][d]
SP	**0.28**[***][e]	**−0.23**[***]	−0.15[*]
DP	−0.02	0.00	−0.14[*]
HR	**−0.21**[**]	**−0.32**[***]	**−0.25**[***]
Body temperature	−0.02	**−0.27**[***]	−0.12
Ambient temperature	**−0.21**[**]	**−0.21**[**]	−0.14[*]
Ambient humidity	−0.05	−0.09	−0.02
Air pressure	0.16[*]	0.16[*]	0.16[*]

[a]Systolic pressure.
[b]Diastolic pressure.
[c]Heart rate.
[d]Significance level: *:$p < 0.05$; **:$p < 0.01$; ***:$p < 0.001$.
[e]Bold font highlights the absolute value of the Pearson's correlation coefficient $r > 0.20$ (indicating at least weak correlation).

pressure slightly decreases as the true systolic pressure, the true heart rate, body temperature or ambient temperature goes up. The APE of heart rate slightly increases as blood glucose increases or heart rate decreases. We also observed that device placement and arm position during measurement could all affect measurement accuracy. In contrast, salivary cortisol, the true diastolic pressure, ambient humidity and air pressure were not related to device accuracy. One possible way to improve the accuracy of the HeartGuide^{TM} is to consider these association factors in designing correction algorithms.

6   Conclusion

Compared to the upper arm blood pressure monitor HEM-1022, the Heart-Guide^{TM} significantly underestimated systolic pressure and diastolic pressure by an average of 16 mmHg and 6 mmHg respectively. In addition, lower discrepancy between two devices was observed when diastolic pressure increased. The HeartGuide^{TM} agreed well to HEM-1022 in measuring heart rate. We also found weak but statistically significant correlations between measurement errors and physiological or ambient conditions. High systolic pressure, low heart rate and low ambient temperature were associated to greater measurement errors on systolic pressure. Low systolic pressure, low body temperature, low ambient temperature and low heart rate were associated to greater measurement errors on diastolic pressure. High blood glucose and low heart rate were associated to greater measurement errors on heart rate. These factors should be taken into consideration to design algorithms for wearable blood pressure monitors in the future.

References

1. Zhang, Y., Vittinghoff, E., Pletcher, M.J., et al.: Associations of blood pressure and cholesterol levels during young adulthood with later cardiovascular events. J. Am. Coll. Cardiol. **74**(3), 330–341 (2019)
2. Satoh, M., Asayama, K., Kikuya, M., et al.: Long-term stroke risk due to partial white-coat or masked hypertension based on home and ambulatory blood pressure measurements: the Ohasama study. Hypertension **67**, 48–55 (2016)
3. Forouzanfar, M.H., Liu, P., Roth, G.A., et al.: Global burden of hypertension and systolic blood pressure of at least 110 to 115 mm Hg, 1990–2015. J. Am. Med. Assoc. **317**(2), 165–182 (2017)
4. Tucker, K.L., Sheppard, J.P., Stevens, R., et al.: Self-monitoring of blood pressure in hypertension: a systematic review and individual patient data meta-analysis. PLoS Med. **14**(9), e1002389 (2017)
5. Bray, E.P., Holder, R., Mant, J., McManus, R.J.: Does self-monitoring reduce blood pressure? Meta-analysis with meta-regression of randomized controlled trials. Ann. Med. **42**(5), 371–386 (2010)
6. Uhlig, K., Patel, K., Ip, S., et al.: Self-measured blood pressure monitoring in the management of hypertension: a systematic review and meta-analysis. Ann. Intern. Med. **159**(3), 185–194 (2013)
7. Smolensky, M.H., Hermida, R.C., Portaluppi, F.: Circadian mechanisms of 24-hour blood pressure regulation and patterning. Sleep Med. Rev. **33**, 4–16 (2017)
8. Briasoulis, A., Androulakis, E., Palla, M., et al.: White-coat hypertension and cardiovascular events: a meta-analysis. J. Hypertens. **34**(4), 593–599 (2016)
9. Kario, K., Thijs, L., Staessen, J.A.: Blood pressure measurement and treatment decisions masked and white-coat hypertension. Circ. Res. **124**(7), 990–1008 (2019)
10. Hansen, T.W., Thijs, L., Li, Y., et al.: Prognostic value of reading-to-reading blood pressure variability over 24 h in 8938 subjects from 11 populations. Hypertension **55**, 1049–1057 (2018)
11. Asayama, K., Satoh, M., Kiyuya, M.: Diurnal blood pressure changes. Hypertens. Res. **41**, 669–678 (2018)
12. Piper, M.A., Evans, C.V., Burda, B.U., et al.: Diagnosis and predictive accuracy of blood pressure screening methods with consideration of rescreening intervals: a systematic review for the U.S. preventive services task force. Ann. Intern. Med. **162**, 192–204 (2015)
13. Appel, L.J.: The effects of dietary factors on blood pressure. Cardiol. Clin. **35**(2), 197–212 (2017)
14. Gómez-Pardo, E., Fernández-Alvira, J.M., Vilanova, M., et al.: A comprehensive lifestyle peer group-based intervention on cardiovascular risk factors: the randomized controlled fifty-fifty program. J. Am. Coll. Cardiol. **67**(5), 476–485 (2016)
15. Babbs, C.F.: Oscillometric measurement of systolic and diastolic blood pressures validated in a physiologic mathematical model. BioMed. Eng. OnLine **11**, 56 (2012)
16. Geddes, L.A., Voelz, M., Combs, C., et al.: Characterization of the oscillometric method for measuring indirect blood pressure. Ann. Biomed. Eng. **10**, 271–280 (1982)
17. Heyen, N.B.: From self-tracking to self-expertise: the production of self-related knowledge by doing personal science. Public Understand. Sci. **29**(2), 124–138 (2020)
18. Liang, Z., et al.: SleepExplorer: a visualization tool to make sense of correlations between personal sleep data and contextual factors. Pers. Ubiquit. Comput. **20**(6), 985–1000 (2016). https://doi.org/10.1007/s00779-016-0960-6

19. White, G., Liang, Z., Clarke, S.: A quantified-self framework for exploring and enhancing personal productivity. In: Proceedings of CBMI 2019, pp. 1–6 (2010)
20. Liang, Z., Chapa-Martell, M.A.: Framing self-quantification for individual-level preventive health care. In: Proceedings of HEALTHINF 2015, pp. 336–343 (2015)
21. Majmudar, M.D., Colucci, L.A., Landman, A.B.: The quantified patient of the future: opportunities and challenges. Healthcare **3**, 153–156 (2015)
22. Liang, Z., Chapa-Martell, M.A.: Validity of consumer activity wristbands and wearable EEG for measuring overall sleep parameters and sleep structure in free-living conditions. J. Healthcare Inf. Res. **2**(1–2), 152–178 (2018)
23. Liang, Z., Ploderer, B., Chapa-Martell, M.A.: Is fitbit fit for sleep-tracking? Sources of measurement errors and proposed countermeasures. In: Proceedings of Pervasive Health 2017, pp. 476–479 (2017)
24. Liang, Z., Ploderer, B.: "How does Fitbit measure brainwaves": a qualitative study into the credibility of sleep-tracking technologies. Interact. Mobile Wearable Ubiquit. Technol. (IMWUT) **4**(1), 17 (2020)
25. Liang, Z., Ploderer, B.: Sleep tracking in the real world: a qualitative study into barriers for improving sleep. In: Proceedings of the 28th OzCHI, pp. 537–541 (2016)
26. Li, Y., Guo, Y.: Wiki-Health: from quantified self to self-understanding. Future Gener. Comput. Syst. **56**, 333–359 (2016)
27. Bland, J.M., Altman, D.G.: Statistical methods for assessing agreement between two methods of clinical measurement. Lancet **1**(8476), 307–310 (1986)
28. Higgins, P.A., Straub, A.J.: Understanding the error of our ways: mapping the concepts of validity and reliability. Nurs. Outlook **54**(1), 23–29 (2006)
29. Fay, M.P., Proschan, M.A.: Wilcoxon-Mann-Whitney or t-test? On assumptions for hypothesis tests and multiple interpretations of decision rules. Statist. Surv. **4**, 1–39 (2010)
30. Friendly, M., Denis, D.: The early origins and development of the scatterplot. J. Hist. Behav. Sci. **41**(2), 103–130 (2005)
31. Park, S.-H., Park, Y.-S.: Can an automatic oscillometric device replace a mercury sphygmomanometer on blood pressure measurement? A systematic review and meta-analysis. Blood Press. Monit. **24**(6), 265–276 (2019)
32. Joukar, F., Naghipour, M.R., Yeganeh, S., et al.: Validity and inter-observers reliability of blood pressure measurements using mercury sphygmomanometer in the PERSIAN Guilan cohort study. Blood Press. Monit. **25**(2), 100–104 (2020)

Artificial Empathy for Clinical Companion Robots with Privacy-By-Design

Miguel Vargas Martin[1(✉)], Eduardo Pérez Valle[2], and Sheri Horsburgh[3]

[1] Ontario Tech University, Oshawa, Canada
miguel.martin@ontariotechu.ca
[2] Instituto Tecnológico y de Estudios Superiores de Monterrey (ITESM),
Culiacán, Mexico
edupv10@hotmail.com
[3] Ontario Shores Centre for Mental Health Sciences, Whitby, Canada
horsburghs@ontarioshores.ca

Abstract. We present a prototype whereby we enabled a humanoid robot to be used to assist mental health patients and their families. Our approach removes the need for Cloud-based automatic speech recognition systems to address healthcare privacy expectations. Furthermore, we describe how the robot could be used in a mental health facility by giving directions from patient selection to metrics for evaluation. Our overarching goal is to make the robot interaction as natural as possible to the point where the robot can develop artificial empathy for the human companion through the interpretation of vocals and facial expressions to infer emotions.

Keywords: Companion robots · Mental health · Privacy-by-design · Automatic speech recognition · Artificial intelligence · Artificial empathy

1 Introduction

This paper outlines a prototype and methodology to enable a commodity humanoid robot for use as a non-pharmacological intervention to support care of individuals with dementia by enhancing the robot with privacy-by-design applications. Our use case utilizes the ASUS Zenbo (see Fig. 1), an Android-based humanoid robot with a number of built-in artificial intelligence (AI) functions that rely on the Cloud by default.

The proposed robot enhancements include the following:

1. Enhance Zenbo with privacy-enabled face expression sensing capabilities to recognize human emotions of dementia patients, off-line.

E. Pérez Valle worked on this project while at Ontario Tech, supported by a MITACS Globalink Research Internship.

J. Ye et al. (Eds.): MobiHealth 2020, LNICST 362, pp. 351–361, 2021.
https://doi.org/10.1007/978-3-030-70569-5_23

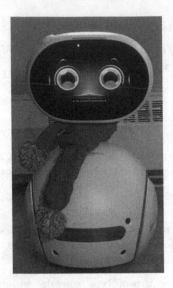

Fig. 1. ASUS' Zenbo.

2. Enhance Zenbo with privacy-enabled vocals sensing capabilities to recognize human emotions of dementia patients, off-line.
3. Identify other potential privacy-enabled functions that can be performed by Zenbo to address the needs of dementia patients and their families, such as programming individualized messages, provide lighting changes to promote calm and safe atmosphere, music therapy, reminiscence therapy and motion tracking to assist in monitoring safety of individuals.

Thus, we propose to enable Zenbo with privacy-preserving capabilities to infer human emotions by combining facial expression and voice vocals using deep learning techniques of AI through the means of specialized automatic speech recognition (ASR) hardware such as Snips [1]. In other words, we are proposing to address the area of interest involving the use of AI companions for patients and family members through systems that learn and adapt based on interactions with a situation through speech, gestures, and physical and physiological measures, amongst others. In our proposed enhanced robot, Zenbo will be able to respond when particular emotions are inferred such as sadness, anxiety, anger, etc., and will act according to clinical guidelines. For example, Zenbo may be programmed to offer the patient to show photos of the last vacation with his or her kids to make them feel better, or provide lighting changes to promote calm and safe atmosphere, offer music therapy, or even engage in a conversation with the patients.

Contributions. Our contributions are twofold: (1) We provide the technical details of our prototype privacy-by-design enhancement of ASR in Zenbo. (2) Furthermore, we describe a proposal to use a private-by-design robot to assist mental health patients and their families within the context of an inpatient mental health facility.

2 Related Work

The use of acoustic clues has been used to identify anxiety manifestations in patients with dementia (see e.g., [2]). Human-AI interaction is a growing field of research due to a persistent uncertainty about AI capabilities, and the complexity of AI's output, among other factors [3,4]. Research indicating potential benefits of assistive robots includes improving mood, communication and stress reduction [5–7]. However, many of these studies have focused on the use of robotic pets and research and functionality of humanoid robots is more limited. In a controlled clinical study [8], therapy using a humanoid robot showed a significant reduction in apathy of patients with dementia suggesting further research and development of these devices is likely of benefit to this population. Humanoid robots can include AI functions that are anticipated to provide additional support beyond those of robotic pets.

One of these robots, the Android based ASUS Zenbo is a 62 cm tall, round white body on concealed wheels, long metallic neck, with a 10″ touch screen face, no extremities, and rechargeable battery. Zenbo is a commercial humanoid robot launched in 2016 in Taiwan, marketed as a companion robot. Zenbo runs the Android operating system, and ships with a number of interactive interfaces including camera, microphone, speakers, touch sensor, drop sensor to avoid falls, range sensor to measure forward distance, and an ultrasonic sensor to avoid obstacles. The Zenbo robot has been alluded in a number of healthcare initiatives in Ontario (see e.g., [9,10]).

The factory settings of Zenbo include a number of apps, some of the most interesting ones relying on the Cloud for AI functions such as ASR. Running Android, Zenbo can be programmed through apps to perform additional functions with great flexibility by using Cloud services. Unfortunately, there has been a number of concerns regarding privacy of Cloud services, and devices like Amazon's Alexa or Google Home aren't the exception, with a number of privacy breach incidents making the news [11–14].

Privacy-preserving hardware like Sonos' Snips [15], a powerful Raspberry Pi card shipping with built-in specialized ASR software, provide a solution to privacy concerns of ASR Cloud services as they are capable of performing all the computations off-line, removing the need for the Cloud. Snips can thus be trained with intents to create voice assistants that understand spoken languages (English, French, Spanish, German, Italian, Japanese, and Korean).

Finally, we note that ASR systems are susceptible to a number of attacks that can seriously hinder the technology. For example, it has been demonstrated how hidden voice commands can be effectively interpreted by voice recognition systems while being imperceptible by humans [16,17]. A hidden voice attack, then, may trigger unwanted and unexpected robot behaviour which could be found unacceptable within certain contexts.

3   Prototype Private-By-Design ASR in Zenbo

The prototype in our Human Machine Laboratory uses Snips, which offers private-by-design ASR, to listen and process voice commands and send them to Zenbo for execution. The prototype includes commands such as "tell me a joke" or "how's the weather?" or "make a happy face". To achieve this, it was necessary to (1) configure Snips to interpret voice commands and create a secure connection with Zenbo, and (2) develop an Android app within Zenbo which can interpret the commands received from Snips.

3.1   Configuring Snips

There are several platforms where Snips can be installed; our prototype used Raspberry Pi. The configuration steps can be found in the Snips documentation [18]. Once Snips is configured for Raspberry Pi, we use the Snips Console to create different types of assistants which will allow us to create a connection with Zenbo. Figure 2 depicts an assistant called *HelloSnips*. Then we can create apps inside the assistant; we called our app *Zenbo*, as illustrated in Fig. 3.

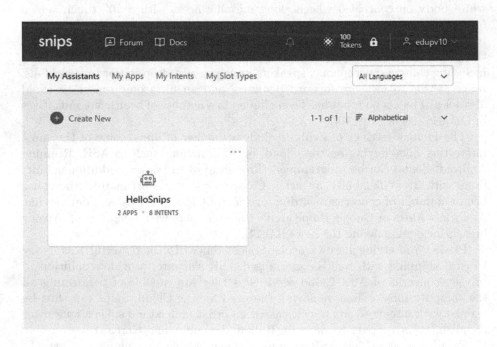

Fig. 2. The assistant shown is called *HelloSnips*.

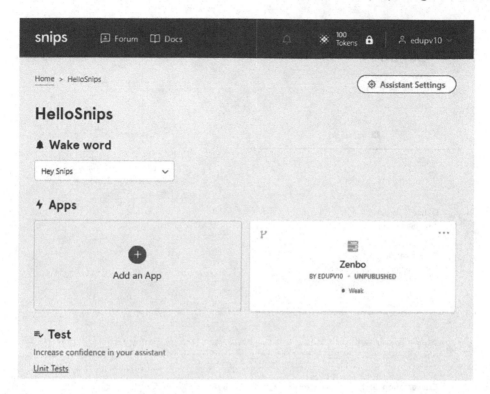

Fig. 3. An application called *Zenbo* within an assistant.

The applications for the Snips assistant are composed of intents and actions, where for every action there can be one or more intents. Intents are the sentences that Snips recognizes and can trigger some action on Zenbo. Figure 4 illustrates some intents.

Within the intent *Faces* we used 7 examples, as shown in Figure 5. So, when Snips identifies the intent it will send the appropriate command to Zenbo to trigger the corresponding action on the robot. The words marked in blue are called *Slots*, which are benchmarks used to recognize intents and link them to the corresponding action. Actions are coded in Python inside *Code Snippets*, as illustrated in Fig. 6. In our prototype the action is the establishment of a secure communication channel with Zenbo where commands are then sent to the robot.

3.2   Android App in Zenbo

In our prototype, Zenbo receives commands via sockets through the WiFi network. The sockets are established with Zenbo as a server, and Snips as a client. To develop the Android app in Zenbo, we used Zenbo's SDK available at [19]. Once the app is built, it can be seamlessly installed in Zenbo. We leave the underpinnings of the app outside the scope of this paper but suffice to say that the app receives the text of the intent from Snips, and then cross-check it against a set of possible actions (Zenbo commands); and execute the one that matches the intent.

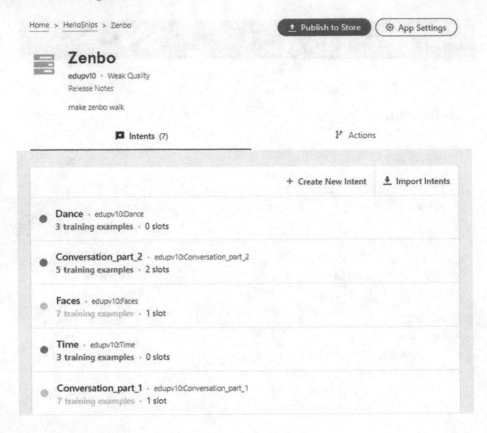

Fig. 4. Examples of intents used in our prototype.

4   Proposed Enhancements and Methodology for Use in a Clinical Environment

The prototype described in the previous section proves the viability of a private-by-design ASR robot. Now we describe two constructs that will make Zenbo a feasible clinical robot.

4.1   Technical Aspects

One construct involves the technical aspects of training a sufficiently large number of intents for every action in such a way that Zenbo can understand a large range of voice commands. Another aspect of this construct is related to vocals and face expression recognition (FER). The second construct is the effectiveness in identifying dementia-specific needs and being able to address these with our technology, and having our solution tested by real patients.

Faces

Zenbo Shows different faces

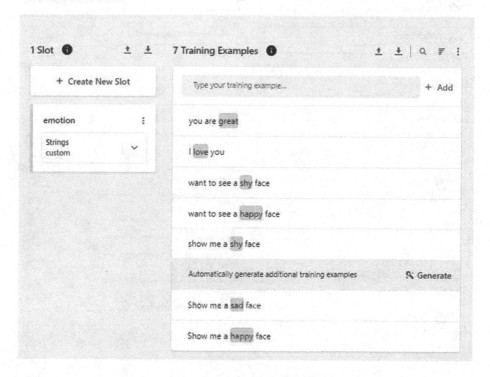

Fig. 5. Some training examples within the *Faces* intent.

Vocals and Face Expression Recognition. It's been generally accepted in the research community that acoustic profiles of vocals are associated to emotions of anger, fear, happiness, and sadness. The profiling of vocals includes pitch, intensity, and speed of speech [20]. We will use deep learning to train a vocals engine to recognize these emotions. And although these vocal profiles are generally accepted, we are aware that emotions may manifest differently on individuals, so we will further consider the possibility to customize and refine the training with the vocals of the dementia patient the robot will serve. As per FER, different techniques have been proposed in the literature to detect expressions such as smile, sad, anger, disgust, surprise, and fear [21]. While FER feature extraction is one of the most difficult challenges of our project, Zenbo comes with pre-installed basic face recognition features that we hope can be adapted for our purposes. We plan to complete the vocals recognition and combine that with FER to infer emotions of the dementia patient. This, combined with the NLP engine in a privacy-enhanced environment will make of our approach a powerful tool with great potential to assist dementia patients.

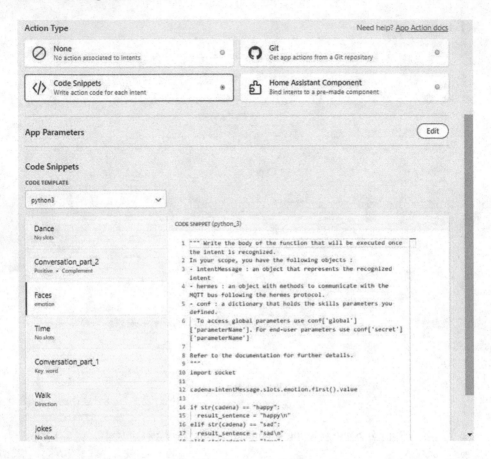

Fig. 6. Snips code template to develop the commands to execute corresponding actions.

Emotions. We will use a dimensional theory of emotion based on the "PAD theory" [22] for pleasure (a measure of valence), arousal (a measure of affective activation), and dominance (a measure of control), termed the valence-arousal model. This model classifies emotions such as sad, happy, and calm, and is able to associate intensities to these [23]. We will be particularly interested in detecting emotions that are deemed as requiring attention of a human caregiver. For example, after using vocals and FER, our system could trigger an alert to the floor nurse if unusual sadness emotions are detected. In addition, our system will be able to pick significantly different vocal features that may be an indication of pain or any other condition such as skipping medications, or sudden changes in the patients' condition.

4.2   Clinical Trials

The second construct of this proposal is the effective identification of dementia patients needs that can be addressed with the physical limitations of the Zenbo robot.

Test Group. The ideal test group would be patients with a primary diagnosis of dementia and behaviours and psychological symptoms of dementia (BPSD). BPSD can include agitation, aggression, restlessness, lability, exit seeking, impulsivity and sexual disinhibition. A trigger for BPSD can be boredom or social isolation, therefore supporting activities and increasing non-pharmacological interventions is critical to stabilizing behaviours in this population. Common non-pharmacological interventions include the use of robotic pets, doll therapy, aromatherapy, therapeutic sensory chair, sensory room (Snoezelen room), SPA-based therapy (e.g., manicure), iPads/iPods, live pet therapy, hand massage, and group activities.

Patient Identification. To identify patient needs, we will look to partner with facilities caring for individuals with dementia, conduct focus groups with frontline staff, as well as individual patients and/or their caregivers. Themes from these focus groups will be reviewed by the research team for exploration of the capabilities of Zenbo to support these activities. Upon enhancement of the Zenbo robot, we will look to pilot the device with a number of dementia patients, determined by the Test Group assessment described above.

Evaluation. To evaluate the effectiveness of the intervention, baseline measures for each patient including DSM-V (Diagnostic and Statistical Manual of Mental Disorders' Working Group 5) diagnoses, Folstein Mini-Mental state Examination (MMSE) on admission, Alzheimer's Disease-related Quality of Life (QoL-AD) scale on admission, baseline measures on the neuropsychiatric inventory, number of incidents of aggression/threatening/sexually inappropriate behaviour and average number of hours slept per night during the week prior to the intervention will be reviewed. Outcome measures will include neuropsychiatric inventory, number of incidents of aggression/threatening/sexually inappropriate behaviour, and average number of hours slept per night the week post the intervention, for comparison. In addition, the QoL-AD will be completed post-intervention as well.

5   Conclusions and Directions for Future Work

The research study will enable Zenbo with privacy-preserving capabilities to infer human emotions by combining facial expression and voice vocals using deep learning techniques of AI. When Zenbo is enabled with these capabilities they will serve as a meaningful companion for individuals with dementia, thus improving the quality of life of these individuals. This will also provide an additional non-pharmacological intervention to support stabilization of BPSD, which will be transferable across acute care, tertiary care, and community care settings (e.g., long-term care homes). In addition, confirming the privacy-preserving capabilities will allow for adaptation of this model to potentially meet the needs of individuals with dementia who continue to live at home. Given the prediction that in 20 years' time over 1.5 million Canadians will be living with dementia and the significant economic burden associated with providing meaningful support and care to these individuals, identifying cost-effective ways to support independence and quality of life will be crucial.

The Zenbo private-by-design approach also has the potential to combine several non-pharmacological interventions into one device as through this study we will be able to investigate incorporation of light therapy, music therapy, reminiscence therapy and potential safety monitoring which negates the expense and space requirements of having multiple devices to provide these interventions.

Improvements to our current prototype include training the private-by-design ASR with sufficiently large number of intents and samples per intent, which will make Zenbo recognize speech in a more natural way. To this end, we could choose to use transfer learning [24], making sure to protect against potential backdoor attacks [25]. Alternatively, the Snips device could be replaced by a fully-fledged ASR that works locally without Cloud services, although this would require expensive equipment which may affect the portability of the hardware set.

References

1. Coucke, A., et al.: Snips voice platform: an embedded spoken language understanding system for private-by-design voice interfaces. ArXiv abs/1805.10190 (2018)
2. Hernandez, N., et al.: Prototypical system to detect anxiety manifestations by acoustic patterns in patients with dementia. PHAT **5**(19) (2019)
3. Yang, Q., et al.: Re-examining whether, why, and how Human-AI interaction is uniquely difficult to design. In: Conference Human Factors in Computing Systems (CHI), Honolulu, USA (2020)
4. Long, D., et al.: What is AI literacy? Competencies and design considerations. In: Conference on Human Factors in Computing Systems (CHI), Honolulu, USA (2020)
5. Murdoch, E., et al.: Use of social commitment robots in the care of elderly people with dementia: a literature review. Maturitas **74**, 14–20 (2013)
6. Broekens, J., et al.: Assistive social robots in elderly care: a review. Gerontechnology **8**(2), 94–103 (2009)
7. Bemelmans, R., et al.: Socially assistive robots in elderly care: a systematic review into effects and effectiveness. JAMDA **13**(2), 114–120 (2012)
8. Soler, M.V., et al.: Social robots in advanced dementia. Front. Aging Neurosci. **7**(133), 1–12 (2015)
9. Perkins, J.: Toronto charity creates robot to entertain, educate kids who can't go to school due to severe illnesses. The Globe and Mail, 31 January 2020. https://www.theglobeandmail.com/canada/toronto/article-toronto-charity-creates-robot-to-entertain-educate-kids-who-cant-go/. Accessed 23 Nov 2020

10. Students using AI to teach robot how to recognize human emotions. CTV News, 19 August 2019, http://ctv.news/6JsxuKV. Accessed 23 Nov 2020
11. Brown, J.: The Amazon Alexa eavesdropping nightmare came true. Gizmodo. https://gizmodo.com/the-amazon-alexa-eavesdropping-nightmare-came-true-183-1231490. Accessed 23 Nov 2020
12. Valinski, J.: Amazon reportedly employs thousands of people to listen to your Alexa conversations. CNN Business. https://www.cnn.com/2019/04/11/tech/amazon-alexa-listening/index.html. Accessed 23 Nov 2020
13. Paul, K.: Google workers can listen to what people say to its AI home devices. The Guardian. https://www.theguardian.com/technology/2019/jul/11/google-home-assistant-listen-recordings-users-privacy. Accessed 23 Nov 2020
14. Barack, L.: Google Home security breach sends your location to hackers. GearBrain. https://www.gearbrain.com/google-home-location-hack-found-2579276699.html. Accessed 23 Nov 2020
15. Snips: Using voice to make technology disappear. https://snips.ai/. Accessed 23 Nov 2020
16. Chen, Y., et al.: Devil's Whisper: a general approach for physical adversarial attacks against commercial black-box speech recognition devices. In: 29 USENIX Security Symposium (2020)
17. Abdullah, M., et al.: Practical hidden voice attacks against speech and speaker recognition systems. In: Network and Distributed System Security Symposium (NDSS), San Diego, USA (2019)
18. Quick Start Raspberry Pi. https://docs.snips.ai/getting-started/quick-start-raspberry-pi. Accessed 23 Nov 2020
19. ASUS Developer. https://zenbo.asus.com/developer/tools/. Accessed 23 Nov 2020
20. Juslin, P.N., et al.: Communication of emotion in vocal expression and music performance: different channels, same code? Psychol. Bull. **129**, 770–814 (2003)
21. Revina, I.M., et al.: A survey on human face expression recognition techniques. Psychol. Bull. (2018). https://doi.org/10.1016/j.jksuci.2018.09.002
22. Albert, M., et al.: An Approach to Environmental Psychology. The MIT Press, Cambridge (1974)
23. Russell, J.A.: A circumplex model of affect. J. Pers. Soc. Psychol. **39**(6), 1161–1178 (1980)
24. Hernandez, N., et al.: Literature review on transfer learning for human activity recognition using mobile and wearable devices with environmental technology. SN Comput. Sci. **1**, 66 (2020)
25. Yao, Y., et al.: Latent backdoor attacks on deep neural networks. In: ACM Conference on Computer and Communications Security, London, UK (2019)

Author Index

Printed in the United States
By Bookmasters